Oxford American Handbook of
Gastroenterology
and Hepatology

D1132122

About the Oxford American Handbooks in Medicine

The Oxford American Handbooks are pocket clinical books, providing practical guidance in quick reference, note form. Titles cover major medical specialties or cross-specialty topics and are aimed at students, residents, internists, family physicians, and practicing physicians within specific disciplines.

Their reputation is built on including the best clinical information, complemented by hints, tips, and advice from the authors. Each one is carefully reviewed by senior subject experts, residents, and students to ensure that content reflects the reality of day-to-day medical practice.

Key series features

- Written in short chunks, each topic is covered in a two-page spread to enable readers to find information quickly. They are also perfect for test preparation and gaining a quick overview of a subject without scanning through unnecessary pages.
- Content is evidence based and complemented by the expertise and judgment of experienced authors.
- The Handbooks provide a humanistic approach to medicine – it's more than just treatment by numbers.
- A "friend in your pocket," the Handbooks offer honest, reliable guidance about the difficulties of practicing medicine and provide coverage of both the practice and art of medicine.
- For quick reference, useful "everyday" information is included on the inside covers.

Published and Forthcoming Oxford American Handbooks

Oxford American Handbook of Clinical Medicine
Oxford American Handbook of Anesthesiology
Oxford American Handbook of Cardiology
Oxford American Handbook of Clinical Dentistry
Oxford American Handbook of Clinical Diagnosis
Oxford American Handbook of Clinical Pharmacy
Oxford American Handbook of Critical Care
Oxford American Handbook of Emergency Medicine
Oxford American Handbook of Gastroenterology and Hepatology
Oxford American Handbook of Geriatric Medicine
Oxford American Handbook of Nephrology and Hypertension
Oxford American Handbook of Neurology
Oxford American Handbook of Obstetrics and Gynecology
Oxford American Handbook of Oncology
Oxford American Handbook of Ophthalmology
Oxford American Handbook of Otolaryngology
Oxford American Handbook of Pediatrics
Oxford American Handbook of Physical Medicine and Rehabilitation
Oxford American Handbook of Psychiatry
Oxford American Handbook of Pulmonary Medicine
Oxford American Handbook of Rheumatology
Oxford American Handbook of Sports Medicine
Oxford American Handbook of Surgery
Oxford American Handbook of Urology

Oxford American Handbook of
Gastroenterology and Hepatology

Edited by

Adam S. Cheifetz, MD
Assistant Professor of Medicine, Harvard Medical School
Director, Center for Inflammatory Bowel Disease
Beth Israel Deaconess Medical Center
Boston, Massachusetts

Alphonso Brown, MD
Assistant Professor of Medicine, Harvard Medical School
Co-Director, Pancreas Center
Beth Israel Deaconess Medical Center
Boston, Massachusetts

Michael Curry, MD
Assistant Professor of Medicine, Harvard Medical School
Director for Liver Transplantation, Liver Center
Beth Israel Deaconess Medical Center
Boston, Massachusetts

Alan C. Moss, MD
Assistant Professor of Medicine, Harvard Medical School
Director of Translational Research
Center for Inflammatory Bowel Disease
Beth Israel Deaconess Medical Center
Boston, Massachusetts

with

Stuart Bloom
George Webster

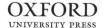

OXFORD
UNIVERSITY PRESS

OXFORD
UNIVERSITY PRESS

Oxford University Press, Inc. publishes works that further
Oxford University's objective of excellence
in research, scholarship and education.

Oxford New York

Auckland Cape Town Dar es Salaam Hong Kong Karachi
Kuala Lumpur Madrid Melbourne Mexico City Nairobi
New Delhi Shanghai Taipei Toronto

With offices in

Argentina Austria Brazil Chile Czech Republic France Greece
Guatemala Hungary Italy Japan Poland Portugal
Singapore South Korea Switzerland Thailand Turkey Ukraine Vietnam

Published by Oxford University Press Inc.
198 Madison Avenue, New York, New York 10016

www.oup.com

Oxford is a registered trademark of Oxford University Press

First published 2011
UK version: 2006

Library of Congress Cataloging in Publication Data

Oxford American handbook of gastroenterology and hepatology / edited by Adam S
Cheifetz ... [et al.] ; with Stuart Bloom, George Webster.
p. ; cm.
Other title: Handbook of gastroenterology and hepatology
Includes index.
ISBN 978-0-19-538318-8
1. Gastroenterology–Handbooks, manuals, etc. 2. Hepatology–Handbooks,
manuals, etc. I. Cheifetz, Adam S. II. Title: Handbook of gastroenterology and
hepatology.
[DNLM: 1. Gastrointestinal Diseases–Handbooks. WI 39]
RC802.O94 2011
616.3′3–dc22
2010028005

**Oxford American handbook of
gastroenterology and**

Preface

The *Oxford American Handbook of Gastroenterology and Hepatology* is intended for medical students, residents, and gastroenterology fellows. It is by no means a complete referendum on gastroenterology but a place to start your learning. Nor is it meant to replace full literature searches or the experience of direct patient care. It will, however, provide you with an accessible and convenient reference and help build a fund of knowledge about gastroenterology at a time when you are most likely to retain it—on the wards or in the clinic, working directly with patients. The handbook is designed to fit in your pocket and organized to make your life easier. We hope you find it helpful. The rest of the advice we will leave to Sir William Osler:

"He who studies medicine without books sails an uncharted sea, but he who studies medicine without patients does not go to sea at all."

Adam S. Cheifetz
Alan C. Moss
Alphonso Brown
Michael Curry

Acknowledgments

We would like to thank our friends and family and those physicians, patients, and nurses that have helped to train us and make us the physicians we are today.

Special thanks go to Martin Smith, MD and Robert Najarian, MD for providing the majority of the radiology and pathology images shown within this handbook.

We also thank the authors of the original British edition, Stuart Bloom and George Webster.

Contents

Detailed contents

3   Upper gastrointestinal tract

6.2   **Rectum**   **297**

9.2   Nutrition   **417**

Appendix   **429**

Abbreviations

BM	in glucose BM, i.e., blood monitoring for glucose or bowel motion
BMD	bone mineral density
BMI	body mass index
BMR	basal metabolic rate
Bn	bilirubin
BP	blood pressure
Bx	biopsy
cAMP	cyclic adenosine monophosphate
CBC	complete blood count
CBD	common bile duct
CDAI	Crohn's disease activity index
CDC	Center for Disease Control
CDEIS	Crohn's disease endoscopic inflammation score
CEA	carcinoembryonic antigen
CF	cystic fibrosis
CFTR	cystic fibrosis transmembrane conductance regulator
CGD	chronic granulomatous disease
CLO	*Clostridium*-like organisms (test for)
CMV	cytomegalovirus
CNS	central nervous system
CO	carbon monoxide *or* cardiac output
COX-2	cyclo-oxygenase 2
CREST	calcinosis–Raynaud's–oesophageal dysmotility–sclerodactyly–telangiectasia (syndrome)
CRP	C-reactive protein
CSF	cerebrospinal fluid
CSU	catheter specimen of urine
CT	computerized tomography
CTD	connective tissue disease
CVA	cerebrovascular accident
CVP	central venous pressure
CXR	chest X-ray
DAEC	diffusely adhering *E. coli*
DBE	double-balloon enteroscopy
DCC	deleted in colorectal cancer (gene)

DEXA	dual energy X-ray absorptiometry
DF	discriminant function
DIC	disseminated intravascular coagulation
DT	delirium tremens
DU	duodenal ulcer
DVT	deep vein thrombosis
EAggEC	entero-aggregatory E. coli
EBV	Epstein–Barr virus
EGC	early gastric cancer
EGD	esophago-gastro-duodenoscopy
EGF	epidermal growth factor
EGG	electrogastrography
EHEC	enterohaemorrhagic E. coli
EIA	enzyme immunoassay
EIEC	enteroinvasive E. coli
EKG	electrokardiogram
ELISA	enzyme-linked immunosorbent assay
EMR	endoscopic mucosal resection
ENT	ear, nose, and throat
EPEC	enteropathogenic E. coli
ERCP	endoscopic retrograde cholangiopancreatography
ESR	erythrocyte sedimentation rate
EST	endoscopic sclerotherapy
ESWL	extracorporeal shock wave lithotripsy
ETEC	enterotoxigenic E. coli
EUS	endoscopic ultrasound
FAP	familial adenomatous polyposis
FDG	2-fluoro-2-deoxy-D-glucose
FE1	faecal elastase type 1
FFP	fresh frozen plasma
FNA	fine needle aspiration
FNH	focal nodular hyperplasia
FOBT	fecal occult blood test
FSH	follicle-stimulating hormone
5FU	fluorouracil
GABA	γ-aminobutyric acid
GAVE	gastric antral vascular ectasia
GBS	Guillain–Barré syndrome
GDA	gastroduodenal artery
GERD	gastro-esophageal reflux disease

GGT	gammaglutamyl transpeptidase
GH	genetic hemochromatosis
GI	gastrointestinal
GIST	gastrointestinal stromal tumors
GMP	guanosine monophosphate
G6PD	glucose 6-phosphate dehydrogenase
GTN	glyceryl trinitrate
GU	gastric ulcer
GvHD	graft versus host disease
HAART	highly active antiretroviral therapy
H & E	hematoxylin and eosin
HAS	human albumin solution
HAV	hepatitis A virus
Hb	haemoglobin
HBcAg	hepatitis B core antigen
HBeAg	hepatitis B envelope antigen
HBsAg	hepatitis B surface antigen
HBV	hepatitis B virus
HCC	hepatocellular carcinoma
β-HCG	beta human chorionic gonadotrophin
HCV	hepatitis C virus
HDL	high-density lipid
HDU	high-dependency unit
HDV	hepatitis D virus
HE	hepatic encephalopathy
HELLP	hemolysis–elevated liver enzymes–low platelets (syndrome)
HEV	hepatitis E virus
HGD	high-grade dysplasia
HGV	hepatitis G virus
5-HIAA	5 hydroxy indole acetic acid
HIDA	hepatobiliary iminodiacetic acid (hepatobiliary scintigraphy)
HII	hepatic iron index
HIV	human immunodeficiency virus
HNIG	human normal immunoglobulin
HNPCC	hereditary non-polyposis cancer
HOCM	hypertropic obstructive cardiomyopathy
HP	*Helicobacter pylori*
HPV	human papillomavirus
HR	heart rate

H2RA	H2-receptor antagonist
HRQL	health-related quality of life
HRS	hepatorenal syndrome
HRT	hormone replacement therapy
HSV	herpes simplex virus
5-HT	5-hydroxytryptamine (serotonin)
HV	hepatic vein
HVPG	hepatic venous pressure gradient
IBS	irritable bowel syndrome
ICP	intracranial pressure
ICU	intensive care unit
IF	intrinsic factor
IFN-α	interferon alpha
IL	interleukin (IL-2, etc.)
IM	intramuscular
INR	international normalized ratio
IPAA	ileal pouch–anal anastomosis
IPMT	intraductal papillary mucinous tumor
IPSID	immunoproliferative small intestinal disease (alpha chain disease)
IU	international units
IV	intravenous
JVP	jugular venous pressure
KS	Kaposi's sarcoma
LBx	liver biopsy
LC	laparoscopic cholecystectomy
LCHAD	3-hydroxyacyl coenzyme A dehydrogenase
LCT	long-chain triglyceride
LDH	lactate dehydrogenase
LDL	low-density lipid
LES	lower esophageal sphincter
LFT	liver function test
LGD	low-grade dysplasia
LH	luteinizing hormone
LKM1	liver–kidney microsomes, type 1
MAC	*Mycobacterium avium complex*
MAI	*Mycobacterium avium intracellulare*
MALT	mucosa-associated lymphoid tissue
MAP	mean arterial pressure
MARS	molecular absorbance recirculation system

MCH	mean corpuscular hemoglobin
MCHC	mean corpuscular hemoglobin concentration
MCN	mucinous cystic neoplasm
MCT	medium-chain triglyceride
MCTD	mixed connective tissue disease
MCV	mean corpuscular volume
MDP	muramyl dipeptide
MELD	model for end-stage liver disease (score)
MEN	multiple endocrine neoplasia (e.g. MEN-1)
MI	myocardial infarction
MIBG	metaiodobenzylguanidine
6-MP	6-mercaptopurine
MRCP	magnetic resonance cholangiopancreatography
MRI	magnetic resonance imaging
MS	multiple sclerosis
MSU	midstream urine
MTB	mycobacterium tuberculosis
NADPH	nicotinamide adenine dinucleotide phosphate (reduced form).
NAFLD	nonalcoholic fatty liver disease
NASH	nonalcoholic steatohepatitis
NBM	nil by mouth
NET	neuroendocrine tumors
NF	neurofibramotosis
NG	nasogastric (tube)
NHL	non-Hodgkin's lymphoma
NRH	nodular regenerative hyperplasia
NSAID	nonsteroidal anti-inflammatory drug
OATP	organic anion transporting polypeptide
OC	open cholecystectomy
OCP	oral contraceptive pill
od	once a day
OHCM	*Oxford Handbook of Clinical Medicine*
OLT	orthotopic liver transplantation
ORS	oral rehydration solution
PA	postero-anterior *or* pernicious anemia
PABA	para-aminobenzoic acid
PAN	polyarteritis nodosa
PaO_2	arterial oxygen tension
PAS	para-aminosalicylic acid

PBC	primary biliary cirrhosis
PBG	porphobilinogen
PCR	polymerase chain reaction
PCT	porphyria cutanea tarda
PDAI	pouchitis disease activity index
PDT	photodynamic therapy
PE	pulmonary embolism
PEG	percutaneous endoscopic gastrostomy *or* polyethylene glycol
PET	positron emission tomography *or* pancreatic endocrine tumour
PHG	portal hypertensive gastropathy
PICC	peripherally inserted central catheters
PMC	pseudomembranous colitis
PNS	peripheral nervous system
PO	by mouth (*per os*)
PPI	proton pump inhibitor
PPPD	pylorus-preserving pancreaticoduodenectomy
PR	by (per) rectum
prn	as required
PSA	prostate-specific antigen
PSC	primary sclerosing cholangitis
PT	prothrombin time
PTD	percutaneous transhepatic drainage
PTH	parathyroid hormone
PTLD	posttransplant lymphoproliferative disorder
PUD	peptic ulcer disease
PUO	pyrexia of unknown origin
PV	by (per) vagina
PVT	portal vein thrombosis
qds	four times a day
RA	rheumatoid arthritis
RCT	randomized control trial
RIBA	recombinant immunoblot assay
SAAG	serum to ascites albumin gradient
SACE	serum angiotensin-converting enzyme
SAMe	S-adenosylmethionine
SBE	subacute bacterial endocarditis
SBP	spontaneous bacterial peritonitis
SBT	Sengstaken–Blakemore tube

SCA	sickle cell anaemia
SCC	squamous cell carcinoma
SCFA	Short-chain fatty acids
SD	standard deviation
SeHCaT	selenium-75 labelled homotaurocholic acid test
SLA	soluble liver antigen
SLE	systemic lupus erythematosus
SMA	superior mesenteric artery
SOD	sphincter of Oddi dysfunction
SOM	sphincter of Oddi manometry
SSRI	selective serotonin reuptake inhibitor
SVC	superior vena cava
SVR	sustained virological response *or* systemic vascular resistance
TACE	transcatheter chemoembolization
TB	tuberculosis
tds	three times a day
TEF	tracheo-esophageal fistula
TG	triglyceride
TGF	transforming growth factor
Th1	T helper cell type 1
TIBC	total iron binding capacity
TIPSS	transjugular intrahepatic portosystemic shunt
TMP-SMX	trimethoprim–sulphamethoxazole
TNF	tumor necrosis factor
TNM	tumor–node–metastasis (staging system for cancer)
TPMT	thiopurine methyltransferase
TPN	total parenteral nutrition
TSH	thyroid-stimulating hormone
UC	ulcerative colitis
UDCA	ursodeoxycholic acid
U & E	urine and electrolytes
UGT	uridine diphosphate glucuronyl transferase
ULN	upper limits of normal
U/S	ultrasound
UTI	urinary tract infection
VBL	variceal band ligation
VIP	vasoactive intestinal polypeptide
VOD	veno-occlusive disease
VTEC	verocytotoxin-producing *E. coli*

WCC	white cell count
WDP	Wilson's disease protein
WE	Wernicke's encephalopathy
WHO	World Health Organization
ZES	Zollinger–Ellison syndrome

Top 10 clinical problems

Anemia and occult GI bleeding

Anemia (Hct less than 36%) is common in GI practice and also a common reason for referral to gastroenterologists by other specialists. Often a gastroenterologist is asked for an opinion on the cause of a macrocytic or microcytic anemia. Careful testing to confirm the presence of various hematinic deficiencies is crucial (see Box 1.1). A classification of anemia related to GI disease is shown in Table 1.1.

Box 1.1 Basic tests for anemia

- Full blood count (Hb, red cell indices—MCV, MCHC, MCH—white count and differential, platelets)
- Blood film examination
- Reticulocyte count
- Iron, TIBC, ferritin
- B12 and folate (red cell folate).
- U&E
- <u>Liver function tests</u> including albumin and GGT

Table 1.1 Classification of anemia related to GI disease

GI bleeding	Iron deficiency
Decreased red cell production	Vitamin B12 (see <u>cobalamin</u>), and <u>folic acid</u> deficiency (deficiency seen in pregnancy, increased cell turnover, inflammation)
	Marrow failure: aplastic anemia, red cell aplasia, marrow infiltration.
Increased red cell destruction	Congenital (hemoglobinopathies, spherocytosis, red cell enzyme defects)
	Acquired (immune/nonimmune)
Abnormal red cell maturation	Sideroblastic anemia, myelodysplasia
Drug-related anemia	See text. May be caused by bleeding (NSAIDs, warfarin), drug-induced hemolysis, or marrow aplasia (e.g., sulfasalazine).
Effect of disease in other organs	Anemia of chronic disease Liver, renal, endocrine disease

Anemia

The most important are **iron, folic acid, and vitamin B12**, but **copper and vitamins A, B6, C, E, riboflavin, and nicotinic acid** are also needed for erythropoiesis. Deficiency can arise through inadequate intake, malabsorption, increased need or use, and loss.

Table 1.2 Causes of iron, B12, and folate deficiency in GI disease

	Iron	B12	Folate
Nutritional	Rarely sole cause	Vegans	Poor diet—elderly, alcoholics, institutionalized
Malabsorption			
Stomach	Anacidity, atrophic gastritis, gastrectomy	Pernicious anemia, food—cobalamin malabsorption, atrophic gastritis	Gastrectomy
Small intestine	Celiac disease, tropical sprue	Stagnant loop with associated bacterial overgrowth, ileal resection, Crohn's, celiac, sprue, fish tapeworm, selective malabsorption	Gastrectomy, celiac, tropical sprue, scleroderma, amyloidosis, Giardia, diabetic enteropathy, lymphoma, Whipple's disease
Other		Chronic pancreatitis, liver disease	Alcohol
Increased loss or utilization	Bleeding		Liver disease, Crohn's disease

For details of treatment of B12, iron, and folate deficiency and further details of individual causes, see iron deficiency: vitamin B12 (see cobalamin) deficiency: folate deficiency.

Increased red cell destruction: hemolysis

Red cell destruction is mainly extravascular in the liver, spleen, and bone marrow. Heme is metabolized to bilirubin, conjugated in the liver, and excreted in the feces and urine.

Congenital causes

- Unconjugated hyperbilirubinemia due to excess hemolysis is seen in the neonate due to:
  - **Congenital spherocytosis** (in the adult spherocytosis indicates antibody-mediated red cell destruction) or
  - **Nonspherocytotic causes** such as inherited red cell enzyme defects (e.g., G6PD deficiency).
- **Hemoglobinopathies**. These include structural hemoglobin variants, such as sickle cell disease and disorders of globin chain synthesis (thalassemias).

Acquired causes

- In adults can be seen in severe liver disease due to abnormal lipid composition of red cells.
- Disseminated cancers (e.g., arising from a gastric or pancreatic primary) can produce disseminated intravascular coagulation and the associated fibrin deposition can produce a microangiopathic hemolytic anemia.

Diagnosis

Plasma haptoglobins bind to hemoglobin and are reduced in intravascular hemolysis and in liver disease. Hemolysis can result in pigment <u>gallstones</u> that can be the presenting feature of illness.

Drug-related anemia

Think of:

- Upper GI irritation causing blood loss: <u>NSAIDs</u> and aspirin. The combination of <u>NSAIDs</u> and <u>CORTICOSTEROIDS</u> is associated with high risk of upper GI bleeding.
- Bleeding due to specific drugs, e.g., warfarin, heparin.
- Drug-induced hemolysis—e.g., oxidative hemolysis due to sulfasalazine or dapsone.
- Production impairment, e.g., aplasia secondary to mesalazine.

Anemia in liver disease

Table 1.3 Causes of anemia in liver disease

Cause	Comment
Dilutional	Increased plasma volume, splenomegaly
Iron deficiency	Bleeding. Iron status can be difficult to establish. Ferritin may be increased as an acute phase protein. Transferrin, accounting for much of TIBC, is often reduced. MCV may be falsely raised due to alcohol.
Vitamin B12 and folate	Liver stores B12 and folate. Folate often deficient in alcoholics due to poor nutrition and effect of alcohol in reducing folate absorption.
Hemolysis	May be autoimmune in association with <u>autoimmune hepatitis</u>. Red cell lifespan reduced, due to abnormal membrane—if severe can produce "spur cell" anemia. Alcohol can cause sideroblastic anemia. Hemolysis is seen in <u>Wilson's disease</u> (probably due to copper toxicity to red cells). <u>Zieve's syndrome.</u>
Aplastic anemia	Viral hepatitis: parvovirus, <u>hepatitis A, B, C</u>, EBV, CMV. Hepatitis is often mild and marrow aplasia severe: damage may be immune-mediated. Alcohol may have direct marrow toxicity effects.

Iron deficiency anemia presumed due to occult GI blood loss

Up to 100 ml blood loss per day can still result in grossly normal looking stools. The source of bleeding is unidentified in about 5% of patients with GI bleeding.

Fecal occult blood testing can be helpful, particularly if menorrhagia is suspected as a cause of anemia in menstruating women. Iron deficiency is diagnosed either by a low ferritin or by a low transferrin saturation (ratio of iron to TIBC). Beware missing iron deficiency because of a normal TIBC; this reflects mostly transferrin synthesis by the liver, which can be impaired in chronic disease or inflammation.

Diagnosing the cause of iron-deficiency anemia

History

- Focus on drugs that injure the GI mucosa (e.g., aspirin, nonsteroidals, bisphosphonates, potassium salts).
- Take a careful family history for bleeding disorders.

Examination

Look for cutaneous stigmata of systemic diseases (dermatitis herpetiformis, neurofibromas, lip freckles suggestive of Peutz–Jeghers, mucosal telangiectasia in hereditary hemorrhagic telangiectasia, osteomas suggestive of Gardner's syndrome).

Investigations

Initial assessment may direct investigations to a particular part of GI tract. For example:

- Dyspepsia or a clear history of NSAID or other irritant drug ingestion directs the need for upper GI endoscopy; and a positive family history of colon cancer, a change of bowel habit, or iron deficiency in an elderly patient with aortic stenosis (suggesting possibility of angiodysplasia) will necessitate colonoscopy.
- In the absence of clear symptoms, upper GI endoscopy and colonoscopy at the same session improves cost effectiveness and results in a significantly increased diagnostic yield over either investigation alone.
- Always consider duodenal biopsy to exclude villous atrophy (see celiac disease) as a cause of unexplained iron deficiency (low iron due to malabsorption and blood loss).

Investigation of the patient with suspected occult GI bleeding or definite blood loss but normal upper GI endoscopy/colonoscopy

This is influenced by the briskness of the bleeding.

- If there is any suggestion of an upper GI lesion, repeat upper GI endoscopy by a senior endoscopist using an enteroscope or pediatric colonoscope has been shown to identify lesions in a substantial proportion of patients.
- In those with active bleeding, radionuclide scanning with Tc^{99}-labeled red cells or angiography can reveal the site of bleeding. Tc^{99} scans

are sensitive at confirming GI bleeding, but evidence on their role in managing patients with GI bleeds is lacking. Angiography is less sensitive (requires bleeding rate of at least 2 ml/min) but can accurately locate bleeding point and in skilled hands allows possibility of therapeutic embolization of bleeding vessel. CT scanning or <u>Meckel's</u> scans may be helpful.

- Evaluation of possible small intestinal pathology by contrast radiology gives a very low diagnostic yield and often results in unhelpful exposure of young patients to ionizing radiation. The suggested sequence of examination is influenced by availability of certain techniques, but available evidence favors <u>enteroscopy</u>, preferably using a dedicated enteroscope with balloons or spiral introducers to ensure adequate depth of insertion. Video <u>capsule endoscopy</u> is another option to detect lesions of the small bowel, providing there are no symptoms of intestinal obstruction.

Ascites

In the developed world, <u>portal hypertension</u> due to cirrhosis accounts for 80%, with intra-abdominal malignancy and heart failure making up most of the rest. Note that ascites rarely occurs due to <u>portal vein thrombosis</u> in isolation, but may develop in setting of systemic sepsis, or low serum albumin.

Table 1.4 Causes of fluid within the peritoneal cavity (i.e., ascites)

Mechanism	Causes
<u>Portal hypertension</u>	Parenchymal liver disease (e.g., <u>cirrhosis</u>, <u>alcoholic hepatitis</u>, <u>acute liver failure</u>); right heart failure; constrictive pericarditis; <u>veno-occlusive disease</u>; Budd–Chiari syndrome; <u>portal vein thrombosis</u>
Peritoneal inflammation	<u>Spontaneous bacterial peritonitis</u>; malignant peritoneal deposits; connective tissue disease (e.g., systemic lupus, <u>sarcoidosis</u>, <u>familial Mediterranean fever</u>), TB; pancreatic ascites
Reduced plasma oncotic pressure	Hypoalbuminemic states (e.g., nephrotic syndrome, malnutrition, <u>protein-losing enteropathy</u>)
Impaired lymphatic drainage	Lymphatic obstruction (e.g., right heart failure, TB, lymphoproliferative disorders); lymphatic tear (e.g., trauma)

Assessment of ascites

Always consider

- Is there unequivocal evidence of ascites (hospital admission and intensive investigation of portal hypertension is rarely effective treatment for central obesity!)?
- What is the cause of ascites?
- What is the optimal management?

History

A full history is essential, especially in those with recent-onset ascites. Focus on:

- Symptoms and risk factors for cirrhosis (see <u>Cirrhosis and chronic liver disease</u>), <u>portal hypertension</u>, and cardiac disease.
- Internal malignancy (including recent weight loss and right upper quadrant discomfort in cirrhotics, suggestive of <u>hepatocellular carcinoma</u>).
- Sepsis (including abdominal <u>TB</u> and <u>spontaneous bacterial peritonitis</u>).

Examination

Look for signs of:

- Chronic liver disease, <u>hepatic encephalopathy</u> (e.g., jaundice, liver flap).
- <u>Portal hypertension</u> (splenomegaly, dilated abdominal veins, caput medusa (superficial veins radiating out from umbilicus)). Ascites due to portal hypertension usually occurs in setting of hyperdynamic circulation (↑HR, peripheral vasodilatation, ↓mean arterial BP).
- Cardiac failure (cardiomegaly, ↑JVP).

Investigation

- Bloods: CBC, BUN & electrolytes, LFTs, ESR, CRP, clotting. Full assessment of causes of liver disease as appropriate (see <u>Recent-onset jaundice</u>).
- Imaging. <u>Ultrasound</u> + Doppler or contrast <u>CT scan</u> allow <u>portal vein flow</u> to be assessed, as well as intra-abdominal organs. 'Internal echoes' or 'septae' within ascites may suggest infection or lymphatic cause.
- Diagnostic ascitic tap is essential in all cases, including in patients with known cirrhosis and ascites in hospital (who have a high rate of <u>spontaneous bacterial peritonitis</u>. See <u>paracentesis</u>. 20 ml of fluid should be drawn, and assessed for:
  - **Color** (see Fig. 1.1). Usually yellow/straw color. Blood suggests "blood tap" or malignancy; white/milky suggests chylous ascites.
  - White **cell count**: (normal <500 white cells/µl, <250 neutrophils/µl).
  - **Ascitic albumin**. This allows calculation of serum to ascites albumin gradient (SAAG), which accurately differentiates ascites due to <u>portal hypertension</u> (SAAG >11 g/l) from nonportal hypertension in > 97% of cases.
  - **Microscopy and culture**. Always inoculate into blood culture bottles. Acid fast bacillus (AFB) is positive in the fluid of <20% of cases of peritoneal TB.
  - **Cytology**. In suspected malignancy, providing larger volumes of fluid to the cytopathologist (e.g., > 100 ml) may increase the chance of making a diagnosis.
- Urinalysis +24 hour urine collection if proteinuria.
- Further investigations will be tailored to the results of these tests, and clinical picture (e.g., ECG, CXR, echocardiogram if possible heart failure). Ascitic amylase >2000 IU/l suggests pancreatic ascites (e.g., following <u>pancreatic pseudocyst</u> rupture), and ascitic bilirubin. > serum bilirubin supports diagnosis of a biliary leak (e.g., post-<u>cholecystectomy</u>). Microbiological diagnosis of TB ascites varies significantly (10–70% positive cultures). Chylous ascites is diagnosed by a measured ascitic triglyceride (TG) level of > 110 mg/dl (and always with ascitic TG > plasma TG).

See Fig. 1.1 for diagnosis on basis of ascitic fluid analysis.

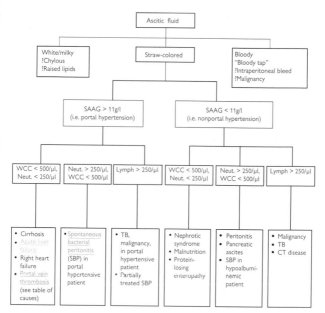

Figure 1.1 Diagnosis of cause of ascites using serum-ascites albumin gradient (SAAG) and cell count. Although SAAG strongly predicts whether ascites is due to portal hypertension, interpretation of WCC results necessitates incorporation of clinical information and other results (e.g., culture, cytology).

Ascites: Management

Vital to treat the underlying cause, not just manage ascites (see Cirrhosis and chronic liver disease).

Portal hypertensive ascites

- **Salt restriction**. No added salt to food should be specified, and low salt diet preferred, but patient compliance with <1.5 g/day (60 mmol/day) is poor. However, salt restriction alone may lead to resolution of ascites in 20% of patients.
- **Restriction of fluid** to 1.5 l is a standard component of management, but as fluid loss in ascites is directly related to negative Na^+ balance, fluid restriction is rarely effective in absence of salt restriction.

- **Diuretics**. Combination of spironolactone and furosemide usually required. Commence spironolactone 100 mg/day and furosemide 40 mg/day. Increase dosages every 4–5 days, to maximum spironolactone 400 mg/day and furosemide 160 mg/day, titrated against body weight (aim ↓0.5 kg/day) and body weight. Monitor BUN & electrolytes to exclude renal impairment.
- In 10% of patients this approach does not work, defining them as having "refractory ascites." Treatment options then include large volume therapeutic <u>paracentesis</u>, surgical shunting, <u>transjugular intrahepatic portosystemic shunt (TIPSS)</u>, or <u>liver transplantation</u>.
- Surgical portosystemic shunts and peritoneovenous shunts are now rarely used, because of high complication rate and availability of alternatives.
- TIPSS is effective at controlling ascites in most patients, but high occlusion rate (30–50% at one year) and risk of <u>hepatic encephalopathy</u> (up to 30%) raise concern about its long-term role, particularly in those with poor liver synthetic function (i.e., ↑ bilirubin, ↑INR, ↓serum—albumin see Child–Pugh score).
- <u>Liver transplantation</u> is the definitive treatment of patients with cirrhotic ascites, who otherwise have a 5-year survival of 20% with medical therapy alone.

Nonportal hypertensive ascites

Malignant ascites is usually refractory to diuretics, and requires repeated therapeutic <u>paracentesis</u>. It generally indicates a very poor prognosis. Biliary peritonitis requires endoscopic or percutaneous biliary stenting ± surgery, dependent on cause. Similarly, management of pancreatic ascites depends on exact site and cause of pancreatic leak, with approaches including pancreatic rest (e.g., with nasojejunal feeding), percutaneous drainage, endoscopic <u>pancreatic stent</u> insertion, surgical pancreatic resection (e.g., <u>Whipple's procedure</u> or distal pancreatectomy) ± <u>OCTREOTIDE</u> to reduce pancreatic fluid output. TB ascites is treated with appropriate chemotherapy.

Chronic or recurrent abdominal pain

Abdominal pain is a very common cause of patients presenting to doctors. **Acute abdominal pain** usually has an organic cause and is dealt with elsewhere (see emergencies: acute abdominal pain). Although there are many pathological causes of **chronic abdominal pain**, most are not due to organic disease, so that the symptom can be a source of worry, frustration, and confusion—to both doctor and patient. (See Box 1.3)

Diagnosis depends on interpreting the patient's experience into a medical model of disease: this can be difficult because of:
- Common innervation of many abdominal organs.
- The low concentration of nerve endings in the viscera.
- The patient's lack of previous experience of pain coming from these organs.
- The nonspecific nature of the pain.

Types of abdominal pain

Distinguish:
- **Visceral** pain, originating from noxious stimuli affecting an abdominal viscus and usually felt in the midline.
- **Parietal or somatic** pain arising from stimulation of the parietal peritoneum or abdominal wall and usually located to the site of the lesion.
- **Referred** pain, felt in remote areas supplied by the same neurosegment as the diseased organ because of shared central pathways for afferent neurons from different sites.

Critical features in assessing pain

- The site of the pain, and where it is referred to.
- The **nature** of the pain is important. Ulcers "gnaw," "viscera" "colic," and ruptured aneurysms "tear." A long duration of pain tends to correlate with a nonorganic cause, especially if not associated with weight loss or other alarm symptoms. Estimating severity of pain is very unreliable.

Factors modifying pain can be very helpful in diagnosis:
- Aggravating foods, or more usually the relationship of pain to eating, may be helpful. Genuine food allergy is rare: food intolerance (e.g., to lactose-containing foods in lactase deficient people) is not. Alcohol can aggravate dyspepsia and intestinal spasm, cause pancreatitis, or worsen lymphoma pain.
- Relief by bowel action or passing flatus suggests a colonic source (see irritable bowel syndrome).
- Pain related to menstruation suggests endometriosis or pelvic inflammatory disease.

Physical examination

- **Tachycardia, fever, and sweating** suggest sepsis. Frequent changes of position suggest visceral pain with no or little inflammation.
- **Inspect** for scars, hernias, visible peristalsis.

- **Auscultation** may reveal hyperperistalsis in intestinal obstruction, or ileus, or bruits.
- Do rectal (PR) and if necessary a vaginal (PV) examination (clear prior discussion of the need for internal examination is vital, and the presence of a chaperone is particularly important for the latter). Tenderness on PR or PV examination may not be appreciated by examination of the anterior abdominal wall.
- **Palpate:** rigidity or guarding suggests local peritonism. A palpable mass may result from organ enlargement, inflammation, or a tumor.
- **Percussion** is helpful: tympany suggests excess air, either intraluminal or extraluminal, and light percussion if painful can suggest an area of peritonitis.

Investigations

- Full blood count with MCV (iron studies, B12, and folate if this is abnormal), ESR, and CRP.
- Check renal function and liver function tests.
- Examine urine for pyuria and hematuria, and send sample for microscopy, culture, and sensitivity. If appropriate, check a woman of childbearing age for pregnancy.
- *Do not* use inappropriate radiological tests. An abdominal ultrasound can be highly informative and is noninvasive.
- Other tests depend on the result of the history and examination.

Functional abdominal pain

Functional abdominal disorders account for about half of all patients with abdominal pain seen by doctors and almost all cases with abdominal pain lasting for years. In most cases, a diagnosis of irritable bowel syndrome is possible from the history (see Box 1.2). A small minority of cases have intractable chronic abdominal pain: this may be associated with previous physical or sexual abuse, and the onset may coincide with bereavement.

Box 1.2 The Rome criteria for irritable bowel syndrome

At least three months of continuous abdominal pain or discomfort relieved by defecation, or associated with a change in stool frequency, or associated with a change in stool consistency, plus two or more of the following, at least 25% of the time:

- Altered stool frequency
- Altered stool form
- Straining, urgency, tenesmus
- Passage of mucus
- Bloating or distension

Over investigation can result from impatience or fear of a missed diagnosis. This tends to sustain the disorder, because the patient recognizes the failure of the doctor to grasp the problem, and gets increasingly frustrated by a succession of normal results. The doctor may have to spend time, spread over several visits, if necessary, to explore emotional factors. The general approach is outlined in Box 1.4.

Box 1.3 Causes of chronic or recurrent abdominal pain

Note: Some conditions can present acutely!

Generalized parietal pain due to peritonitis
- Bacterial peritonitis (including <u>spontaneous bacterial peritonitis</u>).
- Ruptured cyst
- <u>Familial Mediterranean fever</u>

Localized peritoneal pain
- <u>Appendicitis</u>, <u>cholecystitis</u>, <u>Crohn's disease</u>, endometriosis, chronic pelvic inflammation
- Infiltration due to abdominal neoplasms

Pain from increased tension in viscera
- Intestinal obstruction (mechanical, intussusception, internal herniation)
- Biliary obstruction (<u>choledocholithiasis</u>)
- Ureteric obstruction

Ischemia
- <u>Intestinal ischemia</u> (stenosis, embolism, inflammation)

Retroperitoneal causes
- <u>Chronic pancreatitis</u>

Extra-abdominal
- Neurological (neurogenic tumors, spinal degenerative disease, herpes zoster
- Metabolic (diabetic ketoacidosis, acute intermittent <u>porphyria</u>)
- Hematologic (<u>sickle cell anemia</u>, Henoch–Schönlein purpura)
- Toxic (lead)

Functional causes
- <u>Irritable bowel syndrome</u>
- Nonulcer dyspepsia
- Biliary pain (<u>sphincter of Oddi dysfunction</u>)

Box 1.4 General approach to the patient with functional abdominal pain

Establish rapport and trust
- Acknowledge the symptoms as real
- Maintain a nonjudgmental attitude
- Schedule brief but frequent appointments
- Reassure

Avoid temptation to do more diagnostic tests

Set appropriate goals
- Do not expect cure; focus on adjustment
- Emphasize improvement in function
- Emphasize coping and adaptation
- Allow for setbacks

Consider specialized referrals
- Psychiatric, pain clinic, relaxation training

Drug treatment

Analgesics, especially <u>OPIATES</u>, are often not helpful. <u>ANTISPASMODICS</u> can be helpful if targeted to patients with cramping abdominal pain. Start with peppermint tea, oil, or capsules, then consider mebeverine or other similar agents. Low dose antidepressants can be helpful, but patients are often resistant to the idea of taking antidepressants and it is important to emphasize (in layman's terms) that in low doses these drugs have a visceral analgesic effect rather than psychotropic actions.

Cirrhosis and Chronic liver disease

Background

- A diagnosis of chronic liver disease is usually made in patients under investigation for abnormal <u>liver function tests</u> (LFTs) or with unexplained jaundice (see <u>Approaches to recent-onset jaundice</u>, and <u>well patient with abnormal liver tests</u>), or in those who present with decompensation (see below). (See Box 1.5)
- The most common causes of chronic liver disease in Western nations are related to <u>alcoholic liver disease</u> and <u>hepatitis C</u> (see Table 1.5).
- Cirrhosis is a histological diagnosis characterized by diffuse hepatic fibrosis and nodule formation. Chronic noncirrhotic liver disease and well-compensated cirrhosis can rarely be differentiated on clinical findings and biochemistry alone (LFTs may be normal, even in established cirrhosis).
- <u>Liver biopsy</u> should be considered in all cases of chronic liver disease. Exceptions may include a patient with clear etiology of liver disease who has clinically decompensated cirrhosis (e.g., small, irregular liver on imaging, with markedly impaired liver function ($\uparrow$bilirubin, $\downarrow$albumin, $\uparrow$prothrombin) and evidence of <u>portal hypertension</u> (e.g., ascites, splenomegaly)).
- A clinical distinction is often made between patients with compensated and those with decompensated cirrhosis. Although the distinction may not be absolute, the clinical problems and management of these two patterns differ, and so are discussed separately here.
- See also <u>Child–Pugh score.</u>

Table 1.5 Causes of cirrhosis and chronic liver dis-ease

Alcoholic liver disease	Hemochromatosis
Hepatitis B	Autoimmune hepatitis
Hepatitis C	Wilson's disease
Primary sclerosing cholangitis	α-1-anti-trypsin deficiency
Primary biliary cirrhosis	Budd–Chiari syndrome
Drugs (e.g., methotrexate)	Secondary biliary cirrhosis
Metabolic liver diseases	Cryptogenic (approximately 15%)
Nonalcoholic fatty liver disease	

Compensated cirrhosis

The patient will have good liver synthetic function (e.g., bilirubin, albumin, prothrombin time may be normal) without ascites or hepatic encephalopathy. The focus of management is to prevent progression of liver disease (decompensation) and avoid complications.

Management

Treat the cause. A nihilistic approach to cirrhosis is not justified. Although the natural course is for progressive fibrosis and liver dysfunction, treatment of the underlying cause has been demonstrated to slow down, and even reverse, clinical progression in patients with established cirrhosis (e.g., hemochromatosis, hepatitis B and C). It is vital to address alcohol dependency. Promising data is emerging on the role of antifibrotic therapies in reversing some of the effects of cirrhosis, but no agent approved as yet.

- It is increasingly recognized that osteoporosis is strongly associated with cirrhosis, especially if cholestatic etiology (e.g., primary biliary cirrhosis) or on immunosuppression. Bone densitometry is indicated, and calcium and vitamin D supplements slow progression of bone loss, and bisphosphonates may be needed (although they may cause side effects, including esophagitis).

- The complications of portal hypertension may manifest as acute variceal bleeding (see acute upper GI bleeding), ascites, or hepatic encephalopathy (i.e., 'decompensated'—see next section). After diagnosing cirrhosis, upper GI endoscopy should be considered, as the finding of gastroesophageal varices may merit primary prophylaxis (see portal hypertension).

- The risk of hepatocellular carcinoma (HCC) increases significantly once cirrhosis develops (e.g., yearly incidence of HCC 1–4% in patients with cirrhosis due to hepatitis C). Evidence supports role for 3–6 monthly serum alphafetoprotein (AFP) and ultrasound.

- An additional liver insult may lead to decompensation in patients with cirrhosis. Patients with cirrhosis who may be at any risk of hepatitis A or hepatitis B (e.g., frequent travelers to moderate risk areas; drug users; multiple sexual partners) should be tested for immunity, and vaccinated as appropriate.

- Complications of cirrhosis, including ascites, infection, and metabolic bone disease, are more common in malnourished patient. Give thiamine 100 mg od PO, encourage high calorie and protein intake, and refer for nutritional advice as necessary. Note that patients with alcoholic liver disease may get high proportion of daily calorie intake from alcohol.

- Prescribing medication in patients with cirrhosis may be complex, as there is a risk of precipitating: bleeding (e.g., NSAIDs); worsening liver function (e.g., statins); hepatic encephalopathy (e.g., OPIATES); or renal impairment (e.g., NSAIDs, aminoglycosides). Also see drug-induced hepatotoxicity.

- Pregnancy may occur in patients who are cirrhotic, although 50% of premenopausal women with cirrhosis have secondary amenorrhea. Close liaison between patient, obstetrician, and hepatologist is essential.

Decompensated cirrhosis

- This may be indicated by development of jaundice, <u>hepatic encephalopathy</u>, or ascites. Jaundice and encephalopathy are much more commonly due to acutely deteriorating chronic liver disease than <u>acute liver failure</u>.
- Decompensation strongly predicts death, with 1- and 5-year survival in patients with <u>Child–Pugh score</u> C of 42% and 21%, compared with 84% and 44% for Child–Pugh score A disease.

Table 1.6 Etiology of hepatic decompensation

Progressive loss of hepatic function	Dehydration
Additional liver insult (e.g., alcohol, <u>hepatitis A</u>)	Constipation
<u>Acute upper GI bleeding</u>	Renal failure
<u>Hepatocellular carcinoma</u>	Drugs (e.g., opiates)
Infection (e.g., <u>spontaneous bacterial peritonitis</u>)	Noncompliance with treatment
Increased portosystemic shunt (e.g., <u>transjugular intrahepatic portosystemic shunt (TIPSS)</u>)	Vascular impairment (e.g., acute <u>portal vein thrombosis</u>)

Assessment

- Careful history to identify causes of decompensation is vital (see Table 1.6). Ask about recent binge drinking (see <u>alcohol dependency</u>), any new drugs, infections (common cause, but symptoms and signs of sepsis may be masked in cirrhosis), weight loss or abdominal pain (e.g., <u>hepatocellular carcinoma</u>). Has there been any recent change in bowels (e.g., melena, constipation) or history of hematemesis?
- As well as looking for signs of chronic liver disease (e.g., spider naevi, gynecomastia), are there signs of decompensation (jaundice, liver flap, ascites)? Assess the grade of <u>hepatic encephalopathy</u>. Full general examination to elicit source of possible sepsis (including urine dipstick), and rectal examination to exclude melena or constipation is necessary.

Investigations

- In all cases, blood should be sent for BUN & electrolytes, LFTs, glucose, FBC, clotting profile. See also Recent-onset jaundice.
- Further investigations will depend on initial results and manifestation of decompensation, but must include a search for a precipitant:
  - Alphafetoprotein (AFP).
  - Abdominal U/S with Doppler of hepatic and portal veins.
  - Culture of blood, urine, sputum.
  - Diagnostic ascitic tap, for cell count and culture (see paracentesis).
  - CXR.

Management

Directed towards the particular manifestation of hepatic decompensation (e.g., ascites), and treatment of the precipitants

- In patients with acutely decompensated cirrhosis liver support devices, including Molecular Absorbence Recirculation Systems (MARS), may have a role, necessitating transfer to a regional liver unit offering this facility.
- In patients with decompensation due to hepatitis B, LAMIVUDINE therapy may improve liver function and clinical disease.
- In view of the poor long-term prognosis (e.g., 50% 2-year mortality following episode of ascites with spontaneous bacterial peritonitis), liver transplantation assessment should be considered once an episode of decompensation has occurred.

Box 1.5 Five-point checklist for assessing patient with chronic liver disease

1. Does the patient have cirrhosis, or noncirrhotic chronic liver disease?
2. What's the etiology?
3. In the patient with cirrhosis, is it well compensated or decompensated?
4. What interventions may prevent progression to cirrhosis, or to decompensation in the patient with established cirrhosis?
5. What investigations/interventions are needed to avoid/treat the complications of cirrhosis?

Constipation

Definition

Defining constipation is difficult. In practice, constipation is defined by reduced frequency of defecation—twice weekly or less. Many patients complaining of constipation have, in reality, excessive straining at defecation (with or without hard stools), a sensation of incomplete evacuation, or excessive time spent on the toilet, even though frequency may be in the normal range.

Clinical subtypes and related causes (see Tables 1.7 and 1.8)

Patients may have:
- **Normal transit**, but report hard stools or difficulty in evacuation.
- **Slow colonic transit**, and report a reduced frequency or even absence of the urge to defecate.
- **Incoordination of the rectum, anus, and pelvic floor** present with symptoms of straining, incomplete evacuation, and the need for anal or vaginal digitation in order to empty the rectum.

Evaluation

History
- **Onset**. Constipation from birth suggests congenital cause such as <u>Hirschsprung's</u> or meningocele.
- **Patient age and duration of symptoms**. Constipation may be of recent onset or chronic. A recent change, particularly in adults, needs workup for organic causes. Complaints of several years duration are more likely to be due to functional disorders.
- **Details of bowel habit**. Don't be squeamish. Ask about frequency of defecation, the form of the stool (words like small or hard are subjective; description of stringy or pellet-like stool is more helpful), excessive straining, discomfort, a sense of incomplete evacuation or of "blockage." Take note of any pain or bleeding.
- Associated **abdominal pain or bloating** suggest <u>irritable bowel syndrome</u>. Associated genitourinary symptoms may suggest an underlying central or peripheral neurological disorder.
- Evacuatory difficulty. Patients will often only admit this if asked directly about the need to digitate vaginally or rectally or of the need to apply perianal pressure.
- Ask about **laxative use and duration**, and about similar complaints in other family members.
- Ask for or at least make an assessment of potential **affective disorders**. Depression, emotional stress, and the use of mood-altering drugs including antidepressants can affect bowel function.
- Consider the possibility of **sexual abuse**. Somatic reactions to sexual abuse include abdominal pain, constipation, and appetite disturbance.

Table 1.7 Clinical subtypes of constipation

Secondary to an organic colonic cause or outlet obstruction	Recent onset or the presence of alarm symptoms indicates need to exclude tumors or stenotic lesions of the colon by endoscopy or radiology
Outlet obstruction	Any painful anal condition (e.g., <u>anal fissure</u>, herpes) or <u>anal cancer</u> can cause difficulty in defecation
Irritable bowel syndrome	Consider when it coexists with bloating and pain in a young person
Constipation with gut dilatation	Causes include idiopathic <u>megacolon</u> or megarectum, <u>Hirschsprung's disease</u>, or chronic <u>pseudo-obstruction</u>
Severe constipation with a normal diameter colon	Chronic, often associated with slow colon transit, and most commonly occurs in young women of reproductive age
Drug-induced constipation	See Table 1.8
Constipation secondary to coexisting systemic illness	See Table 1.8
Psychological	<u>Anorexia nervosa</u>, affective disorder, dementia, childhood physical or sexual abuse, loss of a parent through death or separation, or disturbed toileting behavior
Constipation due to immobility/age/diet	Elderly or bedridden patients in hospital as well as out may be unable to respond to toileting signals; this can lead to impaction, incontinence, and acute confusional states. Drugs can exacerbate symptoms in this group.

Table 1.8 Drugs causing constipation

Drug type	Examples
Analgesics	<u>OPIATES</u>
Anticholinergics	Antispasmodics, antidepressants (tricyclics), antipsychotics, antiparkinsonian drugs
Cation-containing agents	Iron, aluminum, calcium, barium, bismuth
Others	Antihypertensives, ganglion blockers, vinca alkaloids, anticonvulsants, calcium channel blockers

Examination

- Examine the abdomen for bowel distension, retained stool, or previous surgery.
- Anorectal and perineal examination is important: look for perineal disease or deformity, wasting of the gluteal muscles, and rectal prolapse. Test for perineal sensation. Digital examination may reveal the pain of an anal fissure, an anal stenosis, or a rectal mass or fecal impaction. Assess the anal tone (even though correlation of this with formal anorectal electrophysiological assessment is poor) and ask the patient to strain as if passing a motion, which can help in the diagnosis of prolapse, a rectocele, or abnormal perineal descent.
- Anismus (a paradoxical increase in anal tone when straining at stool instead of the normal relaxation response) may be seen in victims of rape, incest, or sexual abuse.
- Think of nongastrointestinal diseases that may cause or exacerbate constipation.
- Do a neurological exam to look for central or peripheral causes; consider testing autonomic function. Check perineal sensation.

Diagnostic approach and investigations

Most chronically constipated patients do not need investigation beyond the history, examination, and exclusion of systemic or gastrointestinal causes.

Structural investigations

These are important to exclude organic disease when accompanied by alarm symptoms (recent onset, weight loss, PR blood, family history of colonic cancer) but are overused in patients with longstanding symptoms.

- **Colonoscopy** has relatively little use unless to exclude a colonic cancer.
- **Flexible sigmoidoscopy** can help in showing stenosing left-sided colonic lesions and also can diagnose laxative abuse via melanosis coli.
- **Radiology** is sometimes useful. A plain abdominal film may indicate stool retention and colonic dilatation in megarectum or megacolon and can help assess the efficacy of laxative treatment if there is clinical uncertainty. Barium studies may show colonic dilatation in Hirschsprung's disease but are not as useful as physiological studies.
- **Rectal biopsies** can be helpful in diagnosing Hirschsprung's disease but a full thickness biopsy is needed.

Functional evaluation (see Fig. 1.2)

For the patient with infrequent defecation, a prospective two-week bowel diary and measurement of colon transit time by colon transit studies (see colonic inertia) is useful and can distinguish normal from slow transit constipation. Delayed colon transit can be due to colonic inertia or outlet obstruction. Colonic inertia produces chronic constipation and often responds poorly to medical treatment. If there is excessive straining, then transit studies are of little use, but studies of anorectal function may be very useful.

Anorectal manometry is useful in patients with suspected Hirschsprung's disease (absent anorectal inhibitory reflex) or in patients with evacuatory difficulty—inability to expel a balloon filled with 50 ml water suggests incoordinated defecation. Normal anorectal function with outlet obstruction suggests withholding behavior and is common in children.

Defecography or a defecating proctogram may be useful if there is a suspected structural problem influencing defecation, e.g., a rectocele, prolapse, or intussusception, or to assess functional problems in evacuation.

Table 1.9 Systemic diseases causing constipation

Type	Examples	Comment
Metabolic/ endocrine	Diabetes	Usually mild but common.
	Hypothyroidism	
	Hypercalcemia	
	Hypokalemia	
	Pregnancy	
	Porphyria	
	Pheochromocytoma	
	Glucagonoma	
Central neurological disorders	Multiple sclerosis	
	Parkinson's disease	
	CVA	
Peripheral neurological disorders	Hirschsprung's	
	Neurofibromatosis	
	Peripheral nerve damage	Transection of parasympathetic supply in the sacral nerves in the rectum or cauda equina (injury to lumbosacral spine, meningomyelocele, low spinal anesthesia) produces colon dilatation reduced rectal tone and sensation. Constipation may occur with high spinal cord lesions, but the colon reflexes tend to be intact and defecation can be triggered by digitation of the anal canal.
	Autonomic neuropathy	
	Chronic intestinal pseudo-obstruction	
Collagen vascular	Scleroderma	
	Amyloidosis	
	Dermatomyositis	
Primary muscle disorders	Myotonic dystrophy	

Treatment considerations

General principles include consideration of dietary fiber supplementation, ensuring adequate toileting arrangements, and avoiding chronic use of stimulant laxatives if possible.

Diet and the role of fiber

Increasing dietary fiber leads to increased stool weight and stool frequency in normal people, and constipation may result from dietary fiber inadequacy in some patients. But there is no evidence that constipated people in general consume less fiber that nonconstipated people, and dietary fiber is not usually effective in the management of constipated patients referred to hospital; furthermore it is often poorly tolerated due to bloating and flatulence. Nevertheless, conventional management is to increase dietary fiber to 20–30 g per day.

A top-ten list of dietary sources of fiber is shown in Table 1.10. The bulking effect of fiber is only partly due to water-retaining capacity; colonic microbial ecology is also important. Fiber can be a substrate for colonic bacteria and increase stool bulk by bacterial proliferation and production of stool gases. This partly explains why fiber can provoke abdominal distension and flatulence in patients with slow transit constipation.

Fiber supplementation is not indicated in patients with <u>megacolon</u> or megarectum, patients confined to bed, or patients with neurological disease.

Drugs

Vast amount of laxatives are consumed, especially by the elderly. A working knowledge of these compounds is essential and the main classes are described in detail in Chapter 6-1 (see <u>LAXATIVES</u>; see also <u>laxative abuse</u>). For many, laxatives do not provide sustained relief of symptoms.

Drugs to increase colonic transit are an attractive idea but only partially effective: cholinergic agents or anticholinesterases have been tried in patients with colonic inertia. <u>PROKINETICS</u> include metaclopramide, which has been used in upper GI motility disorders but does not work in the colon. <u>CHLORIDE CHANNEL ACTIVATORS</u> (e.g., lubiprostone) have recently been approved to treat constipation. Opiate antagonists, possibly given orally, have been suggested as being able to counteract excessive endogenous opioids and these, too, are under investigation.

Behavioral treatments

Behavioral therapy including <u>biofeedback therapy</u> (teaching the patient to normalize pelvic floor function while watching real time feedback about sphincter function) is an effective treatment for patients with slow transit constipation or impaired evacuation where traditional treatments have failed (about 2/3 of patients benefit). Behavioral treatments include exercises focused on the gut, psychological support, lifestyle/dietary factors, and help in stopping laxatives and have been shown to improve symptoms, colonic transit, and psychological well-being and reduce the need for laxatives.

A behavioral approach involving bowel retraining is often tried in children with idiopathic constipation with or without soiling. Details can be found in larger texts (e.g., Yamada MD *et al.* (eds) (2003) *Textbook of Gastroenterology* p.920. Lippincott Williams and Wilkins.)

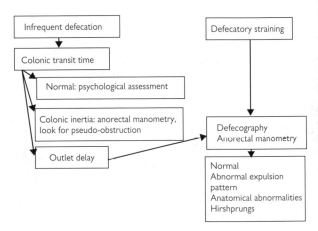

Figure 1.2 Functional evaluation of chronic constipation.

Table 1.10 Food sources of dietary fiber

Food source	Amount of fiber/100 g
Cereals	
All-Bran	26.7
Shredded Wheat	12.3
Cornflakes	11
Whole wheat bread	8.5
Peanuts	9.3
Peanut butter	7.5
Vegetables	
Baked beans	7.3
Peas	6.3
Fruits	
Pear	2.4
Banana	1.7
Apple	1.4

Surgery

Agreed indications

- <u>Hirschsprung's disease</u>.
- <u>Rectocele</u>. About 50% of patients get improvement after repair. Biofeedback is an option in this group.
- Rectal intussusception and prolapse. Surgery is not always curative: intussusception is common in non-constipated people, and its presence in constipated patients is not proof of causation.

Controversial indications

Colonic inertia. The commonest operation is subtotal colectomy with ileo-rectal anastomosis. Segmental resection based on removal of that part of the colon with the greatest hold-up of markers, has not proved effective and there is a high rate of anastomotic leakage. Long-term follow-up data indicates a success rate of less than 50%. Antegrade (ACE) procedure, where a stoma is made in the cecum and water instilled distally, is another possibility in patients with slow transit constipation.

Acute diarrhea (less than 14 days)

Most cases of acute diarrhea are due to infections; in immunocompetent patients these are usually self-limiting and intervention may be limited to oral rehydration if there are no signs of significant fluid loss. Diarrhea lasting more than 14 days is usually described as persistent or chronic and is usually due to some other cause (exceptions in immunocompetent patients include _Giardia_ and _Yersinia_). Diagnosis and management are addressed in chronic diarrhea.

Key questions in the history
- How long is the history?
- Are there systemic symptoms (fever, tachycardia) or vomiting?
- Is there recognizable blood in the stool?
- How frequent are the stools?
- Presence and location of any associated abdominal pain?
- Any contact with possible infected food or water?
- Recent travel history?
- Any contact with similarly ill people? Anyone in the family unwell?
- On examination, always look for signs of dehydration and malnutrition.

Risk factors
- Age. During and after weaning the protective effects of breast milk are lost. The elderly may have declining immune competence, but also reduced acid secretion (e.g., due to pernicious anemia, _Helicobacter_, infection, drugs such as PPIs).
- Immune deficiency: includes patients with HIV (see HIV and the gut), and those on anticancer chemotherapy.
- Medication, including antibiotics: (see antibiotic-associated diarrhea).
- Travel (see later section).
- Infected food and water: either a true infection with ingestion of enteropathogens that multiply in the gut, or ingestion of preformed toxin in food contaminated with an enterotoxin-producing microorganism.
- Known sensitivity to certain foods: see food allergy/intolerance.

Classifying acute diarrhea

Subdivide acute diarrheal diseases into the presence or absence of blood in the stool, since the causes are largely different (but remember *Shigella* and *Campylobacter* can present as acute watery diarrhea).

Box 1.6 Causes of acute diarrhea with blood

- Bacillary dysentery (shigellosis)
- Enterohemorrhagic *E. coli*
- *Campylobacter*
- *Salmonella*
- *Yersinia*
- Amoebic dysentery
- Antibiotic-associated colitis
- Rarely, *Schistosoma* (*mansoni* or *japonicum*) and *Tricuris*

Box 1.7 Causes of acute diarrhea without blood

- Viruses (rotavirus, Norwalk, astrovirus, adenovirus)
- Bacteria
  - Mild infection with *Shigella*, *Salmonella*, or *Campylobacter*
  - *E. coli* (enterotoxigenic, enteropathogenic, enteroaggregative)
  - Cholera, *Clostridia* spp.
- Protozoa: *Giardia*, cryptosporidiosis, *Cyclospora*
- *Strongyloides*
- Food toxins
- Malaria

Also consider whether the process involves mostly the small intestine.

Pathogens targeting the small bowel include toxigenic bacteria, viruses, and the parasite *Giardia lamblia* (see giardiasis). They all produce large volume watery diarrhea and midabdominal pain. Blood and fecal leucocytes are rare.

Pathogens targeting the large bowel are usually invasive organisms like *Shigella*, *Campylobacter*, and enteroinvasive and enterohemorrhagic *E. coli* (EIEC and EHEC). They produce lower abdominal or rectal pain (tenesmus), mucoid or bloody diarrhea with many fecal leucocytes, and inflamed rectal mucosa (see food poisoning).

A few pathogens (e.g., *Salmonella* and *Yersinia*) infect the lower small bowel but can invade the colon as well. They can present with a spectrum from watery diarrhea to colitis (see Box 1.7).

Table 1.11 Infectious agents targeting small bowel

	Agent	Source and incubation period
Viruses	Rotavirus, Norwalk agent, calcivirus, torovirus, enteric adenovirus	Short incubation (1–3 d) for rotavirus and Norwalk agent, longer (8–10 d) for adenovirus. Norwalk occurs in shellfish.
Bacteria that colonize the gut	*Vibrio cholerae*	2–144 hours. See _cholera._
	Vibrio parahaemolyticus	Raw fish or seafood, 2–48 hrs. Usually short illness.
	Yersinia enterocolitica *Salmonella*	Principally invade the lower small bowel but may invade the colon. The clinical spectrum varies from watery diarrhea to colitis.
	E. coli (ETEC, EPEC)	See _Escherichia coli_
	Giardia	See _giardiasis_

Table 1.12 Infectious agents targeting large bowel

Shigella	Highly contagious. Spread usually feco-oral but outbreaks can occur related to contaminated milk, ice-cream, or water. Toxigenic phase of fever, pain, diarrhea starts early after infection.
Campylobacter	Incubation period 24–72 hrs. Usual source is infected animals. Most infections result from improperly cooked chicken (50–70% cases).
Salmonella	Toxic megacolon and perforation due to colitis can occur—commonest when diarrhea has lasted 10–15 d.
E. coli (EIEC, EHEC)	1–14 d, mean 3 d. See _Escherichia coli._
Entameba histolytica	See _amebiasis_
C. difficile	See _clostridial infections in GI tract_

Investigations

Many attacks of acute diarrhea are self-limiting. In general, investigation is indicated in the following circumstances:
- Course more than two weeks;
- Signs of systemic upset including fever;
- Tenesmus or bloody diarrhea;
- Special circumstances:
  - Outbreaks suggesting food poisoning;
  - Male homosexual;
  - Immunocompromised host;
  - Ingestion of raw shellfish;
  - Antibiotic usage.

Stool culture is often requested but few centers offer tests for all pathogens, mixed infections are common, single stool cultures are insufficient for some pathogens, and results often come back too late to influence management. In practice, apart from the investigation of outbreaks and surveillance, stool culture in uncomplicated cases should be limited to exclusion of those pathogens for which antibiotic treatment is indicated (parasites, *Shigella*, *V. cholerae*) or where there are other possible causes of acute diarrhea (e.g., inflammatory bowel disease).

Stool microscopy for fecal leucocytes can be very helpful in diagnosing an inflammatory diarrhea (see Box 1.8).

> **Box 1.8 Fecal leucocytes in intestinal infections**
>
> **Present:** _Shigella_, _Campylobacter_, EIEC, EHEC
> **Variable:** _Salmonella_, _Yersinia_, *C. difficile*
> **Absent:** cholera, ETEC/EPEC, viral diarrhea, _Giardia_, amoebiasis

Identifying microbial antigens ELISA tests for _Giardia_ and serology for amoebiasis are more accurate than stool microscopy and should be ordered given the appropriate history even in the absence of fecal leucocytes. Serology/antibody testing is useful for _Yersinia enterocolitica_. ELISA kits are available for _strongyloides_ and _schistosomiasis_.

Abdominal CT should be taken if the patient is toxic, to look for evidence of diffuse colitis, ileus, or toxic megacolon.

Treatment

Fluid replacement

- **Oral rehydration** is nearly always the preferred route, but if the patient is vomiting or intravascularly depleted (resting tachycardia with postural drop in blood pressure) **intravenous fluids** may be necessary.
- Unlike the situation in patients with intestinal resection or jejunostomy, where sodium concentration of 90–120 mM provides maximum salt and water absorption, the optimal sodium concentration for rehydration in cases of mild to moderate acute diarrhea is probably around 50 mM. The substitution of starch from rice or cereal for glucose is associated with less diarrhea and more rapid resolution.

Diet

Eating during an attack of acute diarrhea can be uncomfortable because any food can provide an additional stimulus to defecation. There is no benefit to fasting, but dairy products should be avoided because of the risk of lactose intolerance. Alcohol, caffeine, and sodas should be avoided. The BRAT diet is often recommended (Bananas, Rice, Apple Sauce & Toast).

Drugs. **Antimotility agents** can be very useful but should not be used if there is an acute severe colitis because of the risk of precipitating toxic megacolon. LOPERAMIDE is the drug of choice.

Indication for antibiotics

- Pathogens: *Shigella*, *Vibrio cholerae*, *Salmonella typhi*, *Clostridium difficile*.
- Community-acquired diarrhea: more than four stools/day for over three days with one or more of pain, fever, vomiting, myalgia, headache. A quinolone such as CIPROFLOXACIN 250–500 mg bd is suggested. Optimal duration is not known; a single dose if given early is very effective.
- Laboratory proven cases of *Giardia intestinalis*.
- Antibiotic treatment of enterohemorrhagic *E. coli* is controversial and expert advice should be sought (see hemolytic–uremic syndrome).
- Laboratory proven enteropathogenic *E. coli* infection, especially in the very young or old.
- Traveller's diarrhea in adults: the duration of diarrhea is reduced when a quinolone such as CIPROFLOXACIN is used. RIFAXIMIN is another alternative.

Table 1.13 Antibiotic therapy of dysentry

	Drug of choice	Alternative
Bacteria		
Shigella spp.	Ampicillin	Cefixime[1]
	500 mg qds, 5 d	400 mg od, 5–7 d
	TMP-SMX	Nalidixic acid
	2 tabs bd, 5 d	1 g qds, 5–7 d
	Ciprofloxacin[3]	
	500 mg bd, 5 d	
Salmonella spp.	Ciprofloxacin[2,3]	
	500 mg bd, 10–14 d	
EIEC	? as Shigella spp.	
EHEC	?	
C. jejuni	Erythromycin	Ciprofloxacin[3]
	250–500 mg qds, 7 d	500 mg bd, 5–7 d
Y. enterocolitica	Tetracycline	
	250 mg qds, 7–10 d	
Y. enterocolitica	Ciprofloxacin[3]	
	500 mg bd, 7–10 d	
	TMP-SMX	
	2 tabs bd, 7–10 d	
C. difficile	Metronidazole tds	
	400 mg, 7–10 d	
	Vancomycin	
	125 mg qds, 7–10 d	
Protozoa		
E. histolytica	Metronidazole	Paromomycin
	400 mg tds, 5 d	25–35 mg/kg tds, 10 d
	Diloxanide furoate	
	500 mg tds, 10 d	

[1]And other third-generation cephalosporins.

[2]Usually only for bacteremia.

[3]And other fluoroquinolones such as ofloxacin, norfloxacin, fleroxacin, and cinoxacin.

EIEC; enteroinvasive E.coli.

EHEC; enterohemorrhagic E.coli.

TMP-SMX;Trimethoprim–sulphamethoxazole.

Adapted from Bloom S (2001). *Practical Gastroenterology: A Comprehensive Guide.* Reprinted with permission from Taylor & Francis Group Ltd.

Diarrhea in travelers

- 30–50% of travelers to developing countries have an episode of infective diarrhea.
- Episodes are usually of mild-to-moderate severity and self-limiting.
- Investigation and treatment may be needed for individuals with bloody diarrhea, when invasive organisms are involved, or when diarrhea persists after their return home.

Causal organisms

- Enterotoxigenic _E. coli_ (ETEC) is the commonest cause worldwide (also leading bacterial cause of gastroenteritis on cruise ships), but _Shigella_ accounts for increasing proportion, and _Campylobacter_ is important in travelers to Asia.
- Other bacterial pathogens: _Aeromonas_, _Plesiomonas_, and _Vibrio_.
- Viruses (rotavirus, Norwalk virus) are common causes (up to 30% of cases).
- Parasitic causes are uncommon, but _Giardia_ is found in 5%. _Cyclospora_ is seen occasionally. _Cryptosporidium_ can be a problem for the immunocompromised.
- Consider amoebiasis caused by _Entamoeba histolytica_ in people with bloody stools.
- Geography affects the likely cause. Although ETEC and _Shigella_ account for the majority of isolates in Africa and the Middle East, over 50% of people affected in Asia have _Campylobacter_.

Natural history, mode of infection

- Most cases occur 5–15 days after arrival. Malaise, anorexia, abdominal cramps, watery diarrhea, and sometimes nausea with vomiting are the hallmarks. Fever occurs in about one-third of cases. Most cases resolve in 6–10 days.
- Gastric hypoacidity and immunosuppression increase the risk. Risk is also increased in patients with ulcerative colitis, Crohn's disease, and celiac disease.
- Careful selection of food and drink to minimize infection reduces but does not eliminate risk: two other approaches include chemoprophylaxis or dispensing medication to be taken if diarrhea develops.

Chemoprophylaxis

The Center for Disease Control does not recommend routine use of prophylactic antibiotics, because of concerns about side effects and selection of resistant strains. Two settings where prophylactic antibiotics are used include:

- Short-term travelers (two weeks or less in an endemic area) whose business or vacation schedule would be severely disrupted by an episode of diarrhea.
- Patients with an underlying medical condition or the immunocompromised.

Where ETEC, _Shigella_, or _Salmonella_ predominate a quinolone antibiotic (ciprofloxacin 500 mg od) is the drug of choice. For travelers to Asia, _Campylobacter_ is common and frequently resistant to quinolones: azithromycin 500 mg od should be used.

Self-medication with antibiotics. A single dose of <u>CIPROFLOXACIN</u> 500 mg taken at the first sensation of impending upset can reduce the duration and intensity of infection.

Other aspects of self-treatment. The benefit of adding antidiarrhea agents, such as loperamide (see <u>ANTIDIARRHEAL AGENTS</u>) to antibiotics is unclear. It is very important to ensure adequate fluid and electrolyte replacement using an oral rehydration solution, such as the World Health Organization (WHO) rehydration solution.

Diagnostic approach to diarrhea in the returning traveler

- Initial approach is the same as that for self-treatment of traveler's diarrhea (three days of quinolone or azithromycin, plus loperamide and adequate fluid/electrolyte replacement).
- Diarrhea can be a prominent symptom of **malaria**. Examine blood film for *Plasmodium* in travelers returning from malarious areas with fever and diarrhea.
- Watery diarrhea persisting for longer than 10 days is most commonly due to <u>giardiasis</u>. Send stool to be examined for *Giardia*, *Cryptosporidium*, *Cyclospora*, and *Isospora*.
- Empirical treatment with <u>METRONIDAZOLE</u> or tinidazole for *Giardia* is often reasonable. If this fails to improve the diarrhea, further investigation with upper GI endoscopy and small bowel biopsy, sigmoidoscopy, and rectal biopsy is required. If symptoms and biopsies are consistent with <u>tropical sprue</u>, tetracycline with folic acid is indicated.

Chronic diarrhea

Definition

Acute diarrhea (less than 14 day's duration) is usually due to infection (see Acute diarrhea).

A patient's perception of diarrhea needs to be clarified (increased looseness of stools; increased frequency of stools; urgency; abdominal discomfort; fecal incontinence). Stool weight (>235 g/day in men, > 175 g/day in women) has been used to define diarrhea but weighing the stool is unpleasant, disliked by patient, nurse, and laboratory, and in any case stool weight above the upper limit of normal with normal consistency is not necessarily diarrhea. A working definition of chronic diarrhea is the abnormal passage of ≥3 loose stools per day for over 4 weeks.

Clinical classification into **watery diarrhea (osmotic or secretory), fatty diarrhea (steatorrhea), or inflammatory diarrhea** is useful, but there is considerable pathophysiological overlap.

Pathophysiology and causes

Osmotic

Occurs due to presence in the gut of an excess amount of poorly absorbable, osmotically active solutes. Stool water content directly relates to fecal output of solutes exerting an osmotic pressure across the intestinal mucosa. (Electrolyte composition may vary according to the electrical charge on poorly absorbed anions or cations, which is why measuring stool electrolytes is rarely useful. Just as well for junior doctors and lab technicians: but see later for a role in evaluating difficult diarrheas.)

This explains two clinical hallmarks of osmotic diarrhea:
- Diarrhea stops when the patient fasts or at least stops eating the poorly absorbed solute causing the diarrhea.
- Stool analysis, if necessary, will reveal an osmotic gap: that is {2 × [Na^+] + [K^+]} (to account for anions) is less than fecal osmolality (usually assumed to be isotonic to plasma, i.e., 290 mOsm/kg).

Secretory

Results from abnormal ion transport by intestinal epithelial cells. Four main categories of disease involved:
- Congenital defect in ion absorption.
- Intestinal resection.
- Diffuse mucosal disease damaging/reduced epithelial cell numbers.
- Abnormal mediators (including neurotransmitters, bacterial toxins, hormones, and cathartics) that can affect intestinal chloride and water secretion through changes in intracellular AMP and GMP.

Secretory diarrhea is characterized by two features:
- Stool osmolality is accounted for by Na^+ + K^+, and related anions, so the osmotic gap is small.
- Diarrhea usually persists during a 48–72 hour fast.

Inflammatory (exudative)

Inflammation and ulceration may lead to loss of mucus, proteins, pus, or blood into the bowel lumen. Diarrhea accompanying intestinal inflammation may be due to impairment of normal colonic absorptive function.

Altered motility

Little experimental proof that increased motility causes diarrhea, but it has been implicated in:
- The diarrhea of irritable bowel syndrome.
- Postgastrectomy diarrhea.
- Diabetic diarrhea.
- Bile salt induced diarrhea.
- Diarrhea associated with hyperthyroidism.
- Drug-related, e.g., erythromycin as a motilin agonist.

Box 1.9 Causes of osmotic diarrhea

Carbohydrate malabsorption
- Congenital
  - Specific (disaccharidase deficiency, glucose–galactose malabsorption, fructose malabsorption)
  - Generalized (abetalipoproteinemia, congenital lymphangiectasia, enterokinase deficiency, pancreatic insufficiency [e.g., due to cystic fibrosis])
- Acquired
  - Specific (e.g., postenteritis disaccharidase deficiency)
  - Generalized malabsorption—(pancreatic insufficiency/biliary obstruction, bacterial overgrowth, celiac disease, parasitic disease, short-bowel syndrome, mucosal damage or disease, postmucosal obstruction in lymphangiectasia, previous surgery including gastrectomy or intestinal resection leading to bile acid malabsorption)

Excess ingestion of poorly absorbed carbohydrate
- Lactulose therapy, sorbitol in elixirs or "sugar-free" sweets, fructose in soft drinks or dried fruits, mannitol in sugar-free products, excess bran or fiber
- Magnesium-induced diarrhea from antacids and laxatives
- Laxatives containing poorly absorbed anions, such as sodium sulphate, phosphate, or citrate

Functional (IBS)
- Consider food hypersensitivity

Box 1.10 Causes of secretory diarrhea

- **Congenital** (microvillus inclusion disease, absent Cl/HCO_3 exchanger)
- **Endogenous**
  - Bacterial enterotoxins (<u>cholera</u>, ETEC, <u>*Campylobacter*</u>, <u>*Clostridium*</u>, *Staph. aureus*) or hormones (VIPoma, medullary carcinoma of thyroid (calcitonin, prostaglandins), <u>gastrinoma</u>, villous adenoma, small bowel <u>lymphoma</u>)
  - Stimulant laxatives: phenolphthalein, anthraquinones, castor oil, cascara, senna
  - Drugs: antibiotics, diuretics, theophyllines, thyroxine, anticholinesterases, colchicine, prokinetics, ACE inhibitors, antidepressants (SSRIs), prostaglandins, gold
  - Toxins: plant (*Amanita*), organophosphates, caffeine, monosodium glutamate

Box 1.11 Causes of inflammatory diarrhea

- Infection: bacterial, viral, parasitic
- Inflammatory bowel disease: <u>ulcerative colitis</u>, <u>Crohn's disease</u>, ulcerative jejuno-ileitis, <u>microscopic colitis</u> (often related to NSAIDs)
- Cytostatic agents: chemotherapy, radiotherapy
- Hypersensitivity: <u>eosinophilic gastroenteritis</u>, nematodes, food allergy
- Autoimmune: <u>micoscopic colitis</u>, <u>graft versus host disease</u>
- <u>Diverticular disease</u>/diverticular colitis
- Ischemia
- Radiation
- Neoplasia (<u>colonic cancer</u>, <u>lymphoma</u>)

Note: some causes of diarrhea do not fit easily into this classification e.g., ischemic colitis (see <u>intestinal ischemia</u>, <u>amyloidosis</u>).

History and examination

Taking a history of diarrhea

- Clarify what the patient means by diarrhea (see definition earlier) and distinguish acute from chronic diarrhea.
- After this, the aims of the history are:
  - To distinguish organic (e.g., duration < 3 months; weight loss; nocturnal symptoms; continuous symptoms) from functional causes (absence of organic symptoms + long history and presence of positive symptoms as defined by Rome II criteria—see irritable bowel syndrome).
  - To distinguish malabsorptive diarrhea (bulky, malodorous, difficult to flush, pale stools) from other causes (liquid/loose stools with blood or mucus).

Stool character and associated symptoms

- Consistently large volume diarrhea is likely to come from small bowel or proximal colon.
- Bloody diarrhea indicates an infectious, neoplastic, or inflammatory process; accompanying lethargy or anorexia may suggest mucosal cytokine release. Pale, floating stools suggest steatorrhea and are commonly due to pancreatic insufficiency (stools float because of gas content due to carbohydrate fermentation, not fat malabsorption).

Assess for specific causes of diarrhea

- Family history of inflammatory bowel disease, celiac disease, colon cancer.
- Previous GI surgery leading to increased transit, bacterial overgrowth or bile salt malabsorption.
- Systemic disease such as diabetes mellitus, thyroid disease—heat intolerance and palpitations may suggest hyperthyroidism, carcinoid (with associated flushing), systemic sclerosis.
- Drugs (see lists in text/boxes of causes of diarrhea—alcohol, caffeine, and nonabsorbable carbohydrates such as sorbitol are often missed and don't forget surreptitious laxative abuse, as factitious diarrhea occurs in 4% of those diarrhea cases in general hospitals, but up to 20% in tertiary referral units).
- Foreign travel, exposure to contaminated water or potential pathogens, e.g., *Salmonella* in food handlers, *Brucella* on farms.
- Evidence of chronic pancreatitis.
- Sexual history is important: anal intercourse is a risk factor for proctitis (causes include *Gonoccocus*, Herpes simplex, *Chlamydia*, amoebiasis).
- Always ask about fecal incontinence: it is common (2% of the population) and not always reported spontaneously. If present, take obstetric history for perineal trauma and possible sphincter damage.
- Ask about diet and stress as aggravating factors. There is a link between physical/sexual abuse and functional bowel disease.
- Ask about illness in companions or family members.

Likely causes of diarrhea in common clinical categories

- **Acute diarrhea:** infection (see advice to returning travelers in <u>Acute diarrhea</u>); drugs/food additives; ischemic colitis; fecal impaction.
- **Diarrhea in homosexual HIV-negative men:** <u>amebiasis</u>, <u>giardiasis</u>, <u>Shigella</u>, <u>Campylobacter</u>, syphilis, gonorrhea, <u>Chlamydia</u>, Herpes simplex.
- **Diarrhea in HIV:** *Crytosporidium, Microsporidia, Isospora,* <u>amebiasis</u>, <u>Giardia</u>, Herpes, <u>CMV</u>, Adenovirus, MAI, <u>Salmonella, Campylobacter</u>, *Cryptococcus, Histoplasma, Candida,* lymphoma, AIDS enteropathy (see <u>HIV and the gut</u>).
- **Chronic or recurrent diarrhea in the patient not previously investigated:** <u>irritable bowel syndrome</u>, <u>Crohn's disease</u>, <u>ulcerative colitis</u>, parasite or fungal infection, malabsorption, drugs or food additives, <u>colonic cancer</u>, diverticulitis, previous surgery, endocrine causes (e.g., thyroid disease), fecal impaction.
- **Chronic diarrhea in patients previously seen and investigated:** surreptitious laxative abuse, <u>fecal incontinence</u>, <u>microscopic colitis</u>, unrecognized malabsorption, <u>neuroendocrine tumors</u>, <u>food allergy</u>.
- **Nosocomial (hospital-acquired) diarrhea.** Diarrhea is among the most common nosocomial illnesses (occurs in 30–50% of patients on ITU) and one-third of patients in chronic care facilities have at least one significant diarrheal illness per year. Two classes of patients need particular consideration:
  - **Diarrhea in patients on ITU:** drugs, especially those containing magnesium and sorbitol, <u>antibiotic-associated diarrhea</u> (*C. difficile* but also reduced salvage of carbohydrate by colonic bacteria leading to osmotic diarrhea—see <u>clostridial infections of the GI tract</u>), enteral feeding, intestinal ischemia, pseudo-obstruction, fecal impaction, defective anal continence.
  - **Patients with cancer or on chemotherapy.** The incidence of GI toxicity with chemotherapy or radiotherapy can approach 100% with some regimens. <u>Radiotherapy enterocolitis</u> occurs at total body doses of 6 Gy or greater or pelvic irradiation of 3–4 Gy (see <u>radiation damage and the GI tract</u>). Toxic chemotherapeutic agents include cytosine, daunorubicin, 5FU, methotrexate, 6-mercaptopurine, irinotecan, and cisplatin. Some biological treatments such as anti-IL-2 therapy are associated with watery diarrhea. <u>Typhlitis</u> (neutropenic enterocolitis) is a potent cause of diarrhea in cancer patients.

Diagnostic tests

Do not accept a diagnosis of diarrhea without some attempt to examine the stool, even if only on the glove after a rectal exam, to look for blood, mucus, oil, or signs of steatorrhea.

- 75% of chronic diarrheas can be diagnosed by a careful history and examination, coupled with basic hematology and biochemical tests, stool examination for pathological infection and fat, and sigmoidoscopy with biopsy.
- Three tests lead to definitive diagnosis in most of the remaining patients.
  - Quantitative stool fat.
  - Colonoscopy with biopsies.
  - Response to fasting with measurement of stool volume and osmotic gap.
- Indicators of a functional rather than organic etiology are a long history (over 1 year), lack of significant weight loss, absence of nocturnal diarrhea, and straining with defecation. These indicators, taken together, are about 70% specific for functional symptoms.

Basic investigations

- Send three stool samples for **culture** (including ova cysts and parasites). Unless there is obvious blood or pus, ask for **stool microscopy** as the presence of fecal leucocytes is a hallmark of inflammatory diarrhea. Consider sending stool for *C. difficile* culture and toxin. If you suspect factitious diarrhea or laxative abuse, send the stool and urine for a laxative screen.
- **Blood tests**. Full blood count, ESR, CRP, iron, B12, folate, thyroid function, glucose, BUN & electrolytes, calcium, liver function tests including albumin, celiac serology.
- In most cases of diarrhea where histology helps to make a diagnosis, **sigmoidoscopy** is sufficient rather than full colonoscopy—the exception is when ileal histology is needed, or the changes are patchy throughout the colon. Where there is significant weight loss or bleeding to suggest lower GI malignancy, full **colonoscopy** is needed.
- **Radiological imaging** may be helpful: a plain abdominal X-ray can show fecal impaction, suggest colonic inflammation, pancreatic calcification, or intestinal dilatation.

Stool fat

This can be a very useful test but is difficult to get done well (and often difficult to get done at all).

- Adults absorb about 99% of ingested triglyceride, but only about 90% of phospholipid derived from endogenous sources like bile, sloughed enterocytes, and bacteria (this is not true for neonates where stool fat can exceed 10% of intake).
- About 5–6 g of normal fecal fat excreted per day is unabsorbed phospholipid from the endogenous pool, and about 1 g comes from the diet. **More than 7 g stool fat per 24 hours is abnormal.**
- Stool fat can be assessed qualitatively or quantitatively.

Response to fasting and stool osmotic gap

- Rarely of practical use in most cases of chronic diarrhea, but may be useful in difficult cases.
- Steatorrheic stools are usually >700 g per 24 h, and stool weight returns to normal on fasting. Inflammatory diarrheas respond variably to fasting, but like steatorrhea stool osmotic gap is usually not helpful.
- Measuring stool electrolytes and osmotic gap may help to classify chronic watery diarrheas. Analysis is done on a centrifuged stool sample, so results are possible from spot stool samples or 24–72 h collections.
- Assume that fecal osmolality is the same as plasma (290–mOsm/kg): this is true of freshly passed stool, but with time measured fecal osmolality can become falsely raised due to bacterial degradation of carbohydrate. Large measured deviations below 290 mOsm/kg indicate contamination of stool with urine or water, or a gastrocolic fistula, or hypotonic fluid intake. In principle, stool sodium/potassium is high in secretory diarrhea (unabsorbed electrolytes retain water in the gut lumen) and low in osmotic diarrhea (nonelectrolytes retain water in the gut lumen). Interpretation of stool osmotic gap and fecal electrolytes is shown in Table 1.14.

Table 1.14 Stool osmotic gap and fecal electrolytes in the investigation of diarrhea

Plasma osmolality (approx. 290 mOsm/kg) − 2 X (stool [Na]+ + stool [K+]) =	= Stool osmotic gap
Stool Na > 90 mM and osmotic gap < 50 mM	Secretory diarrhea: or osmotic diarrhea caused by sodium sulphate or phosphate ingestion
Stool sodium < 60 and osmotic gap > 125 mOsm	Osmotic diarrhea: if stool volume does not return to normal on fasting, suspect surreptitious magnesium ingestion
Stool sodium > 150 and stool osmolality > 375–400	Suspect contamination with urine
Stool osmolality < 200–250 mOsm	Suspect contamination of stool with dilute urine or water

Other tests used in investigating diarrhea

Specific tests for malabsorption.
- **Small bowel biopsy**. Duodenal biopsy, which may be combined with small bowel aspirate for microbiological analysis, can be useful in diagnosing <u>Crohn's disease</u> (especially in children), <u>celiac disease</u>, <u>Whipple's disease</u>, <u>giardiasis</u>, <u>lymphoma</u>, <u>eosinophlic gastroenteritis</u>, hypogammaglobulinemia, <u>amyloidosis</u>, mastocytosis, <u>lymphangiectasia</u>, and various parasitic and fungal infections.
- **Barium studies/small bowel imaging**. These may be useful in fistula, strictures, and previously undetected surgical bypasses.
- <u>Celiac disease</u>. serology.
- <u>Pancreatic function tests</u>.
- <u>Schilling test for assessing B12 malabsorption</u>.
- <u>Breath tests</u> for fat, carbohydrate, and bile salt malabsorption, and <u>bacterial overgrowth.</u>
- SeHCAT test (see <u>bile acid malabsorption</u>).

Specific tests for watery diarrhea
Blood and urine hormone levels. Blood levels of certain hormones produced by <u>neuroendocrine tumors</u> such as gastrin, VIP, somatostatin, pancreatic polypeptide, calcitonin, and glucagon may be useful. Urine levels of 5 HIAA can help in diagnosing <u>carcinoid</u>. See <u>gut hormone profile</u>.

Specific tests for inflammatory diarrheas
In addition to upper and lower GI endoscopy and small-bowel studies, <u>Indium-labeled leukocyte scanning</u> may be useful particularly in children.

Specific tests for enteric protein loss
Fecal α_1-antitrypsin.

Antidiarrheal therapy

These can be divided into those agents useful for mild to moderate diarrheas and those useful for secretory or severe diarrheas. Most agents in current use work by reducing motility rather than reducing secretion. See <u>ANTIDIARRHEAL AGENTS</u> for further details.

Dyspepsia and gastro-esophageal reflux

Definitions and common causes

Current definition of dyspepsia stems from Rome consensus meeting in 1999:

- "Pain or discomfort in the upper abdomen for at least 12 weeks of the preceding 12 months." Includes patients with symptoms of gastro-esophageal, reflux, as well as heartburn, nausea, and vomiting.
- However many other conditions satisfy above definition—e.g., cardiac disease, sphincter of Oddi dysfunction, and pancreatic disease.
- Subdivisions of dyspepsia include "ulcer-like" (epigastric pain), "reflux-like" (heartburn and regurgitation), and "dysmotility-like" (bloating and nausea).
- Common causes are:
- Gastro-esophageal reflux disease.
- Peptic ulceration.
- Nonulcer dyspepsia.

Most causes of dyspepsia are recurrent and intermittent. Only curative treatments are *Helicobacter pylori* eradication and surgery (including treatment for gallstones).

Epidemiology

- Average prevalence in the community is 39% when patients with mainly reflux symptoms are included, and 23% when they are not.
- 5% of the population consult a GP because of dyspepsia.
- 1% of the population are referred for upper GI endoscopy per year.

When and how to investigate

- Decide if the patient needs urgent referral for investigation (see Box 1.12). If no alarm symptoms, then treat first, investigate later (if necessary).
- Review medications for possible causes of dyspepsia: calcium antagonists, nitrates, theophyllines, bisphosphonates (especially alendronate), steroids, NSAIDs.
- Consider cardiac, biliary, or pancreatic disease in the differential diagnosis.
- Consider simple lifestyle advice (see Box 1.13).
- In those patients needing investigation, endoscopy is the preferred investigation because it is more sensitive than barium and allows biopsies. Double-contrast barium meal is an acceptable alternative in patients unwilling to undergo endoscopy (see endoscopic complications).

Box 1.12 **Alarm symptoms prompting urgent investigation of dyspepsia**

- Any sign of chronic gastrointestinal bleeding
- Progressive unintentional weight loss
- Dysphagia
- Persistent vomiting
- Iron-deficient anemia
- Epigastric mass
- Suspicious barium meal

Box 1.13 **Lifestyle advice for dyspepsia: any use?**

All reviews include a section on lifestyle advice but there is almost no evidence it makes any difference—except for **elevating the head of the bed** to decrease nocturnal reflux (not using extra pillows). Other conventional components include:

- Avoiding eating meals within four hours of going to bed
- Avoiding late night alcohol and caffeine, which relax the lower esophageal sphincter
- Weight control, which can reduce symptoms resulting from hiatus hernia

Starting treatment

Initial therapeutic strategies for dyspepsia include:
- Empirical treatment with acid suppressants (patients will often have self-medicated with antacids or alginates).
- PROTON PUMP INHIBITORS (PPIs) are more effective than HISTAMINE RECEPTOR ANTAGONISTS, are safe, and are recommended as first-line treatment.

Testing and treating for _Helicobacter pylori (HP)_

Testing and treating for HP increases response rates compared with antacid therapy alone, and testing and treating reduces the need for endoscopy. At present test and treat appears more effective than acid suppression (the costs of these interventions are similar, because HP eradication prevents future development of peptic ulcers as well as ulcer recurrence). Two weeks off PPIs is necessary before testing for HP using a breath test or a stool antigen test.

Managing gastro-esophageal reflux disease (GERD)

This includes endoscopically determined <u>esophagitis</u> and endoscopy-negative reflux disease (where usually a diagnostic course of acid suppression is needed to make the diagnosis). Esophageal mucosal biopsy does not help in diagnosing reflux disease but does help in diagnosing infection, <u>Barrett's esophagus</u>, and <u>esophageal</u> tumors.

In patients who respond poorly or who have chest pain, 24 hour pH monitoring may be needed.

Treatment of GERD

Most patients are managed with drugs to lower or neutralize gastric acid (see: <u>ANTACIDS</u>, <u>PROTON PUMP INHIBITORS</u>, <u>HISTAMINE RECEPTOR ANTAGONISTS).</u>

- Medical therapy is effective at healing esophagitis and improving reflux symptoms, but drugs do not restore the normal antireflux barrier at the gastro-esophageal junction and stopping medication often leads to rebound acid hypersecretion, which can precipitate relapse.
- Surgery (see <u>antireflux procedures</u>) is often proposed as an alternative and definitive management. Substantial morbidity and frequent need for medical therapy after surgery means that currently surgery is not an ideal solution.
- A variety of endoscopic procedures aimed at improving the barrier function of the lower esophagus have emerged: these are described elsewhere (see <u>antireflux procedures</u>).

Managing peptic ulcer disease

Although the discovery of <u>H. pylori</u> as the causative agent of 90% of duodenal ulcers and 75% of gastric ulcers has led to a declining incidence of hospitalization and surgery rates for uncomplicated peptic ulcer, there remains little change in the number of admissions for bleeding <u>peptic ulcer</u>. Overall mortality remains at approximately 6–8% for the last 30 years, partly due to increasing patient age and prevalence of concurrent illness.

Initial diagnosis and follow-up

Endoscopy accurately diagnoses gastric and duodenal ulceration and allows biopsy for mitotic change. It also allows diagnosis of many upper GI infections including <u>H. pylori</u>.

- In patients with uncomplicated duodenal ulcers whose symptoms resolve on treatment, endoscopic follow-up is not necessary.
- All patients with gastric ulcers need follow-up endoscopy at 6–8 weeks to confirm ulcer healing. If healing has not occurred, further biopsies are needed, to exclude cancer.
- Failure of gastric ulcers to heal by 6 months is held by many to be an indication for gastric surgery.

Drug therapy with full dose <u>PPI</u> or <u>HISTAMINE RECEPTOR ANTAGONISTS</u> will lead to healing of peptic ulcers in the majority of cases.

Helicobacter **and peptic ulceration**

Eradicate *Helicobacter* in *HP* positive patients with peptic ulcer disease.

- HP eradication increases DU healing in HP positive patients, with healing of 74% after 4–8 weeks therapy. HP eradication reduces DU recurrence. Recurrent duodenal ulceration after successful eradication of HP is rare and usually the result of HP re-infection.
- Eradication does not increase gastric ulcer healing but reduces gastric ulcer recurrence. See Helicobacter pylori.
- Retesting after eradication is not suggested as routine, although this information may be valued by individual patients. In patients with persistent or recurrent symptoms, eradication should be confirmed by a carbon-13 urea breath test **more than 4 weeks after the end of treatment**. A positive breath test requires further courses of eradication treatment. Antibiotic sensitivity by biopsy and culture and patient compliance may need to be checked. **Use of serology after treatment is not helpful** as antibody titers may persist long term. If breath testing is not available, repeat endoscopy may be needed.
- In patients with complicated duodenal ulcer disease, HP eradication should be confirmed: some gastroenterologists advocate repeat endoscopy to confirm ulcer healing and biopsies to confirm HP eradication.

Gastric ulceration

Most (over 70%) gastric ulcers are HP-associated. Biopsies must always be taken to exclude malignancy: there is some evidence that gastric brushings for cytology increase diagnostic yield.

NSAIDs and peptic ulceration

The risk of peptic ulceration leading to hospitalization associated with NSAID use is about 1 admission per 100 patient years of use in unselected patients. Patients with previous history of peptic ulcer are at higher risk. There is a five-fold increased risk of clinically significant GI bleeding in patients on NSAIDs for musculoskeletal pain and twofold increased risk for patients taking low dose aspirin for secondary prevention of cardiovascular disease. (Also see nonsteroidal anti-inflammatory drugs (NSAIDS) and the GI tract.)

- For patients taking NSAIDs with a diagnosed peptic ulcer, stop NSAIDs where possible. Treat with full dose PPI or H2RA and eradicate HP if present.
- In patients using NSAIDs who have a peptic ulcer, eradicating HP does not increase ulcer healing compared with acid-suppression therapy. However, eradicating HP reduces the risk of ulcer recurrence
- In patients using NSAIDs who have never had a peptic ulcer, eradicating HP reduces the first incidence of peptic ulceration.
- In patients with previous ulcers and in those at high risk, offer gastric protection with PPI/histamine receptor antagonist (a COX-2 selective NSAID may be less ulcerogenic; most clinicians would still combine them with a gastroprotective agent (see COX-2 selective NSAIDs).
- High dose H2RAs or a PPI reduce the incidence of endoscopically detected lesions in patients taking NSAIDs.

- In those on NSAIDs without peptic ulcers, taking a COX-2 selective NSAID is associated with a lower incidence of endoscopically detected lesions. The promotion of healing and prevention of recurrence in those with existing peptic ulcers is not clear.

Non-HP, non-NSAID associated peptic ulcers

Consider the following causes.
- Failure to detect HP due to PPI or recent antibiotic ingestion.
- Surreptitious or inadvertent aspirin or NSAID use.
- Ulcers related to other drugs: potassium chloride, bisphosphonates, immunosuppressive drugs, and more recently SSRIs have all been implicated in GI bleeding.
- Acid hypersecreting states such as Zollinger–Ellison syndrome (especially if associated with diarrhea, multiple ulcers, weight loss, hypercalcemia).
- Crohn's disease.
- TB.
- Malignancy.
- CMV in immunocompromised.

Managing nonulcer dyspepsia

This includes patients in whom endoscopy has excluded <u>peptic ulceration</u> (including erosive duodenitis and gastric erosions, considered part of the spectrum of peptic ulcer disease), malignancy, or esophagitis. Patients with dominant heartburn or reflux and no esophagitis on endoscopy are classified as "endoscopy-negative reflux disease."

There is uncertainty about the cause or best long-term management of this group of patients. Current recommendations include the following:

Eradicate *H. pylori* if present

In a pooled study of 12 RCTs (2,900 patients) comparing HP eradication compared with placebo in reducing dyspeptic symptoms in NUD, the response in the control group averaged 36% and eradication increased this by 7%, with a number needed to treat for one patient to benefit of 14.

If symptoms continue or recur, PPI or H2RA may be taken on an on-demand basis at the lowest dose needed to control symptoms.

Prokinetic drugs

These have been advocated particularly for the dysmotility-predominant group of patients. Although a meta-analysis of 14 trials involving over 1,000 patients shows a beneficial effect of prokinetics compared with placebo at reducing dyspepsia in short-term (2–8 week) courses, caution has been expressed over the validity of this result because of heterogeneity of patient inclusion (many trials not excluding patients with reflux) and the inclusion in many studies of the drug cisapride, which has been withdrawn from the UK market. Further studies are needed of the effectiveness of <u>DOPAMINE RECEPTOR ANTAGONISTS</u> (e.g., <u>METACLOPRAMIDE</u> and <u>DOMPERIDONE</u>).

The role of *Helicobacter* testing and eradication in managing dyspepsia

Initial testing for HP can include serology, fecal antigen testing, carbon-13 urea breath testing, or endoscopic biopsy. Retesting should use a carbon-13 urea breath test.

HP eradication is appropriate for peptic ulcer disease, nonulcer dyspepsia, and as part of an HP test-and-treat strategy in uninvestigated dyspepsia. A number of eradication therapies are effective (see <u>*Helicobacter pylori*</u>).

Box 1.14 Guidelines for management

American Gastroenterological Association Guidelines 2005 recommend:
1. Age 55 or younger without alarm features*
   a. Test and treat for H. pylori
      - 13c-urea breath test or stool antigen
      - If (+), treat for H. pylori
      - If (−), empiric trial of PPI for 4–8 weeks
   b. If symptoms remain, acid suppression (PPI preferable)
   c. If patients respond, EGD is not necessary

2. Age 55 or older and those with alarm features
   a. Endoscopy
   b. Based on expert opinion
   c. Age cut-off of 55 chosen because of generally low risk of malignancy in most US populations. Not absolute.
   d. Lower age of 45–50 could be considered in U.S. patients of Asian, Hispanic, or Afro-Caribbean descent

*Alarm features include GI bleeding, early satiety, unexplained weight loss, progressive dysphagia, odinophagia, recurrent vomiting, family history of UGI cancer, previous gastric surgery, abdominal mass or lymphadenopathy, and anemia or iron deficiency.

American College of Gastroenterology Guidelines 2005 also recommend testing and treating for H. pylori in patients under age 55 without alarm features.

Lower age cut-off can be used in patients or regions at higher risk of cancer.

Mouth and swallowing problems

Problems with the mouth

Painful mouth ulcers

- Traumatic ulcers.
- Aphthous ulcers: 20% have associated iron, B12, or folate deficiency. Often associated with systemic diseases.
- Malignant ulcers.

Painless mouth ulcers

These are frequently innocuous and caused by dentures or cheek biting. However, remember:

- Lichen planus.
- Leukoplakia.
- Oral candida.
- Oral telangiectasia seen as part of hereditary hemorrhagic telangiectasia (see Color Plate 16).
- Other pigmented lesions (Addison's disease, Kaposi's sarcoma, black tongue in patients on tetracyclines or bismuth).
- Blisters can be caused by pemphigus, pemphigoid, or drugs. Other so-called blistering disorders like epidermolysis bullosa and erythema multiforme tend to cause mouth ulcers rather than blisters.

Halitosis

Common causes are:

- Dental or tonsillar abscesses.
- Gingivitis/stomatitis.
- Any cause of dry mouth (drugs, fever, dehydration, Sjögren's syndrome, radiotherapy).
- Some foods (ethanol, garlic, dimethyl sulphoxide).
- Diseases outside the oropharynx include chronic lung pathology (bronchiectasis, lung abscess), liver failure, uremia, and diabetic ketoacidosis.

Evaluation and management. Ask about diet, medication, and nonoral disease. Emphasize importance of oral hygiene and dental hygiene. Routine tongue brushing can help. Antiseptic mouthwashes can be useful, as can artificial saliva in patients with xerostomia.

Mucocutaneous features of HIV (see HIV and the gut)

- Over 90% of HIV infected patients have at least one oral manifestation.
- The commonest HIV-associated mouth infection is candida (see candidiasis). Most viral causes are secondary to herpes viruses (herpes simplex, cytomegalovirus, varicella zoster virus. Oral hairy leukoplakia is seen in 40% of HIV patients and is associated with Epstein–Barr viral infection.
- Bacterial infection leading to periodontal disease is common and may progress to severe necrotizing stomatitis.
- Neoplasms. Kaposi's sarcoma and lymphoma are important in HIV disease.

Problems with swallowing

Do not confuse **dysphagia** (a difficulty with the act of swallowing or of food proceeding into the stomach) with **globus** (the sensation of a lump or something in the throat). Although globus is often functional, it can be caused by lesions in the neck, pharynx, or larynx. The old term *globus hystericus* is not appropriate: hysterical or histrionic features are nearly always absent. There is little evidence that a high pressure upper esophageal sphincter is associated with globus sensation. Globus is a common somatization symptom.[1]

Odynophagia means pain on swallowing. This suggests esophageal inflammation or ulceration. Two common causes are medications and infections—odynophagia rarely occurs with reflux disease. Pill-induced esophagitis usually has an acute history and a careful history of medication will usually suggest the diagnosis. Infections are becoming more common in immunocompromised patients: symptoms are nonspecific but certain infections are more common in HIV (candida) or transplant patients (herpes or CMV).

Dysphagia: oropharyngeal and esophageal

Difficulty with initiating swallowing is called **oropharyngeal dysphagia**. There are many local, neurological, and muscular causes; the dysphagia is

Table 1.15 Oral manifestations of disease

Disease	Oral manifestation
Vascular disorders	
Hereditary hemorrhagic telangiectasia	Telangiectasia on lips and mouth
Blue rubber bleb nevus syndrome	Dark blue soft compressible nodules
Bullous eruptions	
Epidermolysis bullosa	Mouth involvement most common in the scarring (dystrophic) form
Pemphigus/pemphigoid	Oral lesions are common in pemphigoid and almost universal in pemphigus
Rheumatologic disorders	
SLE	Oral ulcers
Scleroderma	Telangiectasia, microstomia
Behçet's	Oral ulcers
Miscellaneous	
Amyloidosis	Small waxy amber papules on face and lips
Fabry's disease	Angiokeratomas on lips and mouth
Kaposi's	Blue-red macules on oral mucosa
Porphyria	Photosensitivity
Pernicious anemia	Glossitis
Crohn's	Aphthous ulceration
Celiac disease	Aphthous ulceration

1 Othmer, E and De Souza C. (1985) Am. J. Psychiatry 142: 1146

usually part of a wider disease process and diagnosis is usually straightforward (see Box 1.15). Difficulty with the passage of swallowed substances down the esophagus into the stomach is referred to as **esophageal dysphagia**. The causes include motility problems or mechanical lesions (intrinsic or extrinsic to the esophagus) and are listed in Box 1.16.

Box 1.15 Causes of oropharyngeal dysphagia

Neuromuscular diseases
CNS
- Brainstem CVA
- Parkinson's disease
- Wilson's disease
- Multiple sclerosis
- Amyotrophic lateral sclerosis
- Tabes dorsalis *PNS*
- Bulbar polio
- Peripheral neuropathies (diphtheria, botulism, rabies, diabetes)

Motor end plate
- Myasthenia gravis
- Muscular dystrophy
- Metabolic disease (thyrotoxicosis, steroid myopathy)
- Amyloidosis, SLE

Local structural causes
- Inflammatory (abscess, TB, syphilis)
- Neoplastic
- Web
- Plummer–Vinsen syndrome
- Extrinsic compression
- Surgical resection

Disorders of the upper esophageal sphincter
- Hyper- or hypotensive upper-esophageal sphincter

Box 1.16 Causes of esophageal dysphagia

Motility disorders
- Achalasia, scleroderma, diffuse esophageal spasm, secondary motility disorders (collagen vascular diseases, Chagas's disease)

Mechanical, intrinsic
- Peptic stricture
- Esophageal ring
- Esophageal cancer
- Rare causes include webs, diverticula, benign tumors, esophageal hematoma, foreign bodies (e.g., food bolus)

Mechanical, extrinsic
- Vascular compression, cervical osteoarthritis, mediastinal abnormalities

Clinical evaluation

History and examination

Trouble starting a swallow or transferring the food from the mouth into the esophagus suggests oropharyngeal dysphagia. Associated symptoms include nasal regurgitation, dysarthria, and nasal speech. There may be cranial nerve abnormalities. There may be signs of weakness caused by muscular disease or a stroke: careful examination of the pharynx and larynx is important.

In esophageal dysphagia, three questions in the history are important:

- What kind of food (solid or liquid) produces the symptoms?
  - Motility disorders tend to result in slowly progressive dysphagia for solids and liquids, while in mechanical obstruction the dysphagia is worse for solids.
- Is dysphagia intermittent or progressive?
  - Classic causes of intermittent dysphagia are a Schatzki ring or some motility disorders like diffuse esophageal spasm.
- Is there associated heartburn?

The site of localization is of limited value: in particular dysphagia localized to the neck is often referred from below.

Assessment

Although modern endoscopy with intubation under direct vision is safe in most cases, there is a risk of intubating an esophageal pouch, which is one traditional reason for suggesting barium swallow as the initial investigation. More importantly, endoscopy is a crude and inappropriate tool for assessing the dynamic process of swallowing. For oropharyngeal dysphagia, a video barium swallow with a solid or semisolid bolus such as a marshmallow is the best test. If there is any evidence of an obstructing lesion, an endoscopy should be performed, with biopsy of any lesion. If endoscopy is negative or suggests a motility disorder, <u>esophageal manometry</u> should be done.

Therapeutic considerations

- Oropharyngeal dysphagia caused by Parkinson's, hypothyroidism, myositis, and myasthenia is treatable, emphasizing the importance of making a specific diagnosis.
- Dysphagia resulting from degenerative neurological disease can often be helped by a rehabilitation program organized by a speech and language therapist.
- Treatment of mechanical obstruction depends on the cause but may involve surgery, dilatation, or stenting (see <u>esophageal obstruction:</u> treatment).
- Motility disorders are treated medically and sometimes surgically.

Nausea and vomiting

Definitions and neurophysiology

The **vomiting center** lies in the medulla, close to centers controlling respiration and salivation (hence associated hyperventilation and salivation). It receives signals from the chemoreceptor trigger zone (located in the fourth ventricle, also known as the area postrema, with blood supply from posterior inferior cerebellar artery and no blood–brain barrier). This area is the site of action of certain drugs causing vomiting (see Box 1.17) but also receives afferent fibers from stomach, intestines, gallbladder, peritoneum, and heart.

- Nausea is probably mediated by similar pathways, which overlap with those mediating satiety; anorexia, therefore, usually accompanies nausea.
- Distinguish vomiting from regurgitation (latter usually effortless without the muscular activity involved in vomiting, it is associated with a sour or bitter taste, and not associated with nausea).

Clues in reaching a diagnosis

Timing. Early morning vomiting may be associated with pregnancy, but hyperemesis gravidarum is more serious. Vomiting associated with raised intracranial pressure, uremia, or postgastrectomy often occurs in the morning. Vomiting during or soon after a meal is often due to psychogenic causes, while vomiting one to several hours after a meal is more associated with gastric stasis (pyloric stenosis, upper small intestinal obstruction, or functional stasis in diabetic gastroparesis (see Diabetes and GI tract), scleroderma, or celiac disease).

Pain. Think of non-GI causes: severe pain such as renal colic can cause nausea and vomiting, and may be the only sign of a urinary infection. Same may be true of pneumonia, especially in elderly. Pain of peptic ulceration (epigastric, meal-related, causing night-time waking, not peri-umbilical or diffuse) is often relieved by vomiting. Vomiting associated with severe back pain can be caused by posterior duodenal ulcer, pancreatitis, or pancreatic cancer. Central colicky pain associated with gurgling and profuse vomiting of bile-stained fluid suggests small-bowel obstruction. Vomiting with large- bowel obstruction usually occurs late, accompanied by distension and absolute constipation.

Systemic symptoms and signs. Normal appetite should raise suspicion of a psychogenic cause, although can be associated with mechanical obstruction. Weight gain suggests an absence of serious organic disease, but patients with peptic ulcers may put on weight due to eating relieving their symptoms.

Nature of vomitus. Recognizable food suggests gastric stasis. Vomiting that smells feculent suggests small-bowel obstruction, ileus, gastro-colic fistula, or bacterial overgrowth. Blood in the vomit is potentially serious and may require management as for acute upper GI bleeding although "coffee-ground vomiting" is nonspecific, representing the appearance of many different kinds of vomited particulate matter. Blood first appearing after several vomits may be due to damage around the esophagogastric junction (see Mallory-Weiss syndrome).

Past medical history. Details of previous surgery are important. Information on childhood health may be relevant, and gallstones, inflammatory bowel disease, and celiac disease can be familial.

Social factors. Information about home, marriage, job, children, and sexual problems or abuse may be relevant, particularly if no cause can be identified, and if questions in these areas elicit anxiety or emotion.

Approach to investigation

- Blood tests are usually simple and based on the history and examination.
  - CBC may reveal anemia; iron deficiency may suggest peptic or malignant ulceration or disease of the small bowel.
  - ↑MCV may suggest alcohol excess, vitamin B12 or folate deficiency.
  - Electrolytes may be abnormal secondary to vomiting (e.g., ↓K⁺, ↓Na⁺ hyperchloremic metabolic alkalosis) or may reflect underlying primary renal dysfunction; check calcium level and also liver function tests. Send amylase in acute presentation to exclude acute pancreatitis.
- Upper GI endoscopy may help, particularly to exclude peptic ulcer or other mucosal abnormality, and bile reflux. However, endoscopy is a poor test of function and barium studies may be better in assessment of upper GI stasis and obstruction.

Management

- Central goal is to identify cause, as this determines treatment.
- Where psychogenic factors appear important, specialist psychological input may be beneficial.
- Lifestyle advice, including abstinence from alcohol, may help.
- A wide range of drugs is available for nausea and vomiting, which should be used in a step-wise manner, with the knowledge that all carry the risk of side effects.

Box 1.17 Drugs causing nausea and vomiting

- Via chemoreceptor trigger zone: opiates, digoxin, L-dopa, ipecacuanha, cytotoxic drugs
- Antibiotics (tetracyclines, METRONIDAZOLE, ERYTHROMYCIN)
- Sulphonamides (including salazopyrine)
- ASPIRIN, NSAIDS damage the gastric mucosa and may stimulate the vomiting center via ascending afferents
- Alcohol acts directly on the chemoreceptor trigger zone and via gastric mucosal damage

Causes of nausea and vomiting

See Boxes 1.18 and 1.19 for painless causes of vomiting and causes of vomiting without nausea.

Box 1.18 Painless causes of vomiting

Infective
- Viral gastroenteritis
- Food poisoning, possibly infection associated with *Helicobacter pylori*. Infections elsewhere such as UTI or pneumonia in the elderly
- Viral labyrinthitis

Mechanical obstruction
- Pyloric stenosis, or duodenal obstruction due to gastric or pancreatic cancer
- Esophageal cancer
- Biliary reflux, particularly if there has been previous gastric surgery or a gastro-enterostomy

Alcoholic gastritis
- Often causes early morning retching, usually small volumes, often blood stained

Acute liver failure
- E.g., paracetamol overdose, acute fatty liver of pregnancy

Metabolic causes
- Addison's disease (look for postural hypotension, mucosal. pigmentation—↑or normal K^+ particularly important, since ↓K^+ more expected after vomiting)
- Also consider hypercalcemia, uremia, and hyperthyroidism
- Up to 30% of diabetic patients may have intermittent nausea or vomiting—see Diabetes and the GI tract

Box 1.19 Causes of vomiting without nausea

- **Intracranial tumors.**
  - Ask about headache, double vision; examine for gait disturbances
- **Raised intracranial pressure**
  - Look for nystagmus, papilledema, cranial nerve abnormalities
- **Encephalitis**
- **Meningitis**
- **Migraine**
- **Cyclical vomiting**
  - Usually occurs in 2–3 month cycles, in children, teenagers, or young adults. It may accompany migraine and may respond to beta blockers.

Recent onset jaundice

Background

- Jaundice is a yellow pigmentation of the sclerae due to subcutaneous deposition of bilirubin (Bn). Usually detectable when Bn > 1.5 mg/dl. It arises due to either increased Bn production, or decreased hepatobiliary excretion. See bilirubin metabolism.
- In assessment of patients with recent onset of jaundice, four questions need to be answered.
- What type of jaundice is present?
- What is the causative agent or process?
- If due to liver damage, is jaundice a result of acute or acute-on-chronic liver disease?
- Is there evidence of liver failure?

Type of jaundice

On the basis of history, examination, and routine biochemical tests (see Fig. 1.3), it is usually possible to categorize the jaundiced patient into one of three disease groups. Within each group there are a wide range of causes (see Table 1.16).

Disorders of bilirubin production/metabolism ("prehepatic")

Usually asymptomatic hyperbilirubinemia, with few physical findings, and normal transaminases (ALT/AST) and cholestatic liver tests (ALP/GGT).

Liver disease ("hepatic")

- In chronic liver disease, jaundice may present with other evidence of decompensation (e.g., ascites, variceal bleeding, hepatic encephalopathy). Acute liver injury more commonly presents with abdominal discomfort and clinical hepatomegaly.
- Wide variability of LFTs seen, depending on cause of liver injury. Serum ALT > 1,000 U/l is unusual for alcoholic liver disease (even alcoholic hepatitis) or autoimmune liver disease (e.g., autoimmune hepatitis), and suggests acute liver injury due to viruses (e.g., hepatitis A, B), ischemia (? recent hypotension), or drugs (e.g., paracetamol).
- In absence of cause for new-onset jaundice, it may be clinically difficult to distinguish acute from acute-on-chronic disease. Poor/failing hepatic function is not indicated by elevation of liver enzymes, but most reliably by ↑ bilirubin, ↓ albumin, ↑ prothrombin time. ↑ ALP/GGT, in absence of biliary dilatation suggests intrahepatic cholestasis, due to a range of causes (e.g., primary biliary cirrhosis, drugs, TB, lymphoma).

Biliary obstruction ("post-hepatic")

- Jaundice is often associated with pruritis because subcutaneous deposition of bile acids is extremely irritant. Abdominal pain and nausea associated with bile duct stones, and progressive, painless jaundice with malignant obstruction, but history often imprecise.
- Elevation of ALP/GGT classically seen in patients with <u>biliary stricture</u>, but associated marked elevation of transaminases characteristically may occur with biliary obstruction due to stones (<u>choledocholithiasis</u>).

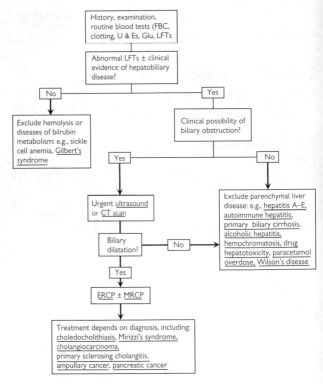

Figure 1.3 Clinical approach to recent-onset jaundice.

Table 1.16 Causes of jaundice

Disorders of bilirubin metabolism	Liver disease	Biliary obstruction
Hereditary hemolysis: e.g., sickle cell anemia	Viral hepatitis A–E	Bile duct stones (choledocholithiasis)
Acquired hemolysis: e.g., transfusion reaction	Alcohol	Primary sclerosing cholangitis (PSC)
Defective conjugation e.g., Gilbert's syndrome, Crigler–Najjar	Drugs (see drug-induced hepatotoxicity)	Intrinsic biliary stricture (e.g., ischemia, or trauma)
Impaired Bn excretion: e.g., Dubin–Johnson syndrome	Ischemia (hypotension, venous/arterial thrombosis)	Cholangiocarcinoma
	Wilson's disease	Extrinsic biliary compression (e.g., aneurysm, hilar nodes)
	Hemochromatosis	Pancreatic carcinoma
	α1-Antitrypsin deficiency	Acute or chronic pancreatitis (and pancreatic pseudocyst)
	Autoimmune hepatitis	HIV cholangiopathy
	Primary biliary cirrhosis (PBC)	Biliary infestation, e.g., Clonorchis
	Nonalcoholic fatty liver disease (NAFLD)	
	Graft versus host disease	
	Pregnancy-related liver disease	
	Granulomatous liver disease (see hepatic granulomas)	
	Budd–Chiari syndrome, veno-occlusive disease	
	Malignant infiltration	
	Bacterial sepsis	
	Viral infection: e.g., EBV, CMV, HSV Leptospirosis	

Clinical assessment

History

Determine the onset of jaundice, and associated symptoms (prodrome, abdominal pain, weight loss?); previous illnesses (autoimmunity?); alcohol intake (amount, type, duration, pattern of drinking); needle exposure (IV drugs, tattoo, transfusions?); drug history (recreational, prescription, over-the-counter, herbal remedies, drug chart?); travel and vaccination history; occupational risks (e.g., health staff, publican?); sexual history; observation charts (hypotension?); family history.

Examination

Look for:
- Hints to cause of jaundice: smells of alcohol, needle marks, self-harm scars.
- Evidence of chronic liver disease: clubbing, Dupuytren's contracture, leukonychia, xanthelasma, Kayser–Fleischer rings, gynecomastia, multiple spider naevi, testicular atrophy, splenomegaly, dilated superficial veins on abdomen.
- Evidence of acute liver failure or hepatic encephalopathy: liver flap, confusion/drowsiness/coma, bruising, ascites and dependent edema.
- Observation chart—low BP?

Investigations

Blood tests

May be tailored according to the clinical setting, but are likely to include tests for:
- **Viruses.** hepatitis A (α-HAV IgM, IgG), hepatitis B (HBsAg, α-HBc, IgM, IgG, HBeAg, α-HBe, and HBV DNA if HBsAg +ve), hepatitis C (α-HCV, HCV RNA), Epstein–Barr virus (α-EBV IgM, IgG), cytomegalovirus (α-CMV IgM, IgG), herpes simplex virus (α-HSV IgM, IgG).
- **Metabolic diseases.** Hemochromatosis (serum iron, TIBC, ferritin), Wilson's disease (serum copper, ceruloplasmin), α₁-antitrypsin deficiency (α₁-antitrypsin).
- **Drug toxicity** (including random blood alcohol level, paracetamol levels, and urine for toxins).
- **Autoimmune liver disease.** Autoimmune hepatitis, primary biliary cirrhosis (immunoglobulins, α-smooth muscle Ab, α-mitochondrial Ab, α-nuclear Ab, α-LKM1 Ab).
- Initial screen for disorders of bilirubin metabolism may include measurement of conjugated and unconjugated bilirubin. Although unconjugated hyperbilirubinemia classically seen in Gilbert's syndrome, mixed conjugated/unconjugated usually seen, and measurement is useful only on occasions.
- Hemolysis is assessed by FBC + film, reticulocyte count, and haptoglobins.
- Culture of blood, urine, and ascites may be relevant, as may *Leptospira* serology for suspected leptospirosis.

- Tests to define degree of liver function impairment and associate disease include: CBC + film, clotting profile (PT, INR, APPT), electrolytes, venous bicarbonate (± arterial blood gases), LFT screen, glucose.
- Markers of impaired synthetic liver function, as mentioned, and which may be seen in liver failure include ↑ serum bilirubin, ↓albumin, ↑PT/INR, ↓bicarbonate/arterial pH.

Imaging

Indicated in all cases.

- Abdominal <u>ultrasound</u> is easily available, with 91% sensitivity, and 95% specificity for biliary obstruction, and allows identification of mass lesions, exclusion of <u>portal vein thrombosis</u>, hepatic vein thrombosis (<u>Budd–Chiari syndrome</u>) and hepatic arterial impairment (if has Doppler facility), evidence of <u>portal hypertension</u>, demonstration of liver texture (?cirrhotic, fatty infiltration), ascites, and splenomegaly.
- CT is of comparable use, but may be less available, and intravenous contrast to define vessels may be nephrotoxic, particularly in patients with associated renal injury (e.g., <u>hepatorenal syndrome</u>).

Liver biopsy

Rarely required in the initial assessment of recent-onset jaundice. Its two roles are as an aid to diagnosis where no cause for jaundice secondary to parenchymal liver injury can be found, and in patients with a proven cause in whom the grade (degree of inflammation) and stage (degree of fibrosis) of liver injury histologically will affect management (e.g., alcoholic hepatitis in patient with established cirrhosis). In the patient with coagulopathy (e.g., INR > 1.3, platelet count < 80 × 10^9/l) a transjugular liver biopsy may be required.

Management

- Effective management is wholly dependent on the prompt identification of the cause of jaundice, and of the severity of any liver disease, as specific treatment will depend on the type of jaundice and its etiology and the presence or absence of liver failure.
- In patients with evidence of biliary disease on initial assessment and imaging, noninvasive modalities should be used for further investigation (e.g., MRI/MRCP), unless there is a high clinical suspicion of large duct obstruction (e.g., biliary stricture, common bile duct stones), in which case ERCP should be planned.

Emergencies

Acute abdominal pain

Acute abdominal pain is a common reason for emergency presentation ("the acute abdomen") and for patients to require review on the wards. The duration of pain that defines it as acute is ill-defined, but would usually be no more than a few days. With a huge range of causes of GI and non-GI causes of abdominal pain (see Box 2.1), many of which may present acutely, the challenge is in making a differential diagnosis on the basis of history and examination, thereby allowing investigations to be tailored to the specific clinical setting.

Clinical assessment

- Ask about the following aspects of the pain:
  - **Site.** Particular intra-abdominal organs and diseases tend to produce pain localized to particular abdominal segments (see figure in Chronic or recurrent abdominal pain).
  - **Character.** Colic tends to wax and wane, in a regular manner, due to spasm in a muscular viscus (e.g., gallbladder, ureter, small bowel); in peritonitis the pain is often constant and unremitting, and the patient wishes to lie still. Pain arising from the abdominal viscera tends to be largely midline, dull in nature, and poorly localized. Inflammation of the parietal peritoneum tends to be sharper, well localized, and exacerbated by movement.
  - **Onset, severity, and duration.**
  - **Radiation.** Right shoulder tip in cholecystitis; through to the back in acute pancreatitis.
  - **Relieving and exacerbating factors.**
- Ask about associated symptoms.
  - Is there a history of feculent vomiting and absolute constipation, suggesting bowel obstruction?
- Take a full genitourinary and gynecological history.
- Have there been previous episodes, and has a diagnosis been made? Any previous surgery (e.g., adhesions, Crohn's disease)?
- Do other medical problems provide hints to diagnosis (e.g., arteriopathy with AF and acute abdominal pain: may suggest intestinal ischemia).

A full **examination** is essential, including assessment of vital signs and evidence of hypovolemia or shock. In generalized peritonitis there may be rigidity, guarding, and rebound tenderness. **Never forget** to examine for inguinal and supraclavicular lymph nodes, hernial orifices, femoral pulses, external genitalia, bowel sounds (may be absent in peritonitis/ileus, tympanitic in obstruction), bruits, and to do a rectal examination.

Box 2.1 Causes of acute abdominal pain

Note: some conditions can present recurrently!

Generalized parietal pain due to peritonitis

- Perforated viscus–peptic ulceration, gallbladder (see gallbladder empyema), diverticulum
- Bacterial peritonitis (and spontaneous bacterial peritonitis)
- Ruptured intra-abdominal cyst
- Familial Mediterranean fever

Localized peritoneal pain

- Appendicitis, cholecystitis, regional enteritis, colitis, abdominal abscess, acute pancreatitis, hepatitis, lymphadenitis, endometriosis, diverticulitis

Pain from increased tension in viscera

- Intestinal obstruction (mechanical, intussusception, internal herniation)
- Intestinal hypermotility
- Biliary obstruction (choledocholithiasis)
- Ureteric obstruction
- Hepatic capsule distension (e.g., liver abscess, hepatocellular carcinoma)
- Renal capsule distension
- Ectopic pregnancy
- Abdominal aortic aneurysm

Ischemia

- Intestinal ischemia (arterial stenosis, embolism, inflammation)
- Splenic infarction, hepatic infarction
- Torsion (gallbladder, cyst, omentum, volvulus, appendix)
- Tissue necrosis

Retroperitoneal causes

- Tumors (e.g., pancreatic cancer)
- Retroperitoneal abscess
- Acute/chronic pancreatitis

Extra-abdominal

- Thoracic (pulmonary embolus, empyema, myocardial infarction, esophagitis, basal pneumonia)
- Neurological (neurogenic tumors, spinal degenerative disease, herpes zoster)
- Metabolic (diabetic ketoacidosis, acute intermittent porphyria, uremia, hypercalcemia)
- Hematological (sickle cell anemia, Henoch–Schönlein purpura, vasculitis)
- Poisoning (e.g., lead)

Investigations

Specific investigations will be tailored to the differential diagnosis arising from initial assessment, but in most cases will include:

- Blood tests
  - CBC + differential (raised neutrophils suggest inflammation, infection, mesenteric infarction, but may be normal in elderly).
  - BUN, creatinine, electrolytes, glucose.
  - <u>Liver function tests</u>: AST/ALT > 1000 IU/l usually due to drugs (e.g., acetaminophen), acute viral <u>hepatiti</u>s, or hepatic ischemia.
  - <u>Amylase</u> (elevated in many causes of abdominal pain; only indicative of <u>acute pancreatitis</u> if > 5 × ULN).
  - ESR/CRP. If significantly elevated suggests inflammation/infection. Also classically elevated in <u>familial Mediterranean fever</u>. CRP of prognostic use in <u>acute pancreatitis</u>.
  - Arterial blood gases (metabolic acidosis?).
  - Blood cultures.
  - Group + save if laparotomy or transfusion requirement possible.
- Urine β-HCG pregnancy test in women of child-bearing age (ectopic pregnancy?).
- Urinalysis ± MSU.
- Upright CXR (air under diaphragm due to viscus perforation?).
- Supine abdominal film (often noncontributory, but may show bowel dilatation (2.5 cm small bowel, 6 cm colon) ± air–fluid levels in obstruction).
- Abdominal U/S. Useful in patients with acute abdominal pain for exclusion of acute cholecystitis and biliary obstruction, detection of abdominal fluid and collections, and assessment of organomegaly, masses, and aortic aneurysms.
- Abdominal CT. More sensitive than U/S in most circumstances (except <u>gallstones</u>), and allows much better views of pancreas and retroperitoneum.
- Diagnostic laparoscopy may have a role in the investigation of acute abdominal pain associated with abdominal trauma, or in women with unexplained right iliac fossa pain, but is contraindicated in peritonitis, obstruction, or intra-abdominal adhesions.

Management

A clear diagnosis may not be possible on the basis of initial assessment and investigations. Specific treatment will be largely determined by differential diagnosis process underlying acute abdominal pain.

- If evidence of peritonitis, viscus perforation, or obstruction, need urgent surgical involvement. If laparotomy may be required, ensure that blood available, and CXR/EKG performed beforehand.
- Keep fasting.
- Obtain IV access and resuscitate with colloid/crystalloid/blood according to degree of hypovolemia, and blood loss. If evidence of

shock, give 500 ml colloid or crystalloid (e.g., 0.9% N saline) stat, and monitor response (HR, BP, CVP). Repeat as necessary.

- Insert central line if evidence of shock, requirement for significant fluid replacement, and/or underlying cardiovascular disease.
- Pass nasogastric tube if evidence of obstruction, and keep on free drainage.
- Insert urinary catheter and monitor hourly output.
- After taking blood cultures, give third- generation <u>CEPHALOSPORIN</u> (e.g., cefotaxime 1 g tds IV) and <u>METRONIDAZOLE</u> 500 mg tds IV.
- Pain of peritonitis may be severe, and analgesia should not be withheld for fear of "masking" clinical features. Opiates (e.g., diamorphine 5–10 mg IV 4 hourly or pethidine 50–100 mg IM 4 hourly, given with <u>METOCLOPRAMIDE</u> 10 mg IV/IM or cyclizine 50 mg IV/IM tds) maybe required.
- Laparotomy is generally indicated for patients with generalized peritonitis related to a viscus perforation (e.g., duodenal ulcer), or following organ rupture (e.g., spleen, aorta).

Where a definitive diagnosis cannot be made, a fundamental aspect of management is patient review and reassessment of clinical course and response to initial treatment.

Acute diarrhea

Diarrhea can constitute an emergency in three clinical situations.

Acute watery diarrhea. This is usually due to infection.

Common causes
- Viruses. <u>Rotavirus</u> in infants and young children can cause profound dehydration. The illness typically lasts about 7 days. <u>Adenovirus</u> infection can last longer.
- In adults, enterotoxigenic <u>*Escherichia coli*</u> (ETEC).
- Food-borne pathogens (see <u>food poisoning</u>).
- Bacteria that colonize the gut: <u>*Salmonella*</u>, <u>*Campylobacter*</u>, enterohaemorrhagic <u>*E. coli*</u>, *Vibrio parahaemolyticus*, <u>*Yersinia*</u>, <u>*Clostridium*</u> *perfringens*.
- Preformed toxins: *Staphylococcus aureus*, *Bacillus cereus*, *Clostridium botulinum*.
- Invasive pathogens and protozoa can produce watery diarrhea in the initial stages.

Diarrhea with blood

Making a diagnosis is important because of the importance of differentiating infection from inflammatory bowel disease and other disorders. Differential diagnosis includes:
- Invasive infectious diarrhea (dysentery): <u>*Shigella*</u>, <u>*Salmonella*</u>, <u>*Campylobacter*</u>, EHEC, and the protozoan <u>*Entamoeba*</u> *histolytica*.
- <u>Inflammatory bowel disease (ulcerative colitis, Crohn's)</u>.
- <u>Ischemic colitis</u>.
- <u>Radiation colitis</u>.
- <u>Colorectal cancer</u>.
- <u>Diverticular disease</u>.
- <u>Intussusception</u>.

Toxic dilatation

Acute dilatation of the colon (**transverse colon diameter > 6 cm on plain abdominal X-ray**) occurs in
- Severe <u>ulcerative colitis</u> or colonic <u>Crohn's disease</u>.
- Infectious colitis.
- Acute distal obstruction (<u>volvulus</u> or carcinoma).
- Acute pseudo-obstruction (see <u>Ogilvie's syndrome</u>).

Management

Resuscitate the patient

- Oral rehydration is the mainstay of managing acute watery diarrhea (see <u>oral rehydration solutions</u>). The World Health Organization oral rehydration solution (sodium concentration 90 mM, osmolality 331 mOsm/kg) is recommended to give adequate glucose source for the sodium–glucose co-transporter and may be necessary if there is a short bowel or jejunostomy: in children with acute diarrhea, the recommendation is for a sodium concentration of about 50 mM.

Making a diagnosis

Clinical examination

This may not yield the diagnosis but it's important to look for signs of **dehydration** and **metabolic acidosis** (textbooks always say look for a dry tongue, loss of skin turgor, and tachycardia, but these are unreliable: the best sign to look for is a **postural drop in BP**). Look also for signs of inflammatory bowel disease (perianal disease, pyoderma, oral ulceration) or signs of immunosuppression (oral candidiasis, Kaposi's sarcoma, leucoplakia). A toxic dilated colon is usually accompanied by fever, tachycardia, and neutrophilia.

Investigations

Blood tests

- Distinguishing infection from nonspecific inflammatory bowel disease is important but can take several days. Most cases of acute infective diarrhea are self-limiting, providing attention is paid to restoring fluid balance.
- **Dehydration:** hemoconcentration with raised hemoglobin, increased packed cell volume, and a raised blood urea.
- **Acidosis:** raised venous bicarbonate, decreased arterial blood pH, and base excess.
- **Inflammation:** anemia, raised neutrophil count, and elevated inflammatory markers (ESR, CRP, platelets).
- **Magnesium and potassium** losses can become significant in severe diarrhea.
- **Eosinophilia** accompanies helminthic infections of the gut, although only stronglyoides, trichinella, and schistosoma are associated with diarrhea (see <u>eosinophilia and the GI tract</u>).

Microbiological examination of the stool

This is the usual way of making a diagnosis of infection, but the delay is always 1–2 days and often longer for slow-growing organisms.

- Fecal antigen ELISAs are available for *Giardia* and rotavirus.
- DNA probes often do not work on crude fecal extracts but can help in characterizing bacterial isolates.
- Stool culture, fecal *Clostridium difficile* assay (ask for both A and B toxins:) and blood cultures should be sent.
- Antimicrobial chemotherapy is indicated for dysenteric infections such as <u>amoebiasis</u>, <u>shigellosis</u>, and <u>pseudomembranous colitis</u>.

Radiological imaging

A **plain abdominal X-ray** can help in assessing intestinal inflammation and is also useful in excluding free air as a result of bowel perforation.

- A gas-filled colon devoid of feces suggests a total colitis.
- Loss of haustration and dilatation indicate severe inflammation.
- There may be mutiple small bowel fluid levels and small bowel dilatation (indicating partial ileus rather than obstruction).

Abdominal ultrasound can reveal bowel-wall thickening and enlarged lymph nodes.

Endoscopy

Sigmoidoscopy can be highly informative, demonstrate colitis, and allows biopsy, which may be of help in differentiating infection from inflammation; appearances of amoebic colitis, ischemic colitis, radiation colitis, and pseudomembranous colitis can be diagnostic. **Total colonoscopy** is usually not necessary and may be risky.

Common mistakes and important points in early management

- Always think of **acute megacolon due to toxic dilatation.** If there is any abdominal tenderness or sign of systemic upset, get a plain abdominal X-ray.
- If the patient is unwell, **frequent review** by a senior clinician is essential, as is a **surgical opinion.**
- Intravenous fluids. Keep **potassium** above 4.0 mmol/L.
- Monitor CBC, electrolytes, and colonic diameter on daily X-rays.
- Stop any drugs that may be contributing to colonic paralysis, especially opiates and antidiarrheal agents.
- **Avoid NSAIDs.** They can aggravate diarrhea and have profound effects on reducing renal cortical blood flow, which can precipitate renal failure in hypovolemia or patients with pre-existing kidney disease.
- In cases of fulminant colitis or toxic dilatation of the colon, the decision to proceed to colectomy can be difficult: useful indicators are:
  - Increasing tachycardia and fever.
  - Failure to improve clinically or radiologically (i.e., colon diameter decreasing) after 24 hours.
  - Signs of perforation (these may be very minimal: steroids mask physical signs of perforation).
  - Mucosal islands seen on X-ray.

Complications

Worldwide the majority of deaths result from dehydration and acidosis. Complications of infection, especially by invasive pathogens, include:
- Hemolytic–uremic syndrome.
- Nonseptic arthritis and Reiter's syndrome.
- Guillain–Barré syndrome.
- Septic arthritis.

Acute liver failure

Definition

Development of <u>hepatic encephalopathy (HE)</u> within 12 weeks of onset of jaundice in patient with no history of liver disease. Subdivided into "hyper-acute" and "subacute" ALF, with intervals from jaundice to HE of < 7 days and 5–12 weeks, respectively. Previous definition of ALF extended only up to 8 weeks, with no subdivision.

Clinical syndrome

ALF is a systemic condition, characterized by:

- **Hepatic encephalopathy/cerebral edema.** All patients with ALF have <u>HE</u> due mainly to poor liver function and cerebral edema (present in > 80% of comatose patients as main causes), rather than <u>portal hypertension</u>.
- **Acute renal failure.** Occurs in > 50% of ALF cases, including toxin-related acute tubular necrosis (e.g., <u>acetaminophen overdose</u>), renal vasculitic injury (e.g., <u>leptospirosis</u>) or type 1 <u>hepatorenal syndrome,</u> as a consequence of the severity of liver injury.
- **Metabolic derangement.** Hypoglycemia is common, and may be confused for encephalopathy. Metabolic acidosis common following <u>acetaminophen overdose</u>, but carries poor prognosis whatever the cause (day 3 Ph < 7.3 predicts > 90% mortality without <u>liver transplantation</u> after <u>acetaminophen</u> overdose). ↑Serum lactate may reflect tissue hypoxemia.
- **Hemodynamic changes.** Characterized by peripheral vasodilatation and hyperdynamic circulation (i.e., ↑HR, ↓systemic vascular resistance (SVR), ↑cardiac output (CO), ↓mean arterial pressure (MAP)). May mask/mimic changes of systemic sepsis.
- **Pulmonary complications** occur in 50% due to range of causes: effects of cerebral edema; gastric aspiration in confused/comatose patient; pneumonia; noncardiogenic pulmonary edema (especially with <u>acetaminophen overdose</u>).
- **Infection** is very common and often clinically masked due to ALF. In patients with ALF and >grade 1 encephalopathy, >80% have bacterial infections, >30% fungal infection (e.g., *Candida albicans, Aspergillus* spp), and infection associated with 50% of ALF deaths.
- **Hematological abnormalities.** Prothrombin time (PT) is one of best indicators of severity of liver failure (after exclusion of vitamin K deficiency); platelets <100 × 10^9/l in 70%.of patients.

Table 2.1 Causes of acute liver failure

Cause	Diagnosis in ALF	Comments
Hepatitis A	Anti-HAV IgM	Possible increased rate of ALF in hepatitis A in association with chronic hepatitis C
Hepatitis B	IgM Anti-HB core (HBsAg may be –ve in ALF)	ALF in 1% of acute infections. May occur with hepatitis D virus infection
Hepatitis C	HCV RNA (anti-HCV Ab often –ve)	Extremely rarely causes ALF
Hepatitis E	Anti-HEV	ALF in 20% of women infected in pregnancy in S. Asia
Other infection (e.g., EBV, HSV, leptospirosis)	e.g., anti-Leptospira IgM, anti-HSV IgM, anti-EBV VCA IgM	
Acetaminophen overdose (acetaminophen)	Blood levels	Common cause of ALF in US
Drug reactions: e.g., NSAIDs, isoniazid, rifampicin, herbal remedies, 'ecstasy'	Drug history, eosinophils Blood/urine analysis	See drug-induced hepatotoxicity
Toxins (e.g., *Amanita phalloides* mushrooms)	History of ingestion	
Acute fatty liver of pregnancy	History, bloods	Mainly clinical diagnosis.
HELLP syndrome	History, bloods	Mainly clinical diagnosis.
Wilson's disease	Urinary copper, ceruloplasmin	Usually presents with ALF <20 years of age
Hepatic ischaemia	↑AST/ALT (> 1000 U/L), imaging	Especially following episode of hypotension
Budd–Chiari syndrome	Imaging	May present with ascites
Autoimmune hepatitis	AutoAbs, Igs	20% of patients present with jaundice, but ALF unusual
Malignant infiltration	Imaging, histology	
'Seronegative hepatitis'	All above excluded	Approximately 20% of cases

Making the diagnosis

- ALF is a clinical diagnosis, based on demonstrating HE in a patient with acute liver disease. Presence of liver disease usually obvious from initial assessment and blood results (↑bilirubin, ↑PT, ↑serum albumin are best blood markers of significant liver disease). Differentiating ALF from an acute presentation of decompensated chronic liver disease may be difficult, but important, as management and prognosis are very different. Is there any history/documentation to suggest more chronic disease (chat to primary physician/review hospital notes/check historical blood results)? Are there physical signs suggestive of chronic liver disease (e.g., spider nevi, Dupuytren's contracture, clubbing, leuconychia). Evidence of <u>portal hypertension</u> (splenomegaly, dilated superficial veins) is unusual in ALF.

Finding the cause (see Table 2.1)
- May be obvious, but information from patient, relatives, medical attendants is vital, including: drugs (prscribed/recreational/herbal); risk of hepatitis (unprotected sex/IVDU/hepatitis contact/foreign travel/ tattoo/piercing); autoimmune diseases (e.g., thyroid/rheumatoid). Any evidence of hypotensive episode (e.g., recent surgery/↓BP on obstetric chart/bleed/adverse cardiac event)? Any history of thrombosis or prothrombotic tendency (e.g., anti-phospholipid syndrome), precipitating <u>Budd–Chiari syndrome</u>?
- Breadth of investigation of cause dependent on clinical scenario (e.g., low yield on leptospira serology in 80-year-old with ALF following prolonged cardiac arrest!).

Management

Optimal management depends on strict general supportive measures; consideration of specific treatments (e.g., N-acetylcysteine); defining prognosis and need for liver unit referral ± <u>liver transplantation</u>.

General approach
- Management in ICU setting.
- Pass urinary catheter and monitor hourly urine output.
- Monitor vital signs (HR/BP/temp) ½–2 hourly.
- Daily bloods for CBC, electrolytes, bicarb, glucose, clotting, LFTs.
- Culture blood, urine, sputum, even if afebrile. CXR.
- Investigate cause of ALF as directed by history (see earlier and Table 2.1). Note that <u>acetaminophen</u> levels may be apparently sub toxic by the time of development of ALF. ↑↑ALT/AST > 1000 U/l most likely due to hepatic ischemia, acute viral hepatitis, or drugs.
- Discuss with specialist liver unit **early**. Detailed referral criteria vary according to cause and type of ALF, but broadly include any of the following: PT > 30 s; hepatic encephalopathy; creatinine > 2.5 mg/dl; hypoglycemia; metabolic acidosis—pH < 7.3. If in doubt, ask: every unit prefers an unnecessary call to a late call for patients with ALF.

- Avoid all potentially hepatotoxic drugs (e.g., NSAIDs), and those that worsen complications of ALF (e.g., ACE-inhibitors, opiates).
- Maintain nutrition, as ALF catabolic state. NG feeding preferable, as may prevent bacterial translocation, but ileus may preclude this.
- CVP for fluid monitoring (correction of coagulopathy not needed if internal jugular approach used and experienced technician).
- Ensure adequate intravascular filling with colloid, crystalloid, blood products. If mean arterial pressure (MAP) < 60 mmHg despite filling consider norepinephrine 0.2–1.8 mg/kg/min, but specialist inotrope management will be required.
- Monitor blood glucose, and give 10–20% dextrose infusions if hypoglycemic.
- N-<u>ACETYLCYSTEINE</u> may be of benefit even in nonacetaminophen-induced ALF, including hepatic ischemia.
- <u>Vitamin K</u> 10 mg IV/day for 3 days (but usually has no effect on PT, unless vitamin K deficiency related to prolonged biliary obstruction). PT/INR very useful markers of clinical course/prognosis, so only give fresh frozen plasma (FFP) if actively bleeding. Maintain platelet count .> 20×10^9/l with infusions.
- Acid suppression reduces risk of hemorrhagic gastritis. Usually give oral/NG PPI (e.g., omeprazole 20 mg od), although clear evidence relates to IV H2-receptor antagonists.
- Prophylactic broad-spectrum IV antibiotics reduce frequency of infections but not mortality, and are associated with resistant organisms, but are nevertheless often given. Prophylactic fluconazole ± liposomal amphotericin reduces risk of systemic fungal infection. Irrespective of use of antimicrobial prophylaxis, meticulous nursing and care of lines/pressure areas, etc. are essential.

Specific management
Cerebral edema/hepatic encephalopathy
- Consider CT brain scan to exclude cerebral bleed.
- 20% Mannitol 0.5 g/kg IV bolus, repeated as necessary (but not if serum osmolality >320 mOsm/l).
- Have a low threshold for intubation/mechanical ventilation in view of risk of aspiration and agitation in patients with cerebral edema/encephalopathy.
- Controlled hyperventilation may help to control surges of raised intracranial pressure (ICP) in patients unresponsive to mannitol.
- In specialist unit, ICP monitor may be inserted in comatose patient, to accurately measure degree of cerebral edema (but risk–benefit ratio of ICP monitoring much debated).
- Avoid sedatives (e.g., benzodiazepines, opiates).
- N-<u>ACETYLCYSTEINE</u> infusion in acetaminophen-related ALF has been shown to reduce signs of cerebral edema.

Renal failure
- Important to involve renal team early.
- Management includes stopping all potentially nephrotoxic drugs; correcting hypovolaemia; excluding and treating infection.
- Patient may require continuous hemofiltration. Standard indications include K^+ >6.0 mmol/l, bicarb <5 mmol/l, creatine >5 mg/dl, but may be considered earlier in patient with liver and renal failure, as associated with less hemodynamic instability.

Artificial liver support
- Range of <u>liver support devices</u> and techniques have been developed over last thirty years to act as "bridge" to <u>liver transplantation</u>, or even to allow time for native liver to spontaneously recover. None reliably effective to date, but search goes on.

Prognosis and liver transplantation

- Spontaneous recovery more likely with hyperacute than subacute presentation. In patients with ALF and grade III–IV hepatic encephalopathy treated with medical therapy alone, survival 10–40%.
- With <u>liver transplantation,</u> survival from ALF now 60–80%. This reinforces need to discuss case early, and consider liver transplantation criteria (see <u>liver transplantation</u>).

Acute lower gastrointestinal bleeding

Definition

Blood originating from below the ligament of Treitz (often quoted landmark: a fibromuscular band that originates from the right diaphragmatic crus and fixes the duodenal–jejunal flexure).

Clinical presentation

- Blood in the stool implies a lower GI cause unless there is very rapid bleeding from an upper GI source (this will produce hemodynamic instability and usually a raised blood urea).
- Blood in the bowel for over about 14 hours is converted to black melena: up to 35% of patients with melena have a bleeding point distal to duodenal–jejunal flexure.
- The patient may be hypotensive and shocked without overt evidence of bleeding; do a rectal exam.

Diagnosis

History

There may be a history of hemorrhoids, inflammatory bowel disease, radiation, or iatrogenic causes (bleeding from polypectomy can be delayed up to 10 days).

- Ask about prior episodes, presence of liver or renal disease, drug usage (antiplatelet drugs, NSAIDs, warfarin).
- Ask whether the blood is mixed with or separate from the stool (bright red blood suggests an anorectal cause) and about an associated change in bowel habit.
- In the West, common causes include bleeding from <u>diverticula</u> (40%), inflammatory bowel disease including infectious and ischemic colitis as well as Crohn's and ulcerative colitis (20%), benign anorectal disease (10%), and arteriovenous malformations, <u>angiodysplasia</u>.

Rare causes include radiation, <u>Meckel's diverticulum</u>, and varices.

Management

Most (90%) lower GI bleeds stop spontaneously: 35% need transfusing; 5% need urgent surgery. Resuscitation is as for <u>acute upper GI bleeds</u>: there is usually time to transfuse if necessary and correct clotting abnormalities. Investigation of a stable patient gives a better chance of effective diagnosis and therapy.

Investigation

In patients who stop bleeding spontaneously, elective colonoscopy after routine preparation is indicated. In continued bleeding, urgent diagnosis is needed. If there is doubt about a lower GI source of the bleeding, upper GI endoscopy can be useful. Simple sigmoidoscopy may be useful if there is a perianal or rectal source, but for most colonic bleeding, colonoscopy is required (more sensitive than barium, and allows biopsy and therapy)

Colonoscopy in acute lower GI hemorrhage. Intestinal lavage using nasogastric intubation followed by giving 2–4 liters of an osmotic laxative such as Golytely allows adequate preparation. The value of emergent colonoscopy in this setting is unclear, due to the wide variation in reported yield from this approach. Angiography offers accurate diagnosis and therapy if the bleeding is brisk (over about 3 ml/min).

Treatment   For in-depth review see Zuckerman, GR and Prakash, C. 1999 *Gastrointest. Endosc.* **49**: 228.

- **Electrocoagulation or mechanical endoscopic techniques** (clipping, placing of loops around bleeding vessels) at colonoscopy can be useful for bleeding angiodysplasia and arterial lesions.
- Intra-arterial **vasopressin** stops bleeding from diverticula and angiodysplasia in 90% but has a complication rate of 5–15% (cardiovascular toxicity, indwelling catheter). Its use is not recommended.
- **Selective embolization** can be very effective in expert hands.
- **Surgery**. The success and postoperative bleeding rate depends on accurate pre-operative localization. Mortality in recent series is 5–10%.

Acute upper gastrointestinal bleeding

Definitions

Hematemesis refers to the vomiting of blood. Occurs in 40–50% of cases of upper GI bleeding, and indicative of bleeding point proximal to jejunum. Melena stool is black, tarry, and smells sickly sweet. Occurs in 70–80% of upper GI bleeds. Usually results from bleeding proximal to cecum, but may sometimes occur in colonic bleeding, particularly from right colon. Hematochezia refers to red blood per rectum.

Box 2.2 Causes of acute upper GI bleeding

- Peptic ulceration (25–50% of cases of nonvariceal upper GI bleeding)
- Gastroesophageal varices (5% of cases, but 80% of deaths due to acute upper GI bleeding—also see portal hypertension)
- Gastritis/gastric erosions
- Esophagitis
- Duodenitis
- Mallory-Weiss tear
- Gastric antral vascular ectasia (GAVE) ("watermelon stomach")
- Dieulafoy lesions
- Hereditary hemorrhagic telangiectasia ("Osler-Weber-Rendu syndrome")
- Gastrointestinal stromal tumor (GIST)
- Angiodysplasia
- Portal hypertensive gastropathy
- Upper GI tumors (e.g., esophageal, gastric cancer)
- Aorto-enteric fistula
- Causes of hemobilia

Initial assessment and management

Estimate extent of blood loss

- Ask about the duration of bleeding; the volume, color, and frequency of melena or hematemesis (e.g., "two cupfuls, bright red vomit"); was there associated dizziness, lightheadedness, shortness of breath, altered consciousness (suggesting large bleed)? 1,000 ml of blood represents 20% of blood volume.
- Has blood loss been witnessed? "Coffee ground vomit"—see it for yourself, as any dark vomitus tends to get this label, and dip-stick tests for blood are useless, as almost always positive. Check what's being meant by "melena" (examine bedpan, do rectal examination), as term often wrongly used to refer to any blood per rectum. Hematochezia in presence of hematemesis suggests large bleed and rapid luminal transit.
- Look for signs of hypovolemia (pallor, cool peripheries, weak pulse, HR > 100 bpm, ↓BP, ↓JVP, confusion, ↑respiratory rate). Measure postural drop in BP (> 10 mmHg fall after standing for 30 s), but not in shocked patient who is hypotensive even when supine, as may precipitate cerebral hypoperfusion.

Initial resuscitation

- Establish good IV access (preferably ×2 14–16G cannulae in antecubital fossae—not a single 20G line in dorsum of the hand).
- Send bloods for: CBC, clotting, BUN & electrolytes, LFTs, glucose, group and save. Note that Hb and hematocrit may not fall immediately, due to loss of whole blood, with fall only occurring after reactive plasma volume expansion and hemodilution. If significant bleed cross-match 2–8 units, according to severity, and always have 2 units available for patient with ongoing bleeding.
- If hypovolemic give 500 ml of crystalloid (e.g., 0.9% saline) or colloid (e.g., Haemaccel®, Gelofusin®), and review hemodynamic response. Repeat if necessary while waiting for blood. Remember that colloid/crystalloid causes hemodilution (approximately 10% fall in Hb for each litre of fluid), and that the patient is hypovolemic due to blood loss, which may need to be replaced. Nevertheless, only in very rare circumstances of massive exsanguinating blood loss and delayed availability of cross-matched blood, does use of uncrossmatched, blood (group O Rh neg), need to be considered.
- Do not attempt CVP line insertion prior to initial volume expansion, as wastes time and failure/complications (e.g., pneumothorax, carotid artery puncture) more likely. Initially use large-bore peripheral cannulae. However, subsequent central line insertion should be considered for those with major hemorrhage at presentation, especially in association with cardiac failure/ischemic heart disease, renal failure, failure to respond to resuscitation, or inadequate venous access.
- Insert urinary catheter in patients with a large bleed, hemodynamic compromise, or evidence of renal impairment. Monitor hourly output.
- Monitor vital signs ¼–2 hourly, dependent on hemodynamic stability.
- Transfuse up to a Hb of 10 g/dl. Ensure repeat clotting is checked after 4 units of blood are given and correct clotting accordingly.
- Ensure that nursing staff knows to keep the patient nil by mouth (NPO).

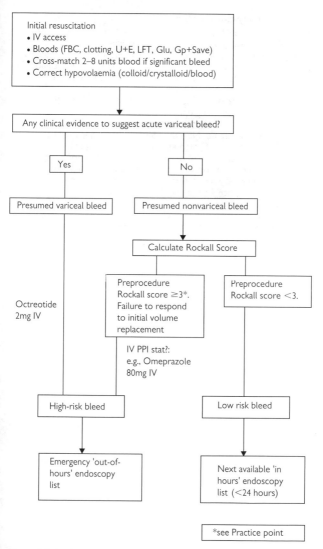

Figure 2.1 Initial management in acute upper GI bleeding.

Establish likely cause of bleed
- Important to identify patients with suspected variceal bleed. (see later).
- Ask about a history of liver disease and varices, or risk factors: alcohol excess; previous jaundice; abdominal surgery/<u>pancreatitis</u>. Thrombophilia may suggest <u>portal vein thrombosis</u>. Unexplained thrombocytopenia may point to hypersplenism due to <u>portal hypertension</u>.
- Consider nonvariceal causes: ask about previous episodes (? <u>angiodysplasia</u>); preceding epigastric pain (? <u>peptic ulceration</u>); reflux symptoms (? <u>esophagitis</u>); weight loss, fatigue (? malignancy); medication (e.g., aspirin, NSAIDs, SSRIs, warfarin, heparin); surgery (? aortic graft, with risk of <u>aorto-enteric fistula</u>); timing of bleeding (e.g., hematemesis after episodes of retching suggests <u>Mallory-Weiss tear</u>).
- On examination look for signs of liver disease (e.g., jaundice, clubbing, palmar erythema, spider nevi, tattoos, splenomegaly, ascites, <u>hepatic encephalopathy</u>). Hints to nonvariceal causes include mucosal telangiectasia (<u>hereditary hemorrhagic telangiectasia</u>), left supraclavicular lymph node (Virchow's node—suggests <u>gastric/esophageal cancer</u>); scars of previous abdominal surgery.

Decide on likeliest cause
- Nonvariceal acute upper GI bleed.
- Variceal acute upper GI bleed.

Suspected nonvariceal acute upper GI bleed

Ongoing management

- 80% of nonvariceal bleeds settle spontaneously.
- Rockall score (see Table 2.2) predicts risk of mortality, and so allows stratification into low- and high-risk bleeds.
- Calculate pre-endoscopy Rockall score. If score 0–2, arrange endoscopy on next available "in hours" list (may even discharge score 0 patients). If ≥3 patient has had a high-risk bleed.
- Inform on-call surgical team early about all high-risk bleeds (and encourage them to witness endoscopy—will focus minds if surgery needs to be considered).

Endoscopy

- Definitive procedure to make diagnosis and treat, and most accurately predicts prognosis (based on final Rockall score and Forrest classification—see later). Do not perform endoscopy before attempts to adequately resuscitate.
- Emergency out-of-hours endoscopy indicated in all high-risk bleeds: pre-endoscopy Rockall score ≥3 (with provisos—see practice point); suspected variceal bleed; or in any patient with large bleed and persistent hypovolemia despite 4 units of blood/fluid.
  - Endoscopic therapy indicated in patients with active bleeding or stigmata of recent hemorrhage (see Forrest classification below).
  - Two modalities of endotherapy are most likely to be better than one (e.g., adrenaline 1:10 000 injection around ulcer + <u>heater probe</u>/haemoclip).
- In patients with bleeding <u>peptic ulcers</u>, antral CLO test biopsy for <u>*Helicobacter pylori*</u> taken (little evidence that "acute" eradication effects natural history of bleeding ulcer, but will reduce recurrence).

Pharmacotherapy

- Debate continues about what proton pump inhibitor (PPI) to use, what route, and when. Clear evidence for PPI efficacy in all suspected nonvariceal bleeders prior to endoscopy is still lacking. In a patient with a significant bleed, primary goal (after resuscitation) is endoscopy, which allows diagnosis and definitive management. Nevertheless, single IV (or high-dose oral) dose of PPI in significant bleeders, prior to endoscopy, is a pragmatic approach used by many, with further PPI determined by endoscopic findings.
- High-dose proton pump inhibitor regimen reduces rebleeding rates, but minimal effect on mortality. In patients with high-risk bleeds, give omeprazole 80 mg in normal saline 100 ml IV over 30 min, then 8 mg/hour in same infusion (i.e., 10 ml/hour) for 72 hours. IV pantoprazole may be an alternative.

- Oral regime (e.g., Lansoprazole 30 mg bd) may be similarly effective, but not directly compared. Expert opinion suggests IV regimens for Forrest I, IIa, and IIb bleeds, and oral regimens for IIc and III endoscopic findings (based on risk of rebleed).
- Tranexamic acid is not used as standard treatment, although meta-analysis has suggested a survival advantage over placebo. Usual regimen is 3–6 g × 1/day IV for 2–3 days, then orally 3–5 days.

Table 2.2 Rockall score

Variable	Score			
	0	1	2	3
Age (years)	< 60	60–79	%80	
Shock	No shock Syst BP > 100 HR < 100	Tachycardia Syst BP > 100 HR > 100	Hypotension. Syst BP < 100	
Comorbidity	Nil major		Cardiac failure, IHD	Renal failure, disseminated malignancy
Post-endoscopy criteria				
Diagnosis	Mallory-Weiss tear, no lesion, no stigmata	All other diagnoses	Upper GI malignancy	
Major stigmata	None, or dark spots		Blood in upper GI tract, clot, visible vessel	

Table 2.3 Predicted mortality related to Rockall score

Score	Pre-endoscopy (%)	Postendoscopy (%)
0	0.2	0.0
1	2.4	0.0
2	5.6	0.2
3	11.0	2.9
4	24.6	5.3
5	39.6	10.8
6	48.9	17.3
7	50.0	27.0
8+		41.1

Box 2.3 Practice point: Rockall score and risk stratification

Don't be a slave to clinical grading systems. The Rockall score is clinically useful, but was never designed to predict who will rebleed or die. For example: an 80-year-old patient with a chest infection and stable angina, who has an equivocal "coffee ground vomit," will have a Rockall score >3. Out-of-hours endoscopy in this situation may not only be unnecessary, but dangerous. Emergency endoscopy is indicated for those with large continuing bleeding. The Rockall score should support, not replace, good clinical assessment.

Postendoscopy care
- Patient can eat and drink at 4–6 hours if hemodynamically stable.
- Daily bloods until stable (FBC, U&Es).
- Rebleeding indicated by new signs of hypovolemia (compensatory tachycardia is an early sign), fall in Hb > 2 g/dl over 24 hours, or development of fresh hematemesis or melena. Decision needed between repeating endoscopy and early surgery (see below).
- No clear role for repeating endoscopy in bleeders who have settled, prior to discharge (but all gastric ulcers need re-scoping ± biopsy in 6 weeks to check for resolution, because of risk that ulcer is malignant).
- See peptic ulceration for treatment after recovery from bleed.

Surgery
- Criteria for surgery are not absolutes, but crucial factors are **the severity of bleed, endoscopic findings, and comorbidity**.
  - High-risk stigmata of rebleeding on endoscopy, and failed endoscopic control (e.g., spurting artery).
  - First rebleed in patient >60 years (elderly patients tolerate further episodes of hypotension and hemorrhage poorly, and so require surgery earlier, not later, than younger patients). But consider patient's "biological age," remembering how many >60- year-olds run the marathon!
  - Second rebleed in patient <60 years (there is rarely a role for a third attempt at endoscopic treatment, unless endoscopist missed the true lesion first time, or treated inadequately, or if surgeon feels that the patient is truly unfit for surgery).
  - Continued bleeding after 6 units of blood in patient >60 years, 8 units in <60-year-olds.
  - Surgery usually involves oversewing the bleeding vessel in the stomach or duodenum, vagotomy with pyloroplasty, or partial gastrectomy.
  - Alternative to surgery, particularly in patients with very poor surgical prognosis, is angiography, with embolization of feeding vessel.

Nonulcer bleeding

- Endoscopic therapy may be effective in controlling bleeding due to <u>Mallory-Weiss</u> tear (although stops spontaneously in 50–80% of cases), and <u>Dieulafoy lesions</u> (96% controlled with primary hemostasis). Bleeding from <u>gastric antral vascular ectasia</u> (GAVE)) may be controlled with <u>argon plasma coagulation (APC)</u>.
- In patient with previous aortic graft, sentinel bleed may precede catastrophic bleed due to <u>aorto-enteric fistula</u>. Emergency endoscopy, with views round to duodeno-jejunal flexure ± CT scan may make diagnosis. Emergency surgery (peri-operative mortality 25–90%) or endovascular stenting may be necessary.

Endoscopy "negative" upper GI bleeding

Further management depends on findings at first endoscopy:

- No blood and no lesion seen: may be explained by:
  - Trivial lesion that has stopped bleeding by the time of endoscopy (e.g., <u>Mallory-Weiss tear</u>). Suggested by no evidence of ongoing blood loss.
  - Bleeding distal to scope view (e.g., small bowel <u>angiodysplasia</u>; <u>gastrointestinal stromal tumor (GIST)</u>; <u>Meckel's diverticulum</u>, <u>aorto-enteric fistula</u>). Further investigations include small bowel ("push") <u>enteroscopy</u>, mesenteric angiography (requires blood loss of 1 ml/min to demonstrate active bleeding) ± embolization of bleeding point, technetium labeled red cell scan, or capsular endoscopy. If bleed is continuous, exploratory laparotomy may be necessary.
- Blood seen, but no lesion: may be explained by:
  - Bleeding arising from "unusual site" (e.g., <u>hemobilia</u> due to bleeding from biliary tree; gastric fundal Dieulafoy lesion).
  - Blood obscuring adequate view on initial endoscopy.
  - Repeat procedure by senior endoscopist within 24 hours. Consider stimulating gastric emptying (e.g., erythromycin 250 mg IV, metoclopramide 10 mg IV 20 min prior to procedure). If possible hemobilia, have duodenoscope available for optimal views of papilla.

Prognosis

- Overall mortality from nonvariceal upper GI bleed approximately 10%. Lack of significant reduction in mortality over last thirty years likely to relate to increasing age of patients, and so worse comorbidity.
- Mortality 3% in patients aged 21–31; 10% age 41–50; 14% age 71–80 years.

Table 2.4 Forrest classification of rebleeding risk

Class	Endoscopic finding	% Rebleeding rate
Ia	Spurting artery	80–90
Ib	Oozing	55–80
IIa	Nonbleeding visible vessel	50–60
IIb	Adherent clot	25–35
IIc	Black spot in ulcer base	0–8
III	Clean ulcer base	0–12

Suspected acute variceal bleed

Varices due to <u>portal hypertension</u> develop in 60% of patients with advanced cirrhosis. First bleed carries 25–50% mortality. Varices in distal esophagus, gastro-esophageal junction, or gastric fundus most usually bleed, but ectopic variceal bleeding (e.g., rectum, stomas, surgical anastomoses) may occur.

- Risk factors for bleeding include:
  - Poor liver function (indicated by <u>Child–Pugh score</u>).
  - Large varices.
  - Endoscopic stigmata (e.g., "red signs" on varices).
  - Bacterial infection.
  - Hepatic venous pressure gradient (HVPG) > 16 mmHg (see <u>portal hypertension</u>).
- Death from variceal bleed related to severity of initial bleed; rebleeding (30–50% within 1 week); infection; comorbid cardiorespiratory/renal disease.

Ongoing management

- If you suspect a variceal bleed, call gastroenterologist on-call immediately, as experienced staff are essential. Involve anesthetist, as risk of aspiration if patient encephalopathic and large bleed, and may need intubation prior to endoscopy.
- Manage in ITU/HDU setting, by staff experienced in care of these patients.
- If still hypovolaemic after initial fluid resuscitation, give blood if ready, otherwise further colloid (e.g., Haemaccel®, Gelofusin®). Avoid overfilling, as may increase risk of rebleeding (↑portal venous pressure), but vital to ensure adequate renal perfusion and urine output. Aim for CVP 4–8 cm H_2O, and Hb 9–10 g/dl.
- Give platelets if <50 × 10^9/l, fresh frozen plasma (FFP) if PT >20 s (and for every 4 units blood). Discuss with hematologists *re* dose.
- Vitamin K 10 mg IV od for 3 days.
- Give cryoprecipitate 10 units if fibrinogen <75 mg/dl.
- Insert central line after initial fluid resuscitation, and preferably (but not essential) after clotting factors given. However, withhold insertion in: agitated patient (e.g., with <u>hepatic encephalopathy</u>); if it will delay essential emergency endoscopy; and in patient with large ongoing hematemesis who risks aspiration on lying supine.
- Give broad spectrum IV cover (e.g., <u>Cefotaxime</u> 1 g bd IV + metronidazole 500 mg tds for 5 days). Bacterial sepsis is common, risk of aspiration is high, and sepsis is associated with initial bleeding/rebleeding.
- Give <u>OCTREOTIDE</u> 50 µg bolus followed by 50 µg/hour by intravenous infusion for 5 days, or until bleeding stops. May cause ischaemia, so contraindicated in patients with ischaemia on ECG, or history of vascular disease. Vasoactive drugs may help to control bleeding (79% of cases in pooled data of patients treated with terlipressin), and may reduce mortality, but their use does not replace necessity of endoscopy.

Endoscopy
- Essential for definitive treatment and investigation. Perform within six hours, ideally after hemodynamically stable.
- Ensure anesthetist present. Have **low** threshold for intubation prior to endoscopy.
- Protect yourself with face mask ± double gloves if any risk of parenteral virus transmission.
- At endoscopy, full examination of upper GI tract performed, as 26–56% of patients with <u>portal hypertension</u> and GI bleed have nonvariceal cause (e.g., <u>peptic ulceration</u>).

Gastro-esophageal varices. Variceal band ligation (VBL) should be performed. This involves placement of rubber bands around the base of the varix (see <u>portal hypertension</u>). Control of bleeding may occur through subsequent tamponade at the gastro-esophageal junction or development of variceal thrombosis. Sclerotherapy, involving a needle puncture in or adjacent to the varix, with the injection of sclerosant (e.g., 5 ml 5% ethanolamine oleate) may be used if VBL fails (or if limited endoscopist experience of VBL). However, VBL associated with a 50% lower rebleeding rate compared to sclerotherapy.

Gastric varices account for approximately 10% of variceal bleeds, with higher rate of uncontrolled and rebleeding, and decreased survival, compared with gastro-esophageal varices. VBL and sclerotherapy with standard sclerosants not effective. Variceal injection of cyanoacrylate ('super-glue') may be effective (90% initial haemostasis, compared with 67% for ethanolamine), but has been associated with cerebral embolism due to glue migration. Thrombin may be effective and safer, but still high rebleeding rates. In view of suboptimal hemostatic control with endoscopy or <u>Sengstaken–Blakemore tube</u> (SBT) inflation (especially if gastric varices not bleeding from high in gastric fundus), contact should be made early with specialist liver unit, for consideration of further management (see later).

Uncontrolled bleeding/early rebleeding
- 10–15% of patients have continuing variceal bleed despite initial medical and endoscopic therapy. Early rebleeding (recurrence of bleeding within 5 days of endoscopy) occurs in 30–50%, and is a strong predictor of death. Little benefit in performing >2 endoscopies in patients with ongoing bleeding.
- In patient with an exsanguinating bleed that cannot be controlled endoscopically, SBT should be inserted. This controls acute bleeding from gastro-esophageal varices in 90% of cases, but recurrent bleeding occurs in 50% on deflation of balloon. Endotracheal intubation should be performed prior to tube insertion. Tube should be deflated and removed within 24 hours, and repeat endoscopy performed.
- If bleeding continues despite repeat endoscopy, or failure to achieve control with SBT, contact liver unit to discuss insertion of <u>TIPSS</u> (transjugular intrahepatic portosystemic shunt).

Further management

- Keep NPO for four hours following VBL.
- NG tube insertion should probably be avoided for 48 hours after VBL (but little evidence of absolute risk of dislodging bands).
- Retrosternal discomfort common after endoscopic therapy, and usually responds to simple analgesia.
- Post-VBL/sclerotherapy ulceration may occur and is treated with <u>SUCRALFATE</u> 1 g qds and PPI (e.g., Lansoprazole 30 mg od). It is also a cause of rebleeding, and then may be difficult to control.
- Prior to discharge, address the following:
  - The cause of varices and severity and etiology of any underlying liver disease. Rebleeding is less common, and less severe, in patients with noncirrhotic portal hypertension (e.g., <u>portal vein thrombosis</u>), and recurrence in those with liver disease is strongly linked to <u>Child–Pugh score</u>.
  - The precipitant to bleed (e.g., recent infection, alcohol binge, NSAID use).
  - Treatment of underlying liver disease, and other manifestations of decompensation (e.g., <u>hepatic encephalopathy</u>).
  - The need for secondary prophylaxis against further bleeds. Don't forget this. See <u>portal hypertension</u>.

Esophageal obstruction

Causes

- Swallowed foreign bodies (see gastrointestinal foreign bodies).
- Sudden occlusion by tumor, e.g., cancer of the esophagus.
- Intramural rupture of the esophagus (see intramural hematoma).
- Acute bolus obstruction. This may occur in a normal esophagus after inadequate chewing, but is more common in patients with pre-existing:
  - Esophago-gastric cancer.
  - Esophageal ring stricture.
  - Motility disorder.
  - Patients with esophageal stents or endoprostheses.

Clinical features

Ask about and look for:
- **Pain**. Esophageal pain can mimic that of acute myocardial infarction, but the close temporal relation to eating, combined with dysphagia, usually helps to distinguish the two.
- The patient's ability to swallow his/her own saliva.
- **Duration of symptoms** before obstruction.
- **Predisposing disease** (stricture, carcinoma, esophageal ring).
- **Triggering factors** (classically steak and bread; also tablets).
- **Dehydration.**
- **Weight loss** (suggests malignancy).
- **Supraclavicular nodes** (e.g., gastric cancer).
- **Complications** (aspiration, perforation).

Management

- Contact the on-call endoscopist.
- Bloods: CBC (anemia may suggest chronic bleeding lesion), BUN & electrolytes to look for dehydration.
- Chest X-ray to look for mediastinal fluid level, or evidence of signs of aspiration pneumonia esophageal rupture.
- Intravenous fluids.

Defining the cause

- Endoscopy is better than barium swallow (which risks aspiration) but must be done by an experienced endoscopist.
- Carbonated drinks can occasionally disimpact a food bolus.
- Endoscopic removal of the bolus can be followed immediately by dilatation of any strictures or biopsy of a suspicious mucosal lesion.
- If there is an esophageal stent or prosthesis in place, assessment of tumor ingrowth, overgrowth, or stent migration is essential.
- Endoscopic placement of a fine-bore feeding tube may be necessary after disimpaction if dilatation is delayed.
- Intravenous antibiotics for aspiration (<u>cefuroxime</u> 750 mg tds, <u>METRONIDAZOLE</u> 500 mg tds).

Esophageal rupture

Causes

- **Spontaneous** (usually caused by vomiting; first described by Herman Boerhaave in 1724: see <u>Boerhaave's syndrome</u>), but also reported with foreign bodies such as bones, batteries, and bottle tops; caustic ingestion; and trauma.
- More than 50% cases are caused by medical procedures (see <u>endoscopic complications</u>). The esophagus is said to be at increased risk because it lacks a serosal layer.
- <u>Intramural hematoma</u> can result from sudden increases in intra-esophageal pressure.

Table 2.5 Cases caused by medical procedures

Procedure	Risk of perforation	Site and comments
Rigid esophagoscopy	1/10	Proximal esophagus (associated with arthritic cervical spine or a pharyngeal pouch)
Flexible endoscopy	<1/1000	Usually at intubation or in attempted passage through narrowings
Balloon dilatation of achalasia	Less that 2% with balloons <35 mm: up to 5% with 40-mm balloon	
Dilatation of malignant strictures	Up to 10% in old series using rigid prostheses: much less with softer expanding stents	

Diagnosis

Early diagnosis is crucial; clinical signs may be minimal as the perforation is usually small, the patient is often fasted (and sedated), and the instruments should be clean if not sterile. Perforation may be apparent at the time of procedure, but surgical emphysema, tachycardia, cyanosis, and pain (especially after swallowing) should arouse suspicion.

Radiology

Plain films may show pneumomediastinum, pneumoperitoneum, or left pleural effusion, but can be normal. Late changes of air–fluid collections are better assessed by CT, but contrast studies using water-soluble media are conventionally used to define the site and length of perforation.

Management

- **Get a surgical opinion**: mortality is high and nonoperative approaches apply only to specific situations and require experience.
- If the perforation is small (<1 cm), recognized early, and not associated with gross contamination, conservative management can be successful and includes NPO, IV broad-spectrum antibiotics (e.g., <u>cefuroxime</u> 750 mg tds, <u>METRONIDAZOLE</u> 500 mg tds), and parenteral feeding. Exceptions are perforations into the abdominal or pleural cavities, which need surgical repair.
- Spontaneous ruptures are usually associated with gross contamination and surgery is usually advised.
- Perforations associated with balloon dilatation are often contained within the esophageal wall and may be managed without surgery.
- **Perforation of esophageal cancer** at endoscopy is a difficult problem, with a higher mortality of up to 50%. The perforation site can sometimes be protected by an endoscopically placed covered metal stent. Give antibiotics and start nutritional support.

Clinical factors determining outcome

- The delay in diagnosis.
- The size of hole.
- The degree of soiling of mediastinum or pleural cavity with stomach contents.

Gastrointestinal foreign bodies

Management in this area is based on experience and not controlled trials. Before intervention, consider the type of object ingested, the organ involved, the patient's condition, and the type of symptoms. Co-operation and sedation are essential for safe removal: general anesthesia is needed for children or the uncooperative. The young, the old, and the mentally impaired are most at risk.

Sharp objects can perforate at a number of sites; the ileocecal region is the most frequent site beyond the esophagus.

Swallowed foreign bodies

Clinical features. The location of any discomfort correlates poorly with anatomical impaction. If the object is impacted in the fauces, get ENT advice. Excess salivation or regurgitation may accompany total esophageal obstruction.

Diagnosis. Plain X-rays (frontal and lateral) can help (look for surgical emphysema) but some objects (aluminum, wood, fish bones) are radiolucent. Remember that foreign bodies may impact in the airway not the esophagus. Gastrograffin studies may help. If pain or symptoms persist, endoscopy (with careful intubation under direct vision) is indicated.

Management. If ingestion is recent and the object needs to be removed (see below) laying the patient in the left lateral position may reduce the chances of passage through the pylorus. Glucagon has been suggested to relax the lower esophageal sphincter: it is rarely effective but relatively safe. Endoscopic techniques are well described [see, for example, Cotton PB and Williams CB (2003). *Practical gastrointestinal endoscopy*, 5th ed. Blackwell Publishing, Oxford]. Small coins, frequently swallowed by children, can generally be left to pass provided they are not lodged in the esophagus (but if still in the stomach after 7–14 days may need endoscopic removal). Sharp objects require an experienced endoscopist and use of an overtube is advised.

Colonic and rectal foreign bodies

The range of objects retrieved is a tribute to the richness of human sexual imagination. Retrieval is usually possible: if an inserted object is beyond reach of sigmoidoscope and there is no evidence of perforation or obstruction, observation for 12–24 hours may allow descent to a reachable level. Do not use enemas or cathartics. Sigmoidoscopy after removal is necessary to exclude mucosal injury.

Special considerations

Alkaline batteries. These can disintegrate with local release of toxic contents. Esophageal impaction should be managed by urgent endoscopic removal. There is less agreement if the button is in the stomach: if a plain X-ray shows separation of button components or if the button remains for more than 24 hours, endoscopic search and rescue is reasonable. Once in the small intestine, it is usually safe to wait for passage of the battery.

Body packers. Illegal drugs can be packaged and swallowed or inserted PV or PR. Intact packets can cause obstruction; burst packets can cause lethal overdose (look for symptoms of opiate or cocaine overdose). It is probably best not to give cathartics and do not attempt endoscopic removal which can rupture packets. Symptoms are an indication for surgical removal.

Ethical considerations. Treat the patient first. Inform the police and hospital administrator. Questioning of the patient must be sanctioned by a senior doctor. The patient must be aware of their right to legal advice, through an interpreter if necessary.

Esophagus

Achalasia

Disorder characterized by failure of relaxation of lower esophageal sphincter and aperistalsis of esophageal body, leading to functional obstruction at lower end of the esophagus, food stasis, and esophageal dilatation. Increased risk of **squamous cell cancer** (see esophageal tumors), presumed due to stasis of food and mucosal irritation.

Etiology. Ganglion cells of myenteric plexus are reduced but cause is unknown: viruses and autoimmune mechanisms have been proposed. The so-called nonadrenergic, noncholinergic inhibitory innervation (mostly nitric-oxide mediated) is impaired, which mediates sphincter relaxation.

Clinical features. Usual symptomatic onset age 30–50 years, with dysphagia, which is often intermittent. Nonbilious, nonacid reflux is common feature, as is chest pain, which may relate to esophageal spasm. Heartburn sometimes reported, but true reflux is (predictably) rare.

Investigation. Diagnosis made on basis of history, radiological, endoscopic, and manometric findings. Chest X-ray may show an air fluid level in a dilated esophagus. Barium swallow shows dilated esophagus with reduced peristalsis (Color plate 1). Endoscopy essential in all patients to exclude mucosal pathology and pseudoachalsia.

Esophageal manometry shows raised lower esophageal sphincter pressure and incomplete or absent sphincter relaxation. Differential diagnosis of achalasia includes esophageal spasm, trypanosomiasis (Chagas's disease), and pseudoachalasia.

Management. Options include drugs, endoscopy, and surgery.

- Drugs do not work well: nitrates and calcium channel blockers provide, at best, short-lived effects on lower esophageal sphincter pressure and have side effects. BOTULINUM TOXIN injected into the sphincter does reduce sphincter pressure and relieve symptoms, but the effects are short-lived and repeated injections are necessary, every 6–12 months.
- Endoscopic dilatation performed using 30, 35, or 40 mm balloons passed over a guide wire, or by direct visualization. The balloon is inflated for 1–2 min. Response is good in 60–70% patients but many patients need more than 1 procedure. Endoscopic complications include perforation (1–5%, commoner with larger balloons) and reflux (about 10%).
- Surgical myotomy effective in 90% but causes reflux in 10%: an antireflux procedure is often done at the same time (see antireflux procedures). Laparoscopic myotomy is the treatment of choice for some patients. Practical approach to treatment is to start with balloon dilatation becaue many patients will do well with this; if there is rapid relapse a myotomy can be offered.

Barrett's esophagus

Definition. Presence of columnar epithelium lining the lower esophagus (see Color Plate 13). Because of imprecision in defining endoscopic landmarks (see Box 3.1.1), definition of classical Barrett's is usually restricted to columnar mucosa extending 3+ cm into the tubular esophagus. Less than this is "short segment Barrett's."

Box 3.1.1 Practice point: diagnosis of Barrett's esophagus

Correct endoscopic identification of anatomical landmarks is vital (also affects interpretation of histology). Diagnosis of Barrett's esophagus is often imprecise because of a failure to document.
- Level of diaphragmatic crus (usually 40 cm in males, 38 cm in females)
- Gastro-esophageal junction (where the gastric rugal folds peter out into the tubular esophagus)
- Squamo-columnar junction

All endoscopy reports should include these values if there is any question of Barrett's esophagus. Failure to do this in so many studies has generated more heat than light over this controversial topic.

Pathogenesis + epidemiology. Usually arises as an adaptive change to reflux esophagitis. Columnar mucosa is more resistant to acid than squamous epithelium, but the price for protection may be high, as epithelium can become metaplasic and premalignant. The incidence of developing adenocarcinoma (see esophageal tumors) is approximately 1 in 100 patient years, representing approximately a 30-fold increase in risk. Frequency studies suggest it is more common than originally thought and moreover may be increasing.

Clinical features. May be entirely asymptomatic, or associated with symptoms of esophagitis.

Diagnosis requires esophageal biopsies showing columnar epithelium. Endoscopy alone is not sufficient.

In general the risk of malignancy seems associated with the presence of intestinal metaplasia on biopsy.

Note. Do not confuse Barrett's with an inlet patch of columnar mucosa in the upper esophagus. This is usually congenital and is not exposed to enough acid to produce significant inflammation. It is not premalignant.

Treatment. No convincing data that either medical or surgical intervention results in clinically meaningful regression of Barrett's epithelium or reduces the risk of it undergoing malignant transformation. Because of the high mortality of surgery (about 7%), some centers are using lasers with or without photosensitizing agents, to ablate dysplastic Barrett's (see photodynamic therapy), or localized resections (Endoscopic Mucosal Resection). This can lead to regrowth with squamous epithelium but long-term follow-up data are awaited. Issue of Barrett's surveillance is controversial.

Barrett's surveillance

Most patients with Barrett's have normal lifespan and die of unrelated disease.[1] Endoscopic surveillance is frequently recommended **if the length of columnar epithelium is 3+ cm and if there is intestinal metaplasia on biopsy.** Surveillance is recommended to detect <u>dysplasia</u> and asymptomatic adenocarcinoma. Cancers in Barrett's evolve slowly and there is some evidence that early resection carries a better prognosis than the 5-year survival of 17% reported for symptomatic adenocarcinomas (see <u>esophageal tumors</u>).

Recommendations (ACG Practice Guidelines, March 2008)

- **No dysplasia.** Survey every three years by taking four quadrant biopsies every 2 cm throughout the length of Barrett's.
- **Low grade dysplasia.** First get a second pathology opinion for confirmation. Give a high dose PPI to minimize inflammation that makes pathological interpretation more difficult; then take repeat biopsies within six months. In established low-grade dysplasia, take biopsies yearly until no dysplasia on two successive occasions.
- **High grade dysplasia**. Should be verified by two experienced pathologists. Any patient with mucosal irregularity should be considered for endoscopic resection for more extensive histological evaluation. Management of patients with high-grade dysplasia is dependent on local expertise, both endoscopic and surgical, and the patient's age, comorbidity and preferences. Endoscopic therapy, continued intensive surveillance, or esophagectomy are options.

Boerhaave syndrome

Herman Boerhaave (1668–1738), Dutch, one of the most revered teachers of his day. Best known for his description of esophageal rupture in the grand admiral of the fleet, Jacob van Wassaenaer. Said to have written a book containing all the secrets of medicine: after he died it was opened and all the pages were blank except one on which was written "keep the head cool, the feet warm and the bowels open."

- <u>Esophageal rupture</u> caused by vomiting against a closed glottis: common after excess alcohol intake. Rupture usually occurs at the weakest point (at the lower end on the left side), but may occur in the mid-esophagus on the right. The lack of serosa in the esophagus may make it more prone to rupture. Gastric contents spill into the thorax. Pain is severe, upper abdominal, and may radiate to the back. Examination may reveal dyspnea, sepsis, hypovolemic shock, and cyanosis. Surgical emphysema may be found in the neck.

---

1 Cameron, A J et al. (1985) *N. Engl. J. Med* **313**: 857

- Early diagnosis reached by clinical suspicion and a gastrograffin swallow. CXR may show air in mediastinum.
- Initial management is to keep patient strictly NPO and give IV antibiotics (e.g., third-generation <u>CEPHALOSPORIN</u> and <u>METRONIDAZOLE</u>), but most patients should be managed surgically. Early surgery (within 6 h) may be life saving. Primary closure may be possible if surgery is not delayed: in late cases alternatives are drainage with a cervical esophagostomy and gastrostomy, or transhiatal esophagectomy. Mortality for cases diagnosed and treated within 6–12 h is 10–15%, rising to over 50% for those diagnosed after that time.

Table 3.1.1 Body weight categories

Category	Body mass index (kg/m²)
Underweight	< 19
Normal weight	19–24.9
Mild overweight	25–29.9
Moderate overweight	30–39.9
Severe overweight	> 40

Caustic injury

80% of caustic ingestions occur accidentally in children; ingestion in adults usually indicates intent of suicide or self-harm. Most ingested corrosives are alkaline (bleach and other household cleaning agents) or acids (toilet cleaners, battery acids, swimming pool cleaners). Risks to the GI tract are of esophageal necrosis and perforation and later sequelae, such as esophageal scarring and stricture formation. However, most deaths following acid ingestion relate to systemic effects (renal failure, liver failure, DIC).

Clinical features can be dramatic: mouth and chest pain, with painful swallowing (odynophagia), dysphagia, excess salivation, and epigastric pain.

Management
- Gastric lavage and induced emesis are contraindicated. Activated charcoal not recommended. Water of no proven use.
- Prophylactic antibiotics are often given parenterally.
- CXR may show free air in the mediastinum or under the diaphragm.
- Water soluble contrast agents such as gastrograffin conventionally recommended over barium, especially if perforation needs excluding, but, in the author's opinion, <u>CT scanning</u> can give the same information.

Endoscopy

- The oropharynx may need to be examined by laryngoscopy, since a supraglottic or epiglottic burn with erythema and edema formation may be a harbinger of airway obstruction and should be seen as an indication for early endotracheal intubation or tracheostomy.
- Endoscopy serves a dual purpose:
  - Patients with no evidence of gastrointestinal injury can be discharged, provided there are no other complications. More than 50% of patients with history of caustic ingestion have no endoscopic evidence of injury.
  - Those with evidence of severe injury can be managed appropriately.
- Endoscopy should preferably be performed <12 hours and generally not >24 hours since ingestion (although some authors state that endoscopy can be safely performed up to 96 hours postingestion). Severity of mucosal damage on endoscopy within 24 hours predicts mortality (overall 2–14%, with increased rate after acid, due largely to systemic complications—renal/liver failure, hemolysis, DIC). Wound softening begins after two to three days and lasts up to two weeks, making endoscopy risky during this period.

Contraindications to endoscopy

- Evidence of full-thickness injury, with possible perforation, shock, or acidosis.
- Third-degree burn of the hypopharynx seen at laryngoscopy.
- Perforation complicating endoscopy is rare but attempts to continue past circumferential burns are associated with increased risk.

Complications of caustic ingestion

- Stricture formation in 15% of cases. Early use of IV CORTICOSTEROIDS may reduce risk of stricture formation, but this is controversial. Endoscopic dilatation rarely provides long-term cure, necessitating surgery in most cases.

Role of surgery

- If there is perforation or gastric necrosis, surgery is mandatory; 50% of patients with esophageal perforation die. Options include esophagectomy and gastrostomy if the stomach is intact, or gastrectomy and jejunostomy if the stomach is necrotic.

Chagas's disease

See: trypanosomiasis.

Diaphragmatic hernia

Can occur through the esophageal hiatus (see <u>hiatus hernia</u>), through other openings (foramina of **Bochdalek,** at the lumbrocosatal margins of the diaphragm posterolaterally or **Morgagni**, at the sternocostal margins of the diaphragm anteriorly) or through posttraumatic defects.

Congenital hernias occur in 0.1 to 0.5 per 1,000 live births. In neonates they are mostly Bochdalek hernias. Morgagni hernias occur mainly in adults and 80% are on the right side. They may contain omentum, stomach, colon, or liver. Repair is possible through open, thoracoscopic, or laparoscopic techniques.

Drug-induced esophagitis

- Many drugs have been reported to cause esophageal injury. See Box 3.1.2. 90% of cases are due to NSAIDs, antibiotics (especially tetracyclines), antivirals, potassium chloride, iron, quinidine, and bisphosphanates.
- Patients with strictures, <u>esophageal tumor</u>, <u>achalasia</u>, scleroderma should take pills upright with plenty of water.
- Chemotherapy esophagitis: adriamycin, 5FU, <u>METHOTREXATE</u>, vincristine can all cause oropharyngeal mucositis and consequent dysphagia. Esophageal damage is unusual in the absence of oral changes. Chemotherapy potentiates radiation damage to the esophagus.

Box 3.1.2 Causes of drug-induced esophagitis

NSAIDs: naproxen, ibuprofen, aspirin-containing pills

Antibiotics: tetracyclines, clindamycin, penicillins

Antivirals: AZT, ddC, foscarnet

Iron and **potassium** formulations

Cardiovascular medications: quinidine, nifedipine, verapamil, captopril

Other common drugs: bisphosphanates, phenytoin, oral contraceptive

Dysplasia

> "Britain and America—divided by a common language"
> George Bernard Shaw 1856–1950

- A question that induces frustration and uncertainty into the hearts of gastroenterologists, particularly when they want a straight answer from the pathologists: "Is it cancer or not?"
- Dysplasia refers to **cellular and architectural changes that are associated with malignancy** (premalignant/adjacent to malignancy) but that, by definition, are not invasive. Differentiate from metaplasia, which refers to the conversion of one type of differentiated tissue into another specialist type (e.g., intestinal metaplasia in stomach related to *Helicobacter pylori*).
  - **Cellular changes** in dysplasia include an increase in cell nuclei size (↑ nuclear:cytoplasmic ratio), loss of nuclear polarity, and loss of cellular differentiation (e.g., mucin production).
  - **Architectural changes** include loss of normal glandular spacing, without intervening stroma.
- In practical terms, high-grade dysplasia on mucosal biopsy suggests significant risk of invasive malignancy developing, or being present at other sites (in view of tiny area of tissue sampled). Unless confident that all affected area is removed (e.g., excised polyp), high- grade dysplasia requires consideration of radical intervention (e.g., colectomy in ulcerative colitis, esophagectomy/photodynamic therapy in Barrett's esophagus).
- Vienna classification of GI epithelial neoplasia (see Table 3.1.2) aims to standardize reporting of dysplasia/neoplasia.

Table 3.1.2 Vienna classification of gastrointestinal epithelial neoplasia

Category	Histological assessment
1	Negative for neoplasia/dysplasia
2	Indefinite for neoplasia/dysplasia
3	Noninvasive low-grade neoplasia (low-grade adenoma/dysplasia)
4	Noninvasive high-grade neoplasia
4.1	High-grade adenoma/dysplasia
4.2	Noninvasive carcinoma (carcinoma *in situ*)
4.3	Suspicion of invasive carcinoma
5	Invasive neoplasia
5.1	Intramucosal carcinoma
5.2	Submucosal carcinoma or beyond

Gastro-esophageal reflux (GERD)

See: Dyspepsia and GERD.

Hiatus hernia

Two types: a **sliding hernia**, when the gastro-esophageal junction and some part of the stomach are displaced above the diaphragm (the commonest type, accounting for about 95%; usually small and of no clinical significance), or **para-esophageal**, when the stomach protrudes through the esophageal hiatus alongside the esophagus.

Most sliding hernias are small but can predispose to gastro-esophageal reflux (see also Dyspepsia and GERD). Large hernias may develop Cameron ulcers, usually on the lesser curve at the level of the hiatus: they can cause upper or lower GI bleeding or be a cause of iron deficiency anaemia.

Treatment. Simple sliding hiatus hernias do not need treatment. Giant or para-esophageal hernias may require surgery (see antireflux procedures).

Mallory–Weiss syndrome

First described by Quincke in 1879, Mallory and Weiss described 15 cases of this syndrome in 1929.

Longitudinal mucosal acerations in the region of the gastro-esophageal junction thought to be caused by retching. They account for 5–10% cases of upper GI bleeding. Bleeding stops spontaneously in 80–90% and rebleeding is rare. Endoscopic therapy to stop bleeding may be necessary but surgical intervention is very rare.

Esophageal motility disorders

Hypermotility disorders
See achalasia. Nonachalasia disorders of hypermotility include:
- Diffuse esophageal spasm.
- Nutcracker esophagus.
- Hypertensive lower esophageal sphincter.
- Nonspecific esophageal motor disorder.

Considerable overlap between these terms exists. All are diagnosed by esophageal manometry.

Pathology is poorly defined but may involve increased esophageal sensitivity to cholinergic stimulation.

Clinical presentation Chest pain occurs in 90%, can be severe, is usually retrosternal, and may radiate to the back. There may be some persisting discomfort after the acute episodes, which may help to differentiate it from angina. Dysphagia occurs in 30–60%, and heartburn is seen in up to 20%.

Diagnosis. Upper GI endoscopy is usually normal, but may show alternative reasons for symptoms such as esophagitis or stricture. Barium studies, especially fluoroscopic studies with swallowing soft solids, can be very helpful because they can link faulty transit with symptoms and also show up features such as nonpropulsive contractions (so-called corkscrew esophagus).

Manometric abnormalities can include:

- **Nonperistaltic contractions after wet swallows.** Diffuse esophageal spasm is diagnosed if abnormal swallows occur more than 20% of the time (with amplitude >30 mmHg) . The term *nutcracker esophagus* is reserved for a subgroup with very high contraction amplitude (pressures exceeding 220 mmHg during 10 or more 5 ml liquid swallows).
- **Abnormal wave of contraction.** This can be variable and is best labeled as a nonspecific spastic disorder; there is no agreed classification.
- **Hypertension or poor relaxation** of the lower esophageal sphincter. This often accompanies spastic abnormalities of the esophageal body. Hypertensive lower esophageal sphincter usually defined as a resting lower esophageal sphincter pressure >45 mmHg
- These manometric findings are not mutually exclusive

Treatment. These disorders are not progressive and not associated with more serious underlying pathology, so symptom reduction is the goal.

- If symptoms suggest abnormal transit (e.g., regurgitation or dysphagia), then treatment similar to that for achalasia may help, especially if manometry shows abnormalities of the lower esophageal sphincter. Botox injections into the LOS or balloon dilatation have been used effectively in this context.
- Treating reflux can be dramatically beneficial, even in the absence of a classical history.
- Therapeutic trial of nitrates, calcium antagonists, and anticholinergics can help and have all been shown experimentally to produce at least short-term improvement in manometry. Remember that nitrates and calcium antagonists will worsen any coexistent esophageal reflux.
- The tricyclic antidepressant trazodone is the only agent found to improve symptoms in a prospective controlled study (although improvement did not depend on any change in manometry).

Hypomotility disorders

This is usually secondary to systemic disease. The clinical manifestations include:

- Dysphagia, secondary to impaired peristalsis or associated sicca syndrome in scleroderma or associated connective tissue disorders.
- Esophageal reflux due to the low pressure LOS. Complications of reflux, such as esophagitis, strictures, and Barrett's esophagus are all more common.

Management of symptoms of impaired GI motility in scleroderma is described elsewhere (see esophageal obstruction).

Esophageal rings

The mucosal ring, located at the gastro-esophageal junction, was first described by Schatski in 1953.

Found in approximately 6–14% of adult population on barium swallow, but causes symptoms in minority. Usually considered a congenital structural variant, although chronic reflux may contribute.

Clinical presentation is classically with intermittent nonprogressive dysphagia to hurriedly eaten solids (classically bread or meat bolus—"steakhouse syndrome").

Diagnosis can be by barium swallow or endoscopy: if using barium, the esophagus must be well distended by getting the patient to perform a valsalva maneuver and including a solid bolus during the exam to identify the lesion.

Management. In symptomatic patients, <u>endoscopic dilatation</u> performed, with intention of splitting ring, using bougies or pneumatic balloons. Repeat treatments may be required.

> ### Box 3.1.3 Causes of impaired esophageal motility
>
> - Usually secondary to multisystem disease
> - 80% of <u>scleroderma</u> patients have altered esophageal motility (second commonest affected organ)
>   - Vascular obliteration, secondary fibrosis
>   - Reflux, esophagitis, and Barrett's all seen
> - Also seen in mixed connective tissue disease, rheumatoid arthritis, and systemic lupus erythematosus
> - Amyloid, alcohol, myxoedema, MS
> - Diabetes: 60% of patients with peripheral or autonomic neuropathy have disordered motility, but symptoms are only seen in a minority
> - Pseudo-obstruction

Esophageal stricture

Commonest benign cause is acid reflux but also seen after caustic injury, after variceal sclerotherapy or band ligation, and after mediastinal chemo/radiotherapy. Prevalence of peptic strictures in patients with reflux <u>esophagitis</u> is 8–20% but may be decreasing with widespread use of PPIs. Strictures can develop weeks to months after sclerotherapy; incidence is 2–13% and the major risk factor is large persistent esophageal ulcers. Can be a feature of esophageal malignancies or due to extrinsic compression of esophagus.

Treatment of peptic strictures centers on <u>endoscopic dilatation</u>, healing esophagitis, and minimizing recurrence. Dilatation can be done with Savary–Gillard graded dilators over a guide wire or using a through the scope balloon. Results are equally effective although the balloon exerts a lower radial force than the rigid dilators. Dilatation to 15 mm generally relieves dysphagia. The schedule varies but repeating the procedure every 1–2 weeks with no more than three step dilatations at any one occasion is advised. More than 50% patients need repeat dilatation: risk factors are number of previous dilatations and persistent esophagitis. Maintenance proton pump inhibitors are advised.

Risks of dilatation
- Perforation (less than 0.5% for benign structures, but higher for malignant structures (2–6%)).
- Bleeding (less than 0.5%).
- Bacteremia (give <u>antibiotic prophylaxis</u> to high-risk patients).

Esophageal tumors

Classified into epithelial or nonepithelial, benign or malignant: see Table 3.1.3.

Malignant epithelial tumors
- Mostly primary esophageal cancers: squamous cell carcinoma (SCC), adenocarcinoma of esophagus, and adenocarcinoma of esophago-gastric junction.
- Worldwide, fifth commonest lethal cancer, with SCC commonest subtype, but in Western countries adenocarcinoma has increased fivefold in last 30 years so that this is now more common than SCC: the rise is particularly marked for cancers of the esophago-gastric junction.

Epidemiology and risks for esophageal cancer are shown in Table 3.1.3.

Clinical features
- SCC occurs in the upper two-thirds of the esophagus; adenocarcinoma occurs in the lower third and at the esophago-gastric junction.
- Symptoms include dysphagia and odynophagia (pain on swallowing), often accompanied by anorexia and weight loss. Both cancer types can infiltrate submucosally but SCC is more locally aggressive, and can cause vocal cord paralysis due to recurrent laryngeal nerve invasion and <u>tracheo-esophageal fistula</u> in 5%. Pulmonary, hepatic, brain, and bone metastasis occurs. Adenocarcinoma is less locally invasive, but hematogenous and lymphangitic spread occurs to regional and distant lymph nodes and to liver. Most patients present with advanced disease because the esophagus has a rich lymphatic supply and lacks a serosa, so that local spread occurs before luminal stenosis causes symptoms.
- Hepatomegaly may be present if there are liver metastases.

Diagnosis
- **Screening** of high-risk groups includes surveillance of patients with <u>Barrett's esophagus</u> (e.g., see <u>Barrett's surveillance</u>).
- **Laboratory** tests may reveal low albumin, anemia (bleeding or chronic disease), and hypercalcaemia due to PTH-related peptide, especially in SCC (seen in 15–30% patients).
- **Radiology.** Chest X-rays can be helpful in diagnosing pulmonary metastases of lung infiltrates suggestive of esophago-bronchial fistula. Contrast radiology with barium can confirm fistulazation or obstruction. Cross-sectional imaging is needed for staging (see later).
- **Endoscopy.** This allows histological diagnosis but also characterization of length and configuration and an opportunity for therapeutic dilatation. Six biopsies are needed for an accuracy of nearly 100%.

Table 3.1.3 Classification of esophageal tumors

Epithelial	Nonepithelial
Malignant	
Squamous cell carcinoma	Lymphoma
Adenocarcinoma	Sarcoma
Adenocarcinoma of the esophago-gastric junction	Metastases
Other rare malignancies e.g., small-cell carcinoma (1–5% of esophageal cancers)	
Benign	
Papilloma	Leiomyoma
Adenoma	Granular cell tumors Others (lipoma, hemangioma)

Table 3.1.4 Epidemiology and biology of esophageal cancer

Squamous cell cancer	Adenocarcinoma
Incidence	
Incidence varies by region: commonest in China, Iran, Turkey, N. Africa. Commoner in black men in 6th and 7th decades	Commoner in white men
Environmental risk factors	
Nitrosamines in the diet, exposure to hydrocarbons from cooking in confined spaces, and chewing of betel nuts have been implicated. Alcohol and tobacco are both linked to SCC	Questionable inverse relation with *Helicobacter pylori*
High risk diseases	
Achalasia (possible due to prolonged stasis of esophageal contents) Caustic strictures	Gastro-esophageal reflux and Barrett's esophagus are associated factors, with most cancers arising from areas of intestinal metaplasia. Annual incidence of cancer in Barrett's quoted as 0.5–1% per annum
Plummer–Vinsen/Patterson–Kelly syndrome	
Tylosis	
Concurrent head or neck SCC	
Human papilloma virus	
Biology	
Associated oncogenes include cyclin D1	P53 and E cadherin are both important tumor suppressor genes.

Staging

Staging is largely based on retrospective Japanese data (most patients had SCC rather than increasingly common adenocarcinoma). Treatment and outcome are stage-dependent (see tumor staging TNM classification) Patients with T1 or T2 lesions who are N0, M0 have significant surgical cure rates. T3N1 patients are potentially curable but do poorly with surgery alone. Patients with local spread into aorta, airway, pleura, and spine and those with hematogenous spread should be treated palliatively, although there is some evidence that patients with positive abdominal lymph nodes can undergo curative resection.

- **Cross-sectional imaging.** CT is accurate at identifying solid organ metastases but less good at identifying lymph node metastases, especially in the chest. MRI has no significant advantage over CT. PET scanning has high sensitivity and specificity for distant metastases but is not widely used at present in staging.
- **Endoscopic ultrasound (EUS)** is probably the most accurate tool for staging; overall accuracy for T stage is 75–85% and N stage is 65–75%. EUS for the guiding fine needle aspiration (FNA) improves diagnosis of malignant lymphadenopathy. EUS has been shown to have high sensitivity and negative predictive value for submucosal invasion of cancer in patients with Barrett's and high-grade dysplasia (HGD) or intramucosal carcinoma.

Treatment

Primary treatment

- Options include surgery alone, chemoradiotherapy, endoscopic mucosal resection, and photodynamic therapy. Combined modality therapy with e.g., surgery plus chemoradiotherapy is under evaluation.
- Surgery is indicated for superficial tumors. Operative mortality is 3–10%. Surgical approach is either transhiatal or involves thoracotomy.
- Squamous cell tumors are more sensitive to radiotherapy than adenocarcinomas, but even in SCC, combined chemo- and radiotherapy is more effective than radiation therapy alone. Results suggest a 75% local control rate, with 18% survival at five years for stage I/II patients.

Endoscopic mucosal resection. Accurate staging and histological diagnosis of HGD or carcinoma limited to mucosa allows endosopic resection using submucosal saline injection and electrocautery techniques. Complete resection appears possible in over 75% but long-term follow-up data are limited at present. Photodynamic therapy (PDT) is being evaluated as a curative modality.

Palliative treatment includes radio- and chemotherapy, intraluminal brachytherapy, endoscopic dilatation or stent placement, contact thermal therapy, endoscopic laser therapy, and PDT. Argon plasma coagulation does not penetrate deeply enough to give relief of dysphagia, and injection of cytotoxic drugs, although theoretically attractive, has not been standardized or compared with other ablative techniques.

Table 3.1.4 Prognosis in esophageal cancer is related to TNM classification

Stage	Five-year survival	Comments
T1	46%	Surgically resectable.
T2	30%	five- year survival is 40% for N0 but 17% for N1
T3	22%	
T4	7%	

- **Chemotherapy.** Objective response rates of 30–50% are seen with platinum-based regimes with 5FU, a taxane, or topoisomerase inhibitor.
- **Endoscopic therapy** aims at palliating dysphagia, although bleeding and esophago-respiratory fistulae can also be treated endoscopically. Endoscopic dilatation can be done using bougies or through-the-scope (TTS) balloons. Advantages include simplicity, low cost, and relative safety. Disadvantages include short duration of efficacy and the frequent need for repeated procedures. It is not adequate palliation for most patients. The best results using thermal ablation are with endoscopic laser, Nd:YAG being the commonest wavelength.
- **Endoscopic stents** offer good palliation of malignant strictures and tracheo-esophageal fistulae. Self-expanding metallic stents have replaced rigid plastic stents because they are easier to place, give better palliation, and are associated with fewer complications.
- **Photodynamic therapy.** This is discussed in detail elsewhere.

Other esophageal tumors

- **Malignant nonepithelial tumors.** The esophagus is a rare site of primary lymphoma and sarcoma: leiomyosarcoma are the most common. Diagnosis can be difficult with conventional biopsy—EUS-guided FNA is the best way of getting a diagnosis.
- **Benign tumors.** Leiomoyomas arise from smooth muscle cells; they have been subsumed into the category gastrointestinal stromal tumors (GIST). There is a risk of malignant transformation into sarcomas that appears to increase with size over 5 cm diameter. EUS is the most accurate diagnostic modality. Surgery should be considered if there are symptoms, uncertainty about the diagnosis, or a suspicion of malignant transformation. Other benign tumors include granular cell tumors, fibrovascular polyps or hamartomas, and lipomas.

Esophagitis

- Most commonly due to gastro-esophageal reflux (see Dyspepsia and GERD) but remember other causes (see Box 3.1.4).
- Diagnostic evaluation of esophagitis is usually by endoscopy, although only 30–40% patients with GERD have endoscopically obvious inflammation. Endoscopic evaluation can be confusing: the commonest classification is the Los Angeles grading system (see Box 3.1.5).

Box 3.1.4 **Causes of esophagitis**

- Infections: fungal (*Candida*, *Aspergillus*), bacterial (staphylococcus, stretococcus), and viral
- Systemic diseases: pemphigus, Behçet's syndrome
- Graft versus host disease
- IBD: esophagus is rarely affected in Crohn's disease
- Pill-induced esophagitis
- Chemoradiation: mucositis can affect esophagel mucosa. Radiation above 30 Gy is associated with esophagitis. Chemotherapy potentiates radiation-induced esophagitis

Box 3.1.5 **Los Angeles grading system for esophagitis**

Grade A: one or more mucosal breaks no longer than 5 mm that do not extend between the tops of two mucosal folds

Grade B: one or more mucosal breaks more than 5 mm long that do not extend between the tops of two mucosal folds

Grade C: One or more mucosal breaks that are continuous between the tops of two or more mucosal folds but involve less than 75% of the circumference

Grade D: One or more mucosal breaks that involve at least 75% of the esophageal circumference

Note that the Los Angeles system does not describe strictures, hiatus herniae, or Barrett's. These have to be described separately.

Los Angeles grading

See: esophagitis.

Pharyngeal pouch ("Zenker's diverticulum")

- Present in 1% of people > 70 years. Diverticulum develops in area of weakness where fibers of cricopharyngeal sphincter meet oblique fibers of the inferior pharyngeal constrictor muscle. Incomplete relaxation of upper esophageal sphincter may lead to   pharyngeal pressure proximal to this during swallowing, with subsequent herniation.
- Symptoms: dysphagia, regurgitation, cough, aspiration, and halitosis.
- Diagnosis usually made by barium swallow. Esophageal rupture is an important complication, often related to endoscope tip penetrating the base of the diverticulum.
- Traditionally, treatment is surgical, with > 90% subsequently symptom-free. Recently, new less invasive and endoscopic techniques are being shown to be effective.

Plummer–Vinson/Patterson–Kelly syndrome

A syndrome characterized by an iron-deficiency anemia, atrophic changes in the buccal, glossopharyngeal, and esophageal mucous membranes, koil-onychia, and dysphagia. The dysphagia is due to an esophageal ring/web formed in the postcricoid region. Squamous carcinoma of the tongue and postcricoid region are complications. It is most common in middle-aged women, rarely in the male. Etiology unknown.

Pseudoachalasia

An appearance usually seen on barium swallow or endoscopy that can mimic achalasia, but in fact is due to malignant compression of the lower esophagus. It accounts for about 5% of cases of manometrically defined achalasia, and should be suspected in the over-50 age group, if onset of symptoms is abrupt (< 1 year), or if there is early weight loss of over 7 kg. It should also be considered if there is a feeling at endoscopy of resistance or stiffness in crossing the lower esophageal sphincter or if the patient tolerates endoscopic dilatation very poorly. Adenocarcinoma of the gastro-esophageal junction is the commonest cause, but other tumors or infiltrative diseases have been reported (see esophageal tumors).

Schatzki ring

See: esophageal ring.

Tracheo-esophageal fistula (TEF)

Background
- Congenital causes.
  - Commonly trachea communicates with abnormal, atretic, distal esophagus (due to failure of lung bud to separate from foregut).
- Acquired causes.
  - Tumor invasion (e.g., bronchial or esophageal tumor).
  - Instrumentation (e.g., endoscopic dilatation or ablation of malignant stricture).

Clinical features
- Congenital TEF usually presents in infancy with regurgitation and aspiration of feed (due to associated atresia as well as TEF).
- In adulthood TEF presents with features of esophageal rupture, recurrent pneumonia, and systemic sepsis.

Investigation
- In congenital TEF diagnosis often confirmed by failure to pass NG tube into the stomach and injection of 1 ml of barium down tube.
- CXR may show air-filled upper esophagus & air–fluid level.
In adulthood, CT may show fistula, with diagnosis confirmed using oral nonionic contrast, if necessary.

Management
- Congenital TEF treated surgically with resection of esophageal atresia and TEF, with end-to-end anastomosis, or interposition of colon, dependent on length of defect. Surgery 90% successful, but patients may develop significant reflux and esophageal motility problems in adulthood.
- Endoscopically placed covered metal stents may be effective in sealing the defect in > 70% of cases of TEFs related to esophageal cancers.

Variceal bleeding

See: Acute upper GI bleeding and portal hypertension.

Video capsule endoscopy

See: enteroscopy

Stomach

Achlorhydria

Defined as failure of intragastric pH to fall below 4 under stimulation with pentagastrin. In absence of gastric acid, negative feedback control of gastrin is lost and hypergastrinemia is seen (see Box 3.2.1).

Gastrinoma (Zollinger–Ellinson syndrome) may be suspected and acid secretory studies may be necessary. Atrophic gastritis may be associated with reduced intrinsic factor secretion (see pernicious anemia).

Box 3.2.1 Causes of achlorhydria

- Atrophic gastritis, either autoimmune, such as pernicious anemia, or environmental, such as *Helicobacter pylori*
- Mucolipidosis type 4 (crippled parietal cells due to absent protein needed for vacuolar trafficking)
- Previous gastrectomy or vagotomy
- Rare tumors that produce hormones inhibiting acid secretion (e.g., somatostatinoma—see pancreatic endocrine tumors)
- Severe hypocalcaemia impairs parietal cell acid secretion
- Acid secretion is also reduced in AIDS

Atrophic gastritis

A histological diagnosis, requiring endoscopic biopsy (2 biopsies from body, 2 from antrum, 1 from incisura). Findings include chronic gastric inflammation with loss of gastric glands and replacement by intestinal-type epithelium and fibrous tissue.

Two main causes:

- **Type A or auto-immune atrophic gastritis**. This is mainly restricted to the gastric corpus, sparing the gastric antrum. It is characterized by auto-antibodies against gastric parietal cells and intrinsic factor, and often leads to pernicious anemia.
- *Environmental factors* usually produce multifocal gastritis, involving antrum and corpus. Examples include dietary factors (e.g., nitroso compounds produced by bacterial metabolism of dietary nitrates) and *Helicobacter pylori*. *Helicobacter*-associated gastritis results from the release of bacterial and inflammatory toxic products, and can result in either antral-predominant gastritis or multifocal gastritis affecting corpus, fundus, and antrum, with partial replacement of gastric-type epithelium by intestinal epithelium. Mucosal inflammation, and, therefore, atrophic gastritis, is more marked with cagA positive strains of HP. Antral-predominant gastritis is commonly found in infected patients with peptic ulcers, whereas mutifocal gastritis and autoimmune gastritis are associated with the development of gastric carcinoma.

Bezoars

From a Persian word for counterpoison, because they were originally thought to be antidotes for snake bites and insect stings.

Defined as persistent concretions of foreign matter found in the GI tract: nearly always in the stomach. Usually composed of plant and vegetable fibers, hair, or medications (aluminium antacids, enteric-coated tablets, bismuth). They are not common but occur when material that enters the stomach cannot exit because of size, indigestibility, obstruction, or poor motility. Symptoms depend on the size and location.

Endoscopy is the most sensitive test. Although surgical removal is sometimes needed, nonoperative strategies include enzymatic digestion, mechanical disruption using endoscopic forceps and snares, and even laser treatment.

Billroth

See also gastrectomy. Christian Billroth (German–Austrian surgeon, 1829–1894).

Billroth pioneered many surgical operations including gastrectomy. Billroth I operation involves directly joining gastric remnant after partial gastrectomy onto the duodenum; Billroth II operation involves closing the duodenal stump and making a gastroenterostomy. Billroth I is preferred because of a lower incidence of dumping and weight loss. Billroth II is used if duodenal inflammation makes a Billroth I technically difficult.

Dieulafoy lesion

First described by Georges Dieulafoy, a French surgeon, in 1898, this lesion is a rare cause of acute upper GI bleeding. It consists of an arteriole that protrudes through a 2–5 mm mucosal defect, and is usually found in the stomach, within 6 cm of the gastro-esophageal junction, in 75–95% of cases. Rarer sites include the distal esophagus, small intestine, colon, and rectum. Diagnosis made on endoscopy, and endotherapy (e.g., electrocoagulation, adrenaline injection, hemoclipping). Results in permanent hemostasis in 85% of cases. See Color Plate 14.

Ectopic mucosa

Refers to the presence of mucosal tissue in sites distant to their normal location. Examples include:

- Meckel's diverticulum (often harboring gastric mucosa).
- Pancreatic rests (islands of pancreatic acinar tissue, lacking anatomic and vascular continuity with main pancreas). Found in 1–14% of autopsies. Most common in stomach and duodenum, where they appear as yellowish subcutaneous nodules. Usually asymptomatic, requiring no treatment.
- Gastric heterotopia also most common in duodenum, (but described in all parts of GI tract) appearing as sessile/polypoid lesion. Usually asymptomatic finding on endoscopy, but histological diagnosis necessary to exclude other causes of lesion.
- Malignancy may rarely occur within ectopic mucosa.

Gastrectomy/gastroenterostomy

- Elective peptic ulcer surgery (see <u>Billroth</u>) is now rare and most often applied to patients with gastric outlet obstruction due to longstanding <u>peptic ulceration</u>. Emergency surgery is still needed, largely when perforation or catastrophic bleeding is the first manifestation of disease. Subtotal gastrectomy to remove the source of gastrin and parietal cell mass has a high rate of complications and is now reserved for treatment of uncontrollable hemorrhagic gastritis and gastric cancer.
- Surgery is the only curative procedure for <u>gastric cancer</u> and is also useful for palliation of symptoms, especially of obstruction. There is controversy about the necessary extent of surgery, with some groups advocating total gastrectomy in all "curative cases, and also the extent of lymph node resection.
- Gastroenterostomy (loop of jejunum anastomosed to stomach) may be performed without partial gastrectomy. Indications include malignant duodenal invasion/stenosis (e.g., due to <u>pancreatic cancer</u>). Long afferent limb makes endoscopic access to duodenal papilla at ERCP difficult, occasionally impossible, and may predispose to a range of complications (see <u>afferent loop syndrome</u>).

Complications of gastrectomy. Peptic ulcer surgery has mortality of 0.3–1%, higher if emergency surgery is required. Morbidity includes postoperative hemorrhage, leakage from anastomoses with abscess formation, <u>postgastrectomy syndrome</u>, <u>biliary reflux</u>, and <u>afferent loop syndrome</u> (e.g., following Billroth II gastrectomy).

Gastric antral vascular ectasia (GAVE)

Vascular lesion of gastric antrum, characterized by tortuous dilated blood vessels radiating proximally from pylorus GAVE (also called "watermelon stomach").

Most commonly seen in middle-aged–elderly women, with autoimmune disease (e.g., Sjögren's syndrome, <u>atrophic gastritis</u>). Association with <u>portal hypertension</u> in 30% of patients. Focal capillary thrombosis, with dilated submucosal venous channels, and fibromuscular hyperplasia of the muscularis mucosa found histologically, but diagnosis made on endoscopic appearance. May cause <u>acute upper GI bleeding</u> or chronic iron deficiency anemia. Iron therapy and transfusions may be required. Endoscopic therapy with laser photocoagulation, <u>argon plasma coagulation</u>, and heater-probe therapy increasingly used. GAVE is not a recommended indication for <u>TIPSS</u>.

Gastric cancer

Definition and epidemiology

Adenocarcinoma accounts for >90% of gastric neoplasms (others include gastric lymphoma, gastrointestinal stromal tumor (GIST), carcinoid). Two broad types of gastric adenocarcinoma: **diffuse form** has the same frequency worldwide, is more common in women, occurs at younger age, and carries a particularly poor prognosis. More common **intestinal form** closely linked to environmental factors. Early gastric cancers (EGC) mainly reported in Japan (accounting there for approximately 35% of cases), and are defined as tumor not extending beyond mucosa. Despite fall in incidence over the last 30 years (particularly in the West), gastric adenocarcinoma remains the second most common cancer worldwide. Large geographical variation, with highest incidence in Far East. Majority of patients > 60 years.

Etiology and pathogensis

- Combination of genetic and environmental factors important. 10% of cases of gastric cancers exhibit familial clustering. Mutations of p53 tumor suppression gene and APC gene appear to be important in tumor development.
- **Risk factors** include: _Helicobacter pylori_ (probably predisposes to cancer by inducing atrophic gastritis, and classified by World Health Organization as class 1 carcinogen); smoking; high intake of salted and/or preserved foods; familial adenomatous polyposis (x10 risk of gastric cancer, related in part to gastric adenomas (found in >30% of cases); hereditary non-polyposis colorectal cancer (11% chance of gastric cancer); Ménetriér's disease; pernicious anemia/atrophic gastritis/postpartial gastrectomy; high grade dysplasia on biopsy. Gastric adenocarcinoma develops in < 1% of gastric polyps, usually in those > 1.5 cm.
- Distribution of cancer within stomach: 40% in antrum, 35% in body, 15% in fundus/cardia, and 10% diffuse (i.e., linitus plastica). Decline in gastric cancer particularly relates to distal tumors, but proximal lesions may be increasing (see also esophageal tumors). Metastases commonly to liver (40%), lung, bone marrow, peritoneum.

Clinical features

Gastric cancer usually presents late, with epigastric discomfort, weight loss, anorexia, nausea, upper GI bleeding, or symptoms of anemia. Symptoms may be indistinguishable from those of peptic ulceration. Vomiting may relate to pyloric obstruction, and tumor bulk may give early satiety. On examination palpable epigastric mass may be found.

Investigation

- Blood results nonspecific (no reliable tumor markers), but iron deficiency anemia may be present.
- Upper GI endoscopy is the most frequently used diagnostic tool. Tumor may have appearance of benign gastric ulcer (repeat endoscopy and biopsies until resolution of even "benign-looking" gastric ulcers is essential), polypoid mass, or diffuse gastric wall involvement (linitis plastica).

- Endoscopic ultrasound (EUS) allows depth of invasion to be determined with 80% accuracy (gastric cancers usually staged according to TNM classification (see tumor staging)). EUS > 90% accurate at distinguishing between stage T1 and T2, so is best modality at determining early from advanced cancer.
- Barium studies are widely used in Japan for detecting EGC.
- CT scanning. Main role in detecting distant metastases and as complement to EUS for determining depth of invasion.
- PET scanning may have an increasing role in detecting lymph node metastases.

Management and prognosis
- Surgery provides only hope of cure for locally advanced gastric cancer. The optimal surgical approach (e.g., total gastrectomy/subtotal gastrectomy/gastrectomy + splenectomy/extent of lymph node resection) is debated.
- Endoscopic mucosal resection (EMR) of early cancers confined to the mucosa (particularly common in Japan). EMR should be limited to those with solitary small tumors (< 2 cm), with no evidence of extension beyond mucosa on imaging, including EUS.
- Gastric adenocarcinoma is poorly responsive to chemotherapy or radiotherapy, but chemoradiotherapy as adjuvant to surgery has recently been shown to provide survival benefit. A range of chemotherapy regimens has been used (e.g., 5-fluorouracil and leucovorin).
- EGC have a 90% five-year survival, but overall, five-year survival in the United States is approximately 20%.

Gastric emptying

A major function of the stomach is to act as a food reservoir and to control food delivery to the intestine. A delay in emptying produces postprandial fullness, bloating, nausea, and vomiting: causes are outlined in Box 3.2.2.

Diagnosis. Mechanical obstruction is best excluded with endoscopy or barium studies. Noninvasive scintigraphic techniques are the principal clinical tools for assessing gastric motor function: different isotopes can be used to study emptying of solids and liquids. Some reports of abnormal electrical rhythms studied with electrogastrography (EGG) and found to be associated with abnormal gastric emptying and its symptoms have recently appeared: clinical application requires further clarification.

Vagotomy impairs receptive relaxation of the stomach and the resulting rapid emptying of hyperosmolar liquids contributes to early dumping. Later phases of solid emptying are impaired.
Diabetic gastroparesis (see Diabetes and the GI tract) can cause disabling and difficult to treat symptoms.

Gastric emptying and functional dyspepsia. Many studies report disturbed motility in a substantial proportion of patients (ca. 40%) with functional dyspepsia. The relation to symptoms and also therapeutic response to prokinetics is imperfect. There is some evidence that viral infection with CMV and HSV results in impaired emptying.[1]

Therapy

Gastric dysmotility can be difficult to treat. Available classes of <u>PROKINETIC DRUGS</u> include <u>DOPAMINE RECEPTOR ANTAGONISTS (METACLOPRAMIDE</u>, domperidone) and <u>MACROLIDES</u> (erythromycin). Cholinergic agonists or <u>ANTICHOLINESTERASES</u> are not widely used, and cisapride, an effective prokinetic belonging to the group of substitute benzamides, has been withdrawn because of concerns about it causing cardiac arrhythmias.

Box 3.2.2 Causes of delayed gastric emptying

Mechanical obstruction
- <u>Pyloric stenosis</u>
  - Adult hypertrophic pyloric stenosis
  - Chronic benign <u>peptic ulceration</u>
  - <u>Gastric cancer</u>
  - <u>Bezoars</u>
- Duodenal tumor
- Pancreatic disease (e.g., <u>pancreatic cancer</u>, <u>chronic pancreatitis</u>)

Impaired motility
- Autonomic neuropathy
  - <u>Diabetes</u>
  - Shy–Drager syndrome
- Infiltrative
  - <u>Amyloidosis</u>
- Collagen vascular disease:
  - <u>Scleroderma</u>
- Postsurgical
  - Vagotomy
  - <u>Roux-en-Y anastomosis</u>
- Drugs
  - Anticholinergics
  - Opiates
  - Tricyclic antidepressants
- Other
  - Postviral (e.g., CMV)
  - Trauma (e.g., head injury)
  - <u>Dermatomyositis</u>
  - <u>Pregnancy</u>
  - Myotonic muscular dystrophy
  - <u>Parkinson's disease</u>
  - Hypothyroidism
  - <u>Anorexia nervosa</u>

---

1 Bityutskiy, LP et al. (1997) *Am. J. Gastroenterol.* **92**: 1501–1504.

Gastric polyps

Uncommon (found in 1% autopsies). Usually asymptomatic and benign. Some authorities recommend biopsy of polyps over 5 mm to exclude neoplasia. Polyps can be snared using electrocautery: bleeding can occur as a complication in about 5%.

Histology. Most common type is the hyperplastic polyp (75% of all polyps). Multiple fundic gland polyps can occur (in the fundus) and are not significant. Adenomas account for 10–20% of gastric polyps, may progress to adenocarcinoma, and may occur in pernicious anemia. The risk of cancer relates to size of polyp and is low in polyps less than 2 cm diameter. Patients with adenomatous polyps require follow-up because of the risk of malignancy.

Gastric ulcers

Pathogenesis, epidemiology, treatment, and complications are discussed in section on peptic ulceration.

Management recommendations. Take six biopsies from the edge of the ulcer and a biopsy remote from the ulcer to look for *Heliobacter pylori* (HP). Eradicate HP if present. Continue antisecretory therapy for a total of eight weeks. Healing rates are higher with a PROTON PUMP INHIBITOR than a H2 RECEPTOR ANTAGONIST. Follow-up endoscopy is widely practiced but current recommendations suggest that this is not necessary if ulcer is clearly benign on histology. Gastric brushings add expense and also provide a small increase in diagnostic accuracy. Follow-up endoscopy is suggested for complicated ulcers (i.e., those that have bled or perforated).

Gastrinoma (Zollinger-Ellison syndrome)

Background

- One of the commonest types of neuroendocrine tumor. Incidence approximately 1/million; > 90% of gastrinomas occur in pancreas or duodenum (equal distribution). Unlike other pancreatic endocrine tumors, majority of gastrinomas are malignant. At presentation, pancreatic gastrinomas are more likely to be > 2 cm and to have metastasized than a duodenal lesion. Multiple endocrine neoplasia (MEN) in 30%.
- Zollinger–Ellison syndrome (ZES) refers to triad of severe peptic ulcer disease (PUD), gastric acid hypersecretion, and gastrinoma.

Clinical features

- Upper abdominal/epigastric pain in 75%, related to peptic ulceration. ZES accounts for 0.1% of cases of peptic ulceration.

- Chronic diarrhea (± steatorrhea) in >70%.
- Large pancreatic primary/liver metastases may present with abdominal pain/palpable mass.

Investigation

- Consider diagnosis in "unusual" PUD (e.g., recurrent multiple ulcers, _Helicobacter pylori_, and NSAID-negative PUD, jejunal ulcers).
- Endoscopy may show single/multiple duodenal ulcers, and prominent gastric folds (may mimic <u>Ménétrier's disease</u>).
- Fasting serum gastrin level >1,000 pg/ml highly specific for ZES (in absence of achlorydia and chronic atrophic <u>gastritis</u>). Gastrin 115–1,000 pg/ml due to range of causes, including gastrinoma (see Table 3.2.1 and <u>Gut hormone profile</u>).
- Secretin provocation test performed if equivocal fasting gastrin (>200 pg/ml increase in serum gastrin after secretin injection is diagnostic).
- Gastric pH less than 2.0, with large gastric fluid volume (>140 ml over 1 h) confirms hypersecretion (but rarely performed in practice).
- Serum hypercalcemia suggests possibility of MEN-1.
- To localize primary and metastases, scintigraphy (e.g., Octreoscan) sensitive (most gastrinomatos are somatostatin receptor positive). CT scan useful for identifying gastrinomas >1 cm. <u>Endoscopic ultrasound</u> increasingly used for small lesions.

Management

- Management in specialist units advised. Aim to control acid secretion and resect primary tumor.
- High dose <u>PROTON PUMP INHIBITORS</u> (e.g., Omeprazole 40–80 mg/day, pantoprazole 80–160 mg/day) effectively control hyperacidity in most patients.
- If localized pancreatic head/duodenal gastrinoma, curative surgical resection possible in majority of cases.
- Management of metastatic disease (often to liver) similar to that of other <u>neuroendocrine tumors</u>. Following resection of liver metastases five-year survival of 85% reported, but cure in < 30%.

Table 3.2.1 Cause of serum gastrin 115–1,000 pg/ml

Gastrinoma	Vagotomy
Proton pump inhibitors (stop for >1 week prior to test)	Small bowel resection
Atrophic gastritis	Renal failure (impaired gastrin excretion)
Primary hyperparathyroidism (?linked to MEN-1)	Hyperlipidaemia (may interfere with gastrinassay)
<u>Gastric cancer</u>	<u>Pyloric stenosis</u>

Gastritis

Histological inflammation of the stomach correlates poorly with endoscopic appearances and clinical symptoms. Some erosive and hyperplastic disorders may not be associated with much inflammation. Diagnosis requires endoscopic biopsy: indications and biopsy protocol are shown in Box 3.2.3.

Classification. There is no universally accepted system: The Sydney system is the best but is apparently too complicated for widespread use. A general classification is shown in Box 3.2.4.

Viruses

Cytomegalovirus (CMV) may affect esophagus and stomach. Biopsy specimens reveal enlarged cells with CMV "owl eye" inclusion bodies. Herpes virus can (rarely) produce multiple small raised ulcers. Biopsies show intranuclear inclusion bodies surrounded by haloes.

Bacteria

- Acute necrotizing gastritis is rare and dangerous. There is an association with alcohol binges, respiratory infections, AIDS, and infected peritoneal shunts. The mucosa appears thickened with a greenish black exudate. Treatment involves extensive resection and penicillin.

Box 3.2.3 When and how to take gastric biopsies

Indications for biopsy
Gastric erosion or ulcer, thickened folds, gastric polyps or masses, possible *Helicobacter*, possible diffuse of chronic gastritis.

Biopsy protocol
Take five biopsies: Antrum (greater and lesser curve) incisura, and gastric body (greater and lesser curve).

Box 3.2.4 Classification of gastritis

Inflammation associated
- Atrophic gastritis
- Infectious: viral, bacterial, *H. pylori*, fungal, parasitic
- Granulomatous: Crohn's sarcoid, TB, foreign bodies
- Distinctive: eosinophilic, lymphocytic
- Graft versus host.

Minimal inflammation
- Aspirin/NSAIDs
- Alcohol, cocaine
- Radiation
- Bile reflux
- Ischemia
- Hiatus hernia
- Hyperplastic: Ménétrier's disease, Zollinger–Ellison syndrome.

- Very rarely the stomach may be infected with TB (usually associated with pulmonary TB), actinomyces, and syphilis.
- Reactive gastropathy (acute erosive gastritis).
- Inflammation is not a major feature. Causes are shown in the box.

Helicobacter pylori (HP)

- A slow-growing microaerophilic Gram-negative spiral rod that is causally linked with gastritis, peptic ulceration, gastric cancer (adenocarcinoma), and gastric lymphoma.
- Usually acquired in childhood, prevalence varies with age, country, and social class. Transmission is usually person to person.
- Acute infection can occur, causing a neutrophilic gastritis that can lead to epigastric discomfort with nausea and vomiting.
- Infection in adults is usually chronic, producing nonatrophic superficial gastritis. The physiological effect of this process on acid and gastrin secretion depends in part on the area of stomach affected: gastritis in the body of the stomach tends to reduce acid output (although there is rebound hypergastrinemia), while antral predominant gastritis is associated with increased acid output and also with duodenal ulcertion.
- Progression to atrophic gastritis may occur and may explain in part the association with gastric cancer.

Diagnosis

Tests not requiring mucosal biopsy

- These include serology, urea breath tests, and stool antigen tests. Tests on saliva, buccal scrapes, or urine are at present unreliable. Serum tests are useful to confirm infection but unreliable in confirming eradication, as antibody titres do not always fall.
- Urea breath tests use urea labeled with ^{13}C or ^{14}C. The more commonly used ^{13}C method requires a mass spectrometer for analysis involving a delay of, at best, several days. The test requires the patient to be off PPI therapy for 14 days, H2 antagonists for 3 days, and at least 14 days after eradication therapy. Accurate method of demonstrating ongoing HP infection.
- Stool antigen testing appears to show comparable sensitivity and specificity for diagnosis to urea breath testing, but the test may need to be delayed for three months after therapy to confirm eradication.

Tests requiring mucosal biopsy

- Biopsy generally unnecessary unless culture and antibiotic sensitivity testing required. Routine H&E histology will show HP if large numbers are present; a special (e.g., silver) stain is more sensitive for smaller number of organisms (Color plate 5). In patient undergoing diagnostic upper GI endoscopy, mucosal biopsies may be tested for urease by agar gel slide tests such as CLO test.

Treatment
- Cure requires combinations of at least two antibiotics and non-antibiotics such as <u>PROTON PUMP INHIBITORS</u> (PPI). Pre-treatment sensitivity testing is not performed so the proportion of failed treatments due to resistant organisms is not known.
- Standard therapeutic strategies include triple therapy as first-line treatment, consisting of a PPI with two antibiotics for 7 days. Failure of eradication is dealt with by changing antibiotics, increasing the length of treatment to 10–14 days, or adding in a fourth agent, usually bismuth, either as subcitrate (De-Nol) or as subsalicylate (Pepto-Bismol).
- Choice of antibiotic regimen.

Table 3.2.2 Accuracy of diagnostic tests for Helicobacter pylori

| Parameter | Percentages | | | |
	Sensitivity	Specificity	PPV	NPV
Serum IgG	91	97	95	85
Urea breath test	90	96	98	84
CLO test	90	100	100	84

PPV= positive predictive value; NPV= negative predictive value.

Box 3.2.5 Recommended regimens to treat *Helicobacter pylori*

PPI triple therapy: PPI twice daily plus amoxycillin 1 g bd plus clarithromycin 500 mg bd **or** metronidazole 500 mg bd

Quadruple therapy: PPI twice daily plus bismuth 2 tabs bd plus metronidazole 500 mg bd plus tetracycline 250–500 qds

- *H. pylori* is sensitive to amoxicillin and resistance is rare, but concomitant antisecretory therapy is essential for activity.
- Tetracyclines are usually effective and resistance is low in Western countries. Contraindicated in children.
- <u>METRONIDAZOLE.</u> Usually effective against *H. pylori*, but the incidence of metronidazole resistance varies widely and is increased in urban areas.
- Clarithromycin. Incidence of resistance is approximately 15%.
- Other antibiotics. There is some empirical evidence on the efficacy of furazolidone but it is not considered a first-line antibiotic for eradication of *H. pylori*.

Follow-up after eradication

- Although routine follow-up testing is not performed, failed therapy in an ulcer patient is very often associated with recurrence of the ulcer. Certainly in patients with complicated peptic ulcer disease (i.e., bleeding or perforation) documentation of eradication is advised before maintenance antisecretory therapy is stopped.
- Confirmation of HP eradication usually performed with urea breath tests six weeks after completing course of eradication therapy.

Intrinsic factor (IF)

- A 50 kDa glycoprotein secreted by human parietal cells, IF is one of two proteins that bind cobalamin (vitamin B12)—the other is called R binder protein. Most B12 initially binds to R binder in the stomach; the complex is cleaved by pancreatic trypsin, and the freed B12 then binds to IF. The IF–B12 complex binds to a specific ileal receptor called cubilin that mediates endocytosis of the IF–B12 complex (autosomal recessive mutation in this receptor causes juvenile megaloblastic anemia, the Imerslund–Graesbeck syndrome). B12 is then transported to tissues bound to transcobalamin II.
- Diagnosis of vitamin B12 deficiency due to loss of functioning IF can be clarified by Schilling test (although no longer available in most locations).
- Secretion of IF is usually in physiological excess. Most patients with hypochlorhydria produce enough IF to prevent B12 deficiency; and H2 blockers and PPIs do not induce IF deficiency.
- Circulating antibodies to IF are found in pernicious anemia.

MALT lymphoma

See: lymphomas in GI tract.

Ménétrier's disease

- Characterized by giant hypertrophic gastric folds, mainly involving gastric fundus (enlarged gastric folds also seen in other conditions, e.g., gastrinoma (Zollinger–Ellison syndrome)). Associated hypochlorhydria, hypergastrinemia, excess mucus production, and hypoalbuminemia due to protein-losing gastropathy. Cause uncertain, but increased expression of the epidermal growth factor (EGF) reported. High prevalence of *H. pylori*.
- Symptoms include epigastric pain (may mimic peptic ulcer), nausea, peripheral edema, anorexia, and weight loss. Premalignant condition, with gastric cancer reported in 2–15%.

- Diagnosis often made on endoscopy, but full thickness biopsy (e.g., with <u>endoscopic ultrasound</u>) required to adequately assess histology.
- Histological changes of marked foveolar hyperplasia, glandular atrophy, and increased mucosal thickness. Little controlled data on treatment, but response to *H. pylori* eradication, acid suppression (<u>PROTON PUMP INHIBITORS</u>, <u>H2-ANTAGONISTS</u>), <u>CORTICOSTEROIDS</u>, <u>OCTREOTIDE</u>, and monoclonal antibodies against the EGF receptor reported. Partial/total <u>gastrectomy</u> reserved for refractory/recurrent bleeding, severe hypoproteinemia, or gastric cancer.

Nonsteroidal anti-inflammatory drugs (NSAIDs) and the GI tract

NSAIDs, even as low-dose aspirin for cardiovascular protection, cause bleeding and ulceration in the GI tract (2–4% users per year: relative risk compared to matched controls 4-fold higher for gastric ulcers and 2-fold for duodenal ulcers).

Site of damage: as well as gastric and duodenal injury, NSAIDs cause small bowel ulcers and are associated with web like small intestinal strictures. In the colon they can cause acute colitis and precipitate relapses of IBD. They may potentiate bleeding from diverticulosis or established vascular malformations.

Mechanism of injury

Topical damage is largely prevented by enteric-coated preparations. It is very common (erosions seen in 30–50% patients on NSAIDs and, although associated with increased blood loss, probably not associated with serious ulcers or perforations).

Systemic damage. Reduced mucosal prostaglandins caused by NSAIDs inhibiting COX-1 result in lowered mucosal defense and reduced mucosal blood flow (this is nitric oxide (NO) dependent and can be reduced by NO donors).

Risk factors for NSAID-associated complications are shown in Box 3.2.6. There is current uncertainty about the role of <u>Helicobacter</u> as a risk factor for NSAID-induced GI damage, but current consensus favors the two being independent risk factors.

Relative frequency of injury with different NSAIDs

Generally this correlates with COX-1 inhibitory efficiency. Ibuprofen and naproxen have the lowest relative risk, and indomethacin and piroxicam have the highest.

Clinical studies with COXIBs

Celecoxib was released in 1999. Rofecoxib was released in the same year but withdrawn in September 2004 because of increased risk of cardiovascular toxicity. Celecoxib produces comparable effects on pain and inflammation to diclofenac in rheumatoid arthritis, with less GI ulceration and withdrawal due to GI side-effects and less admission to hospital in elderly patients due to GI complications. The incidence of endoscopically assessed GI ulceration is comparable to that with placebo. However, COX-2 inhibitors are not cardioprotective and the reduction in GI side-effects is not seen in patients co-prescribed aspirin at cardioprotective doses.

Box 3.2.6 Risk factors for NSAID-induced peptic ulceration **and complications**

- Age over 60
- Previous ulcer disease
- Concomitant corticosteroids
- High dose NSAIDs
- Chronic major organ impairment
- Concomitant anticoagulant use

Box 3.2.7 Methods of limiting GI toxicity of NSAIDs

- Enteric-coated preparations, antacid buffers, histamine receptor antagonists, PPIs, and natural prostanoids all attenuate mucosal injury caused by NSAIDs.
- Agents that include nitric oxide (NO) or induce release of NO exert a protective effect against mucosal injury by vasodilatation and reducing cell-endothelial adhesion. Such agents show reduced GI toxicity but good anti-inflammatory actions.
- Selective COX inhibition: cyclo-oxygenase 1 (COX-1) is involved in control of mucosal blood flow, platelet aggregation, renal tubular function, and regulation of gastric acid. COX-2 is inducible and is the main source of pro-inflammatory prostanoids. This has led to development of COX-2 selective inhibitors.

Nonulcer dyspepsia

See: Top 10 Clinical Problems: Dyspepsia and Gastro-esophageal Reflux.

Obesity surgery

Anti-obesity (bariatric) surgery is now an enormous growth industry in the United States. Of nine million morbidly obese adults, approximately 140,000 undergo weight-loss surgery each year, with the number increasing. According to NIH, patients should be: well-informed and motivated, have a BMI ≥40 kg/m2, have acceptable risk for surgery, and have failed previous nonsurgical weight loss. Adults with a BMI ≥35 kg/m2 who have serious co-morbidities (diabetes or sleep apnea), may also be candidates. Studies have demonstrated that bariatric surgery is effective in reducing obesity-related co-morbidities overall and cause-specific mortalilty. However, bariatric surgery is also associated with significant perioperative complications and mortality. Bariatric surgery needs to be performed in conjunction with an in-depth follow-up plan of nutritional, behavioral, and medical programs. The surgical approaches vary, with commonest operation involving division of the stomach at the fundus, with a loop of small bowel, following <u>Roux-en-Y anastomosis</u>, brought up to the small remnant of stomach (which accommodates <30 g of food). Complications include leaks, bleeding, gastric remnant distention, stomal stenosis, marginal ulcers, <u>gallstones (30%)</u>, and metabolic bone disease (30%), including <u>osteoporosis</u>. Gastric banding procedures are also widely used.

Peptic ulceration

Note. Pathophysiology and epidemiology, treatment, and complications are discussed here. For approach to investigation and specific management recommendations, see <u>gastric ulcers</u>, <u>duodenal ulcers</u>, and also <u>Dyspepsia and GERD</u>).

- Includes all acid-related ulceration: gastric ulcers, duodenal ulcers but also esophageal ulcers relating to gastro-esophageal reflux and ulcers in Meckel's diverticulum. Textbooks and pathologists differentiate **ulcers** and **erosions** according to whether they erode through muscularis mucosae but this is not useful to clinicians or endoscopists because ulcers are diagnosed by morphological or radiological features.
- Before 1980s peptic ulcer was considered a chronic relapsing disease. Since the 1980s most peptic ulcers were shown to be related either to infection with <u>Helicobacter pylori</u> or to nonsteroidal anti-inflammatory drugs (NSAIDs), with hypersecretory states such as <u>gastrinoma</u> (Zollinger–Ellison syndrome) accounting for some others.
- Physiological stress (burns, sepsis, multi-organ failure) can cause multiple superficial erosions. Ulcers arising in burns patients are called Curling's ulcers. Ulcers in head injury patients are called Cushing's ulcers. Unlike other stress–related peptic injuries, Cushing's ulcers are associated with hypergastrinemia.
- Pathogenesis appears related to impaired mucosal resistance due to reduced mucosal blood flow. Stress ulcer prophylaxis should is indicated in patients with mechanical ventilation > 48 hours, coagulopathy, recent history of GI ulceration/ bleeding, and can be considered in multi-organ failure or if there is a history of peptic ulceration, cirrhosis, or renal failure. PPIs, H2RA, and sulcrafate can be utilized.

Pathophysiology

Disordered epithelial defenses. These include factors protecting the epithelial cells against acid, such as mucus and bicarbonate in the unstirred water layer covering cells as well as tight junctions between epithelial cells and also effective mucosal blood flow.

Abnormal acid and motility. Patients with duodenal ulcers are hypersecretors; some of this may relate to increased gastrin stimulated by HP or by an HP-mediated fall in somatostatin secretion. There may be high levels of pepsinogen (again related to HP) and possibly abnormal vagal control or disordered motility with a resulting increased delivery of acid to the duodenum.

<u>*Gastric ulcers*</u> in the body or fundus are associated with gastric atrophy, chronic <u>gastritis</u>, and low acid, whereas antral gastric ulcers and gastric ulcers associated with concomitant duodenal ulcers are associated with high acid output.

Box 3.2.8 Risk factors for peptic ulceration

- **True**: <u>*Helicobacter pylori*</u>; NSAIDs; <u>gastrinoma</u>; cigarette smoking; associated diseases such as COPD and cirrhosis; probably some genetic factors (e.g., Lewis blood group antigens mediate HP attaching to musosa).
- **False**: alcohol in absence of cirrhosis, dietary factors.
- **Uncertain**: emotional stress.

<u>*Helicobacter pylori (HP).*</u> There is a strong association with both <u>duodenal ulcer</u> (DU) and <u>gastric ulcer</u> (GU), but, although experimental data suggests, HP infection produces a gastritis that, if untreated, can progress to gastric atrophy and cancer, still only 20% of infected people get peptic ulcers, so poorly understood host factors and virulence factors must be important. The paradox about HP is why infection in some produces high acid and duodenal ulceration, whereas in others it leads to chronic gastritis, gastric atrophy, and <u>gastric cancer</u>. Although this may relate to different patterns of infection (antral or body), more investigation is needed for proof of this hypothesis.

Nonsteroidal anti-inflammatory drugs (NSAIDS). These damage the GI mucosa by direct and systemic effects. Direct damage occurs within minutes of ingestion and can be reduced by enteric coating or rectal administration. Systemic affects are mediated by reduced mucosal prostaglandin synthesis with consequent effects on secretion of mucus and mucosal blood flow. Ulcers can be shown on endoscopy in 15–30% patients on chronic NSAID therapy. The risk is multiplied with concomitant corticosteroid ingestion. Risk is also increased by previous peptic ulceration, old age, and co-morbidity. There is some evidence that risk of ulceration is also increased by concomitant HP infection.

Other drugs. Peptic ulcers are associated with some chemotherapeutic drugs (intra-arterial 5FU), potassium chloride tablets, crack cocaine, and bisphosphanates, especially alendronate.

Hypersecretory conditions. Suspect in the absence of HP or NSAID use, especially if there is diarrhea, complications (perforation or hemorrhage), or if ulceration extends beyond the duodenal bulb. Relevant conditions include:

- Gastrinoma.
- Systemic mastocytosis and myeloproliferative disorders with increased basophils: both of these produce increased amounts of histamine, which can cause acid hypersecretion—DU is found in 40%.
- Antral G cell hyperplasia—although this is usually a consequence of HP infection.

Epidemiology

Rare before the nineteenth century, it became more common in the early twenieth century, but incidence been declining since the 1960s. Hospitalization rates have not changed, probably because older people consume more NSAIDs. For risk factors, see Box 3.2.8.

Clinical features. See Box 3.2.9.

Investigations

See Dyspepsia and GERD. Remember that endoscopic examination alone is a poor predictor of malignancy and gastric ulcers should always be biopsied (take at least six biopsies). Duodenal ulcers are very rarely malignant. Follow-up endoscopy to confirm ulcer healing is traditional but the tradition dates from the radiological era when diagnosis of malignancy was inaccurate. Repeat endoscopy may not be necessary if the pretest probability of cancer was low, the ulcer endoscopically appeared benign, and pathology was benign on extensive biopsy sampling. If there is any question, follow-up endoscopy and biopsy is recommended at eight weeks.

Box 3.2.9 Clinical features of peptic ulcers

Do not attempt to diagnose peptic ulceration by the history alone despite the classic descriptions of abdominal pain in peptic ulcers:

- **Gastric ulcer.** Pain soon after meals, often not relieved by eating, associated with anorexia and weight loss in 50%.
- **Duodenal ulcer.** Pain 2–3 h after meals, often wakes patient in middle of night, relieved by eating so most patients maintain or increase weight.
- The pain of peptic ulceration can be mimicked by cancer, pancreatitis, cholecystitis, reflux, and mesenteric angina.

Treatments

Test for HP; eradicate if present. Ask about NSAID ingestion.

Histamine receptor antagonists. Used by themselves, healing rate for DU is 70–80% and for GU is 55–65%. They are especially useful at decreasing basal acid output at night, although tolerance can develop rapidly. See H2 RECEPTOR ANTAGONISTS.

PPIs are the most effective inhibitors of gastric acid, but their efficacy is markedly limited in the fasting state when only 5% of the stomach's proton pumps are active. Even patients taking twice daily PPI often experience nocturnal acid breakthrough, which can be helped by nocturnal H2RA. Once daily PPI gives DU healing rate of 80–100%, and GU healing rate of 70–85%. Elevation of gastric pH impairs absorption of ketoconazole and facilitates absorption of digoxin. PPIs can affect levels of other drugs metabolized by cytochrome P450 (warfarin, diazepam, and phenytoin). For discussion of possible adverse effect of PPIs, see PROTON PUMP INHIBITORS.

Antacids. Although antacids can heal ulcers in high doses, they are poorly tolerated and often cause unacceptable GI side effects. See ANTACIDS.

Other drugs. SUCRALFATE and BISMUTH preparations both can heal ulcers but are infrequently used. The prostaglandin analogue MISOPROSTIL has similar efficacy to omeprazole for healing NSAID-induced ulcers.

Surgery (see gastrectomy). The need for surgery to treat uncomplicated peptic ulcers has almost disappeared because of effective drug treatment. Current indications for surgery include bleeding from ulcers not responding to endoscopic therapy, perforated ulcers, and gastric outlet obstruction that cannot be relieved by endoscopic dilatation. Operations for duodenal ulceration include patching a perforation with a tongue of omentum or removing the acid-producing tissue either with antrectomy or by vagotomy (usually highly selective vagotomy). Simple division of the vagus results in pyloric spasm so vagotomy needs to be combined with a drainage procedure such as pyloroplasty or gastro-jejunostomy. Operations for benign gastric ulcers depend partially on the site of the ulcer: an ulcer near the esophageal junction refractory to medical treatment may need a subtotal gastrectomy and Roux-en-Y anastomosis.

Refractory peptic ulcers. See Box 3.2.10.

Complications

Hemorrhage. Use of aggressive antisecretory therapy is reasonable. There is no benefit in using H2RAs in controlling bleeding or preventing rebleeding. An important study from Hong Kong (Lau, J W *et al.* (2000). *N. Engl. J. Med.* **343**: 310) showed that, in patients who had received endoscopic treatment to control acute hemorrhage, a bolus of 80 mg IV omeprazole followed by 8 mg/h infusion for 72 h reduced rebleeding rates and shortened hospital stay. Also see: Acute upper GI bleeding.

> **Box 3.2.10 What to do if a peptic ulcer is not healed by 8 weeks of a PPI (12 weeks for ulcers over 2 cm)**
>
> - Check compliance with drug treatment
> - Is there HP infection?
> - Is there ongoing and possibly surreptitious NSAID use?
> - Smoking? Cigarette smoking delays healing.
> - Is there evidence for a hypersecretory condition?
> - Is the ulcer peptic? Consider <u>gastric cancer</u> (very rarely duodenal cancer), infection, cocaine use, and <u>Crohn's disease.</u>

Perforation. Can be life-threatening. Strong association with NSAIDs, smoking (especially in younger patients), crack cocaine. Diagnose by erect chest X-ray and possibly CT scanning. Avoid endoscopy, which will exacerbate any leak. Sometimes careful radiological exam with water soluble contrast will reveal site of perforation. Usual treatment is broad spectrum antibiotics, surgery to close perforation, and irrigation of peritoneum. Nonoperative therapy (NPO, nasogasric suction, antibiotics, and antisecretory drugs) rarely appropriate; consider in highly selected patients where patient is well and perforation has sealed. **Watch these patients very carefully**—operation is indicated at first sign of clinical deterioration.

Penetration. Posterior DUs can invade the pancreas and GUs can penetrate the left lobe of liver. Choledochoduodenal fistulae and gastrocolic fistulae can occur.

Obstruction. Pain, bloating, early satiety, vomiting after a meal are suggestive. Weight loss can be dramatic. Examine for a succussion splash. A gastric aspirate of over 200 ml after overnight fasting is evidence of delayed gastric emptying. Management is medical and endoscopic using dilatation in 70% of cases, with only 30% needing surgical bypass of the gastric outlet obstruction.

Pernicious anemia (PA)

Called pernicious because it was fatal before treatment became available. Classic pernicious anemia is caused by failure of gastric parietal cells to produce sufficient intrinsic factor (IF) to permit absorption of adequate amount of dietary vitamin B12 (cobalamin); this produces a megaloblastic anemia. For other disorders that can cause cobalamin deficiency, see <u>vitamin B12</u>.

Etiology

In adults, PA is probably an autoimmune disorder (familial association, association with other autoimmune diseases and HLA A2, A3, B8, DR3, blood group A). Antiparietal cell antibodies occur in 90% of patients (5% of healthy controls); also both binding and blocking antibodies to IF are found. In adults, PA is associated with atrophic gastritis and <u>achlorhydria</u>. In children the etiology is different: there is usually a hereditary problem of cobalamin metabolism or of intrinsic factor production. Coexistent iron deficiency is common.

Epidemiology

Most cases occur after age 40, although there is a recognized incidence in children (juvenile pernicious anemia): women outnumber men approx 2:1; prevalence is about 1 per 1,000. 20–30% cases have a positive family history. There is an association with other autoimmune disorders—type 1 diabetes, Addison's, thyroid disease.

Diagnosis

Macrocytic anemia, low B12, antibodies to IF, abnormal Schilling test (not currently available in most areas). Elevated bilirubin due to hemolysis occasionally reported.

Therapy centers on B12 replacement.

- The standard regimen is to give cobalamin IM 1 mg daily for 1 week, weekly for 1 month, and then monthly thereafter. There is some evidence that giving larger doses orally (1–2 mg daily) may be effective.
- After initial parenteral replacement, most people can be maintained on oral supplementation of 250–1,000 µg of B12 daily.

Complications

There is a two- to three fold increased risk of gastric adenocarcinoma. Screening is currently not recommended because of a high cost–benefit ratio. The hypergastrinemia resulting from achlorhydria causes enterochromaffin cell hyperplasia—there is an increased incidence of <u>carcinoid</u> tumors, which respond to antrectomy and are of relatively low grade malignancy.

Postgastrectomy syndromes

Division of the vagal nerve, bypass or destruction of the pylorus, and resection of the stomach result in permanent anatomical and physiological changes resulting in:
- Reduced reservoir function.
- Altered gastric adaptation.
- Altered gastric emptying.
- Duodenal reflux into the stomach.
- Altered absorptive capacity.

Early complications of gastrectomy include:
- Delayed gastric emptying following widespread denervation of the stomach.
- Pain and distension 30–60 min after meals resulting from rapid emptying of the stomach and jejunal distension: this usually settles as the patient learns new eating habits.
- Most changes are long lasting or **late complications.**

Late complications

- **Chronic gastroparesis** can occur following truncal vagotomy, and can be difficult to treat. Metoclopramide and erythromycin may help, but sometimes further surgery with a <u>Roux-en-Y anastomosis</u> is needed to return the patient to oral feeding.
- **Anastomotic ulcers** can occur due to decreased resistance to acid digestion of the jejunum, gastric stasis, and partial obstruction of the anastomosis due to scarring or edema. Biopsy of the ulcer to exclude malignancy may be needed and revisional surgery is often needed.
- <u>Afferent loop syndrome</u> is described elsewhere.
- **Reflux of duodenal contents** (bile and pancreatic secretions) into the gastric remnant can cause pain and vomiting. Endoscopic biopsy may show features of a chemical gastritis. Treatment is operative, requiring conversion to a <u>Billroth I</u> or a <u>Roux-en-Y</u> configuration.
- **Gastric cancer**. There is a twofold risk of gastric cancer 15 years after gastrectomy, probably due to reflux-stimulated increases in cell proliferation.

Rapid emptying

Postvagotomy diarrhea is poorly understood, but patients usually have rapid gastric emptying. Occurs in 30% of patients. Codeine and loperamide can help, as can <u>OCTREOTIDE</u>.

Dumping is discussed elsewhere.

Metabolic complications

- **Iron deficiency** anemia is common. Apart from recurrent ulceration, reduced gastric acid impairs absorption of ferric iron.
- **Intrinsic factor** is absent in patients with total gastrectomy, which can lead to B12 deficiency.
- **Steatorrhea** can result from poor mixing of food with pancreatic enzymes or afferent loop syndrome.
- **Calcium deficiency** with <u>osteoporosis</u> and <u>metabolic bone disease</u> can result from steatorrhea or impaired absorption at less acidic pH.

Proton pump inhibitors

See: <u>PROTON PUMP INHIBITORS</u>.

Pyloric stenosis

Usually associated in adults with <u>peptic ulcer</u> disease or <u>gastric cancer</u>: hypertrophic pyloric stenosis is rare.

Symptoms are nausea, vomiting, early satiety, and epigastric pain after eating. Unlike in infants, physical exam is often not helpful because in adults the pyloric mass is difficult to palpate. A succussion splash may sometimes be elicited. Identical symptoms and signs may be found in gastric outlet obstruction due to duodenal structuring in <u>pancreatic cancer</u>.

Diagnosis can be via barium radiology, although imaging with ultrasound or CT is more effective at revealing any extraluminal pathology that may be contributing to luminal stenosis. Endoscopy is needed to diagnose peptic ulceration or tumor and to make a histological diagnosis.

Treatment. If malignancy has been excluded, <u>endoscopic dilatation</u> with a balloon can be effective, although there is a postprocedure recurrence rate of about 80%. Surgical pyloromyotomy or resection of the involved region can offer a long-term cure. Gastric bypass may be necessary.

Superior mesenteric artery syndrome

The superior mesenteric artery comes off the aorta at a right angle and crosses over the duodenum just to the right of the midline. Rarely, the artery may obstruct the duodenum as it crosses over: an acute angle between the SMA and aorta might be relevant, and it only seems to happen in very thin patients.

Symptoms include epigastric fullness and bloating after meals and bilious vomiting. Barium or CT may reveal a dilated stomach and duodenum with a sharp cutoff to the right of the midline (don't forget other causes of duodenal dilatation: scleroderma, diabetes, distal duodenal stricture).

Treatment is by decompression, possibly surgical—most commonly duodeno-jejunostomy.

Zollinger–Ellison syndrome

See: <u>gastrinoma</u>.

Small intestine

Afferent loop syndrome

- One of a number of <u>postgastrectomy syndromes</u>, usually associated with <u>Billroth II</u> (polya) <u>gastrectomy</u>. The afferent loop (the segment of small intestine leading to the stomach) can fill with bile, particularly when the gallbladder contracts after a meal. This causes upper abdominal pain after meals, often relieved by vomiting bilious fluid. Obstruction may be caused by stenosis of the anastomosis, adhesions, twisting of the intestinal loop, and rarely by tumor, stones, or enteroliths.
- Diagnosis made by showing dilatation of the afferent loop and the site of obstruction. This is possible with barium studies, scintigraphy (HIDA scanning), CT, or MRI.
- The term is sometimes confused with small-bowel <u>bacterial overgrowth</u> (incidence 50% in Billroth II gastrectomy) producing classical symptoms of weight loss, diarrhea, steatorrhea, and deficiency of B12 and fat-soluble vitamins.

Ampullary cancer

- Rare cancer (< 0.5% of GI cancers) that may present with painless obstructive jaundice. May develop in villous adenoma, in association with <u>familial adenomatous polyposis</u> (FAP), or occur spontaneously.
- Abnormal, ulcerated ampulla at ERCP. Dilated pancreatic and common bile ducts ('<u>double duct sign</u>') may mimic <u>pancreatic cancer</u>. <u>CT scan</u> ± <u>endoscopic ultrasound</u> to define local invasion.
- Approximately 50% of ampullary cancers are resectable, with > 80% five-year survival following <u>Whipple's resection</u> in those without local invasion (i.e., much better than for <u>pancreatic cancer</u>). Nonoperative cases treated with endoscopic biliary stenting. Palliative chemotherapy has poor efficacy.

Angiodysplasia (see Color Plate 3)

Gastrointestinal mucosal vascular ectasia not associated with cutaneous lesions, systemic vascular disease, or a familial syndrome (see also <u>gastric antral vascular ectasia</u> and <u>hereditary haemorrhagic telangiectasia</u>).

Most commonly found in patients > 60 years, and in 1–2% undergoing upper GI endoscopy for any indication, 4% if being endoscoped for bleeding (and more if being investigated for anemia), and 3–6% in those undergoing colonoscopy.

Etiology may be degenerative, relating to chronic low-grade obstruction of mucosal veins, or alternatively result from mucosal ischemia. Much quoted (and debated) association of angiodysplasia with aortic valve disease may be linked to an acquired form of von Willebrand disease.

Clinical features. Always through bleeding, which can range from hematemesis to PR bleeding to occult anemia. In majority bleeding not life-threatening, but 15% patients with colonic angiodysplasia have acute massive hemorrhage.

Investigation. Diagnosis usually endoscopic (see Color Plate 3). Although lesions may be indistinguishable from those of <u>hereditary hemorrhagic telangiectasia</u> (Osler–Weber–Rendu syndrome), Turner's syndrome, and the CREST syndrome, the other extra-intestinal signs of these various disorders are not seen. Small intestinal angiodysplasia can be diagnosed by push enteroscopy or wireless capsule endoscopy (see <u>enteroscopy</u>). Colonic lesions can be diagnosed at colonoscopy or at angiography.

Specialized diagnostic tests include radionuclide scanning with labeled red cells, but the intermittent nature of bleeding from angiodysplasia limits utility of this test. Historically intraoperative enteroscopy has been helpful in the diagnosis of distal small bowel lesions, although this will be partially replaced by the advent of wireless capsule endoscopy.

Management most often with endoscopic obliteration procedures (see <u>endoscopic hemostasis</u>), although the rebleeding rate is substantial. In patients unfit for surgery, transcatheter <u>embolization</u> using coils or gelfoam has been successful in stopping acute bleeding. Surgery may be definitive treatment if the bleeding source has been clearly defined. Medical treatment with oestrogen-progestogen therapy (0.05 mg ethinyloestradiol and 1 mg norethisterone given daily) has been unsuccessful in clinical studies.

Aorto-enteric fistulae

Nearly always occur after reconstructive aorto-iliac surgery: frequency is about 1 in 200 patients at an average 3–5 years after operation. Usually affects third part of duodenum, so out of reach of standard upper GI endoscopy. Diagnosis requires enteroscopy or CT. **Always suspect the diagnosis if there is any hint of upper GI bleed** in a patient with appropriate surgical history: there is classically a self-limiting "herald bleed" which may be the only chance to save the patients life, since this is often followed by a second massive life-threatening bleed.

Pathogenesis is usually subtle infection with *Staph. aureus* or *E. coli*, so beware of low grade fever, unexplained fatigue, raised inflammatory markers, or leucocytosis in the right clinical setting.

Bacterial overgrowth

Refers to an increase in the normally low bacterial colonization of the GI tract upstream of the distal ileum. Produces symptoms of vitamin malabsorption, malnutrition, and weight loss. Role of overgrowth in patients with Irritable Bowel Syndrome controversial.

Etiology and pathophysiology

Contributing factors are shown opposite.

- Fat, protein, carbohydrate, and vitamin malabsorption result from poor enterocyte function and bacterial transformation of nutrients into nonabsorbable and toxic metabolites.
- Anerobes deconjugate bile acids, preventing bile acid function and enterohepatic circulation. Deconjugated bile acids induce watery diarrhea.
- Carbohydrate intolerance results from reduction of brush border disaccharidases: increased amounts of osmotically active carbohydrate fragments contribute to the diarrhea associated with bacterial overgrowth.
- Anaerobes compete with the host for vitamin B12, which results in B12 deficiency and macrocytic anemia.

Clinical features. Diarrhea, weight loss, possibly neurological features associated with vitamin B12 deficiency, abdominal pain, and symptoms of impaired absorption of fat-soluble vitamins A, D, E, K.

Investigation Microbiological culture is the most direct method (> 10⁵ colonies/ml after duodenal aspiration and culture). Breath tests are less invasive. The SeHCAT test is useful in testing for bile acid malabsorption. Also see Steatorrhoea.

Treatment

If surgical correction of the underlying abnormality leading to stasis is not possible, antibiotics and treatment of dysmotility are the mainstays of treatment. Antibiotic regimens are usually empirical and involve drugs with activity against aerobic and anaerobic bacteria. Tetracycline 250 mg qds is a traditional choice, with augmentin, trimethoprim sulphamethoxazole (Septrin), and ciprofloxacin as alternatives. Rifaximin has shown good results in patients with Irritable Bowel Syndrome. Often a single 7–10-day course can relieve symptoms for months, but sometimes continuous rotating antibiotics are necessary. So far, trials of probiotic therapy have given negative or inconclusive results.

Box 3.3.1 Causes of bacterial overgrowth

Reduced host defenses
- Hypogammaglobulinemia
- Immunodeficiency (e.g., HIV)
- Old age
- Chronic pancreatitis

Excess bacterial entry to small bowel
- Atrophic gastritis/gastric acid suppression (e.g., proton pump inhibitors)
- Gastrojejunostomy/Roux-en-Y anastomosis
- Gastrectomy
- Enteral fistulae

Delayed small-bowel clearance
- Small-bowel/jejunal diverticula (e.g., scleroderma)
- Strictures (e.g., Crohn's disease, postsurgical)
- Pseudo-obstruction
- Amyloidosis
- Autonomic neuropathy (e.g., diabetes, postvagotomy)

Bile acid malabsorption

Background
- Enterohepatic circulation of bile acids involves excretion from liver into bile of water-soluble conjugated bile acids (cholic and chenoxydeoxycholic acid). Deconjugation by intraluminal gut flora to insoluble dihydroxy bile acids (deoxycholic acid and lithocholic acid) allows 95% reabsorption of bile acids from terminal ileum and, via portal venous system, circulation back to liver. This process conserves bile acids, providing adequate intraluminal bile acids to allow micelle solubilization, and absorption of lipids and fat soluble vitamins (vitamins A, D, E, K).
- Bile acid malabsorption is usually secondary to other causes, including ileal resection/Crohn's disease, ileal radiation enteritis, cholecystectomy (postcholecystectomy diarrhea), chronic pancreatitis, celiac disease, cystic fibrosis. Rare primary disease due to congenital deficiency in sodium–bile acid co-transporter.

Clinical features
- Bloating, abdominal discomfort.
- Steatorrhea: due to fat malabsorption secondary to reduced bile acids in small bowel.
- Diarrhea. Increased concentrations of deconjugated bile acids in colon inhibit carbohydrate transporters, reduce intraluminal pH, and directly damage enterocyte.
- Gallstones: due to bile acid pool and production of lithogenic bile.
- Oxalate stones.

Investigation
- High level of clinical suspicion often raised by associated clinical problems (e.g., terminal ileal <u>Crohn's disease</u>).
- Range of tests available, many of which are cumbersome and impractical (e.g., 72-hour stool collection for bile acid absorption test).
- Other approaches include:
  - Trial of bile acid sequesters. Failure to improve diarrhea within three days of starting <u>CHOLESTYRAMINE</u> makes bile acid malabsorption an unlikely cause of diarrhea. However, cholestyramine may occasionally worsen symptoms if malabsorption severe.
  - Selenium-75 labeled homotaurocholic acid test (SeHCaT). Radioactive taurocholic acid given orally, and serial whole-body scintigraphy over four to seven days used to demonstrate abnormal absorption. Test is time consuming and difficult to standardize.

Management
- Treatment of underlying cause.
- Use of bile acid sequesters such as cholestyramine.
- Maintain adequate fluid intake to reduce risk of <u>oxalate stones</u>.
- Replacement of fat-soluble <u>vitamins A</u>, <u>D</u>, <u>E</u>, <u>K</u> may be necessary.

Blind loop

Surgical alterations of intestinal anatomy with creation of pouches or long segments of diverted intestine (entero-enteric anastomoses, Billroth II, jejuno-ileal bypass, Kock distal ileal pouch for continent ileostomy) interfere with peristalsis and can lead to <u>bacterial overgrowth</u>.

Brush border

The terminal products of luminal stomach digestion, as well as diasaccharides, such as sucrose and lactose, cannot be absorbed intact and must be hydrolyzed by brush-border membrane hydrolases, maximally expressed in the villi of duodenum and jejunum. Impaired activity of these enzymes may occur if the brush border is damaged (by, for example, infective gastroenteritis, chemotherapy, <u>celiac disease</u>, <u>HIV</u>)—although there are also rare congenital causes of carbohydrase deficiency. This results in non-absorbable carbohydrates passing into the colon where they are metabolized by bacterial flora, producing osmotically active short-chain fatty acids. This leads to gaseous distension and diarrhea if the colonic capacity to absorb short chain fatty acids is overwhelmed.

Celiac disease

A disease involving abnormal small-intestinal mucosa that reverts to normal when patients are treated with a gluten-free diet and that relapses when gluten is re-introduced.

Epidemiology and pathogenesis

- Prevalence through Caucasians is about 1:300, and is more common in Celtic populations. It also occurs in non-Caucasians but is very rare in Black populations. Females are slightly more commonly affected than men. Mortality is reduced by a therapeutic gluten-free diet, but remains higher than for a matched control population.
- The disease phenotype is produced in a susceptible host by intestinal atrophy and inflammation due to a T-cell mediated hypersensitivity reaction to a component of gluten.
- The precise structure of the protein antigen remains unknown, but recent studies suggest that enterotoxicity is produced by a peptide corresponding to amino acids 31–49 of A-gliaden. 10–15% of first-degree relatives are affected. Concordance rates for identical twins are 70–100%. There is a strong association with the histocompatability antigen HLA-DQ2, but other genes are also though to be involved in mediating genetic susceptibility. Genome-wide screening to identify susceptibility alleles is being undertaken in a number of centers.

Clinical features

- Celiac disease can present at any age.
- In children, it classically occurs after weaning; there is failure to thrive with pallor, apathy, anorexia, abdominal distension.
- In adults the commonest age of presentation is 20s and 30s. Diarrhea is usually present, as are constitutional symptoms of lassitude, weight loss, glossitis, angular stomatitis, and symptoms relating to anemia. Vitamin D deficiency or <u>osteoporosis</u> may be the presenting problem in adults.
- Other presentations in adults include depression and a Korsakoff-like syndrome. In women of child-bearing age, 30% have amenorrhea. Men with untreated celiac disease have low sperm counts and reduced plasma testosterone levels.
- Although a bowel habit of 3–4 loose, pale, often offensive stools is a typical finding, normally formed and colored stools do not preclude the diagnosis, and bowel habit depends on gluten intake. Severe pain is not a typical feature. Symptoms are often mild and nonspecific. Given the recently recognized high prevalence, a high index of suspicion is appropriate, especially in patients with unexplained mild macrocytic anemia with low serum <u>folic acid</u>.

Disease associations

- Link with organ-specific autoimmune diseases.
- Associated skin conditions include <u>dermatitis herpetiformis</u>, psoriasis, eczema, cutaneous vasculitis, epidermal necrolysis, mycosis fungoides.
- 10–15% of celiacs have abnormal liver blood tests and there is a higher than expected incidence of <u>autoimmune hepatitis</u> and <u>primary biliary cirrhosis</u>.

- There is also an association with <u>inflammatory bowel disease</u>, especially ulcerative proctitis.
- Ulcerative jejunitis can be associated with celiac disease and may be a variant of a T-cell proliferative condition that can result in a T-cell lymphoma.

Investigations

Blood tests may show anemia, classically with iron or folate deficiency. The peripheral blood may show target cells, Howell–Jolly bodies, acanthocytes, and thrombocytosis. Biochemistry may show low calcium, vitamin D, zinc, and albumin. Useful **serological tests** include IgG and IgA gliadin, IgA reticulin, IgA anti-endomysial and tissue transglutaminase antibodies. Anti-endomysial antibodies are 90% sensitive and almost 100% specific. The antigen recognized is tissue tranglutaminase: specific transglutaminase antibodies may be even more sensitive.

In the general population, 2% is IgA deficient, so it is important to exclude IgA deficiency as a cause of false negative serological testing.

Small-bowel biopsy remains essential. Four biopsies from the second part of duodenum using standard or jumbo-sized forceps are recommended (difficulty in interpretation sometimes occurs because of normal villous mucosa overlying Brunner's glands). In severe cases, loss of the normal circular fold pattern of the duodenum can be seen macroscopically, but this is not a reliable method of diagnosis.

Radiology. The barium follow-through can be abnormal, with loss of fine feathery mucosal pattern. Radiology is important in the presence of abdominal pain to exclude a complicating jejunal stricture, lymphoma, or carcinoma. Abdominal CT may show splenic atrophy and an associated low-grade lymphadenopathy.

Treatment

- Diet. A **gluten-free diet** should avoid wheat, rye, barley, and oats (although there is controversy about the toxicity of oats). Supplementation with fiber may be needed. Repeat biopsy at six months is necessary to assess response to diet. Further endoscopy after gluten challenge is not indicated if the patient has responded well to the diet with a corresponding histological response. Failure of response to the diet is usually (but not invariably) due to poor dietary compliance or inadvertent ingestion of gluten. Rarely, failure to respond is due to a small-intestinal lymphoma or the presence of another disorder, such as chronic pancreatitis.
- <u>CORTICOSTEROIDS</u> reduce the diarrhea and facilitate weight gain and reduction in steatorrhoea, but the effects do not persist after stopping the drugs. Steroids may be useful in 10% and in these patients second line steroid-sparing agents, such as <u>AZATHIOPRINE,</u> can also be useful.

Complications. Most patients are lactose intolerant at the time of diagnosis, but this rarely persists after treatment. There are reported but poorly understood neurological complications including demyelination of the posterior and lateral spinal cord columns and cerebellar degeneration that may respond, at least partly, to supplementation with vitamins A, E, B, or calcium.

Dumping syndrome

One of a number of <u>postgastrectomy syndromes</u>, resulting from alter-ation in the storage function of the stomach and the pyloric emptying mechanism. Incidence relates to the extent of gastric surgery and may affect 20–25% of patients. Syndrome is much less common now because of decline in number of operations for peptic ulcer disease and lower incidence of problems with gastric emptying after newer operations such as proximal gastric vagotomy.

- **Early dumping** occurs 30–60 minutes after a meal and is thought to result from accelerated emptying of hyperosmolar gastric contents into the small bowel. This leads to fluid shifts from the intravascular compartment into the bowel lumen, resulting in **vasomotor symptoms**: tachycardia, vasodilatation, sweating, and light headednesss as well as **distension, crampy pain**, and **diarrhea**. Postprandial release of gut hormones (enteroglucagon, peptide YY, pancreatic polypeptide, VIP, neurotensin) is increased in patients with dumping, and some of these may play a part in the pathogenesis of dumping syndrome.
- **Late dumping** occurs 1–3 hours after a meal. The rapid delivery of a meal to the small intestine leads to rapid absorbtion of glucose and a hyperinsulinemic response, causing subsequent hypoglycemia. The diagnosis can be confirmed by an extended glucose tolerance test.

Postoperative dumping is common and tends to improve with time. Dietary manipulation with high protein/low carbohydrate meals can help. Inhibitors of gastric emptying can help, and there is some evidence to support the use of <u>OCTREOTIDE</u>. Acarbose interferes with carbohydrate absorption and may help with late dumping.

Duodenal diverticulum

- Peri-ampullary diverticula are a common finding at <u>ERCP</u>, and it is debated whether they are associated with common bile duct (CBD) stones, pancreatitis, and biliary obstruction. Their presence may make CBD cannulation difficult (and occasionally impossible), and particular care during biliary sphincterotomy is essential, in order to avoid retroperitoneal perforation (see <u>endoscopic complications</u>). Food debris in diverticulum may be confused on U/S or <u>MRCP</u> as an intraductal filling defect.
- Large diverticula may occur elsewhere in small bowel (see <u>jejunal diverticulum</u>), where they may cause abdominal discomfort, diarrhea, and features of <u>bacterial overgrowth</u>. Many are diagnosed incidentally during imaging.

Duodenal ulcer

Pathogenesis, epidemiology, treatment, and complications are discussed in section on peptic ulceration.

Management recommendations. Don't take biopsies routinely at endoscopy because malignancy is extremely rare. Take a CLO test or alternative test to establish *Helicobacter* status and treat if positive. Continue antisecretory treatment with PROTON PUMP INHIBITORS (PPI) for at least six weeks.

If symptoms resolve and compliance with treatment is good, routine follow-up endoscopy and confirmation of HP eradication is not necessary. However, follow-up endoscopy is suggested for complicated ulcers that have bled or perforated or fail to respond to treatment after six weeks of therapy. Studies on maintenance therapy for complicated ulcers are limited, and this issue remains disputed; consider maintenance if recurrence would be high risk (elderly, severe comorbidity).

Embolization

- Radiological embolization of arteries leads to obstruction of flow more distally. Usually achieved through placement of intraluminal coils.
- Indications for embolization include acutely bleeding posterior duodenal ulcer (due to gastroduodenal artery (GDA)); pseudoaneurysm related to pancreatic pseudocyst (often splenic artery); colonic angiodysplasia or postpolypectomy bleed (branch of superior or inferior mesenteric arteries).
- Malignant tumors are often hypervascular, and so embolization may reduce tumor load due to ischemia/infarction (e.g., embolization of branch of hepatic artery in patients with hepatocellular carcinoma).
- Selective ipsilateral portal vein embolization in patients with hepatocellular carcinoma or liver metastases from colonic cancer may produce compensatory hypertrophy of contralateral liver lobe, and provide sufficient liver reserve to allow hemihepatectomy and tumor resection.

Important complications of embolization include vascular compromise of surrounding tissue: duodenal ulceration/stricture following GDA embolization; liver infarction, and acute liver failure following hepatic artery embolization (particular risk in patients with portal vein thrombosis and those with Child–Pugh score B/C.

Fat malabsorption

See: Chronic diarrhea and steatorrhea.

GIST (gastrointestinal stromal tumors)

Etiology and pathogenesis. Subset of mesenchymal GI tumors, previously classified as leiomyomas, leiomyosarcoma. Represent 3% of GI tumors. Intramural, well-demarcated spherical masses arising from muscularis propria. They may project intraluminally, with overlying mucosal ulceration. Malignancy not reliably predicted by tumor size (may be >30 cm), and 10–30% are malignant, with >40% of malignant GISTs metastasized by the time of presentation. GISTs usually arise from upper GI tract (stomach 70%, small bowel 20%).

Clinical features. May be found incidentally, but common presentations include abdominal pain, gastrointestinal bleeding, or a palpable mass. Rarely present with obstruction, and perforation occurs in 20%.

Investigation

- Endoscopy may show smooth mass with central ulceration.
- Endoscopic ultrasound (EUS) allows accurate assessment of GIST, including demonstration that tumor arises from muscularis propria.
- CT scanning and barium meal/follow-through may also delineate mass.
- Histologically graded as benign, borderline, or malignant, with histology showing diffuse sheets of spindle cells. Immunohistochemical staining of biopsy specimens is important, with expression of surface markers CD117 and CD34 characteristic, and vimentin expression in >90%. Correlates with malignancy include tumor size of >4 cm, irregular extraluminal border, and cystic spaces and echogenic foci within GIST. Presence of two or three of these features predicts malignancy with 80–100% confidence.

Management

- Surgical resection is treatment of choice (but complete resection may not be possible due to tumor size).
- Significant recent advance in treatment of metastatic or nonresectable GIST is development of Gleevec (imatinib mesylate), a tyrosine kinase inhibitor. In patients with unresectable GIST, two-year survival increases from 26% with conservative treatment, to 76% with Gleevec. Tumors often become unresponsive after two treatments with Gleevec, and additional treatments are now in development. In patients with malignant GIST, five-year survival postsurgery is 30–35%.

Hereditary hemorrhagic telangiectasia (HHT), (Osler–Weber–Rendu syndrome)

Rendu was first to describe the condition in 1896: should really be Rendu–Osler–Weber.

- Autosomal dominant disorder characterized by telangiectasia of the skin and mucous membranes.
- Commonest presentation is epistaxis at puberty: the cutaneous telangiectasia can appear later, usually before 20 years. Severe

GI bleeds occur, usually after age of 40. Melena is most common manifestation. The telangiectasia are easily seen at endoscopy. Angiography may show the arteriovenous (AV) malformations. Pathologically the disease affects capillaries, venules, and less commonly arterioles. Pulmonary AV malformations occur in 20%, especially those families with HHT1, caused by a mutation in the endoglin gene on chromosome 9; this can lead to high output cardiac failure. Arteriovenous malformations occur less commonly in the cerebral and hepatic circulations. HHT2 maps to chromosome 12, where mutations have been identified in the ALK-1 gene.

- Treatment is difficult; options include estrogens, aminocaproic acid, endoscopic ablation, and bowel resection. Endoscopic ablation including the use of <u>argon plasma coagulation</u> and thermal contact devices is probably the most promising.

Ileus

The failure of forward passage of intestinal contents in the absence of mechanical obstruction. There are several common causes in hospitalized patients—see Box 3.3.2.

Intestinal motility is impaired after abdominal surgery or injury. Small-bowel motility usually returns in 24 h, followed by gastric motility in two days and colonic motility in three to five days. The duration of operation and degree of manipulation do not appear to influence the length of ileus.

Clinical features. Poorly localized abdominal pain, nausea, vomiting, reduced or absent bowel sounds. Differentiation from obstruction is usually possible based on gas in stomach, small intestine, and colon on plain X-ray. Passage of contrast, either on barium or CT imaging can assist in the diagnosis. CT can also show inflammatory processes like pancreatitis, abscesses, or retroperitoneal hemorrhage.

Management. NPO, maintain intravascular volume, correct electrolyte imbalances, avoid narcotics. Pass a nasogastric tube if there is distension or vomiting. Search for a cause (see Box 3.3.2) if it does not resolve quickly.

Box 3.3.2 Causes of ileus

- **Laparotomy**
- **Electrolyte disturbance:** low K or Na, low or high Mg
- **Drugs:** narcotics, phenothiazines, anticholinergics
- **Intra-abdominal inflammation:** <u>appendicits</u>, <u>diverticulitis</u>, perforated DU
- **Retroperitoneal inflammation:** lumbar fracture, <u>pancreatitis</u>, pyelonephritis
- **Intestinal ischemia:** arterial embolus or thrombosis, mesenteric venous thrombosis
- **Thoracic disease:** MI, lower lobe pneumonia
- Systemic sepsis

Intussusception

- The invagination of a proximal segment of bowel (the intussusceptum) into an adjacent distal segment (intussuscipiens). Important cause of small-bowel obstruction in children, and is etiology of 5% of cases in adults. The important point is that in adults, intussusception always needs investigating because there is usually a pathological cause (tumors, inflammatory lesions, <u>Meckel's diverticulum</u>). This usually results in surgical resection of the affected segment.
- Clinical presentation is usually with partial small-bowel obstruction. Occult or overt rectal bleeding may occur.
- Diagnosis is usually by CT.

Jejunal diverticulum

A common location for small-bowel diverticula (also seen in the duodenum and <u>Meckel's diverticula</u>): found in 0.5% to 7% of small- bowel series. Most are asymptomatic but they can cause pain, bleeding, diarrhea, and fever. Malabsorption can arise from stasis and <u>bacterial overgrowth</u>.

Diagnosis is most efficient with a barium contrast radiograph. Can be seen on CT scans. Treatment is surgical for significant bleeding or diverticulitis. Malabsorption can be treated with oral antibiotics to treat bacterial overgrowth.

Lactose intolerance

- Deficiency of brush-border lactase can lead to lactose intolerance. Symptoms are bloating, cramps, gas, and diarrhea after milk or dairy ingestion (although milk protein allergy or fat intolerance are alternative causes).
- Commonest cause is acquired primary lactase deficiency. This is regulated at gene transcriptional level and varies in different populations (most frequent in Asians and Africans). Even in populations where lactase activity persists, levels are lower than for other disaccharidases, making lactose digestion more susceptible to impairment by acute gastrointestinal infections where the brush border is lost.
- Diagnosis can be confirmed by a lactose hydrogen <u>breath test</u>. Treatment consists either of a lactose-free diet or dietary supplementation with lactase.

Lymphangiectasia

Obstruction of lymphatic drainage from the small intestine, resulting in dilatation of small lymphatic channels in serosa and mesentery. Consequences are reduced absorption of chylomicrons and fat soluble vitamins, and excess loss of lymph into the lumen, with hypogammaglobulinemia and lymphocytopenia (especially of T cells): there is a loss of cell-mediated immunity. Blockage of lymphatics can result in chylous ascites or a chylous pleural effusion. GI symptoms are not prominent, although there can be diarrhea, pain, and vomiting. Causes are outlined in Box 3.3.3.

Diagnosis. Suspect in any patient with unexplained hypoalbuminemia, especially if there is lymphopenia and/or steatorrhea. Small- bowel biopsy can demonstrate dilated lacteals. Radiology may reveal edematous bowel folds. Fecal concentrations of ₁-antitrypsin can be used to measure intestinal protein loss (not gastric protein loss, as ₁-antitrypsin is degraded at pH less than 3). The optimal test is to measure clearance during a 72-hour stool collection, with plasma clearance expressed as ml/day.

Treatment. Acquired lymphangiectasia should be treated by correction of the primary disease. Congenital lymphangiectasia can be partially controlled with dietary restriction of long-chain fatty acids with enrichment by medium-chain triglycerides (which do not require lymphatic transport).

Box 3.3.3 Causes of lymphangiectasia

Primary (congenital): asymmetric lymphedema dating from infancy or early childhood.

Secondary (acquired): abdominal or retroperitoneal carcinoma, chronic pancreatitis, mesenteric TB or sarcoid, Crohn's, Whipple's, scleroderma, constrictive pericarditis, congestive heart failure, and systemic lupus erythematosus.

Lymphoma in GI tract

Solid malignancies of lymphoid tissue. The GI tract is very rarely affected by Hodgkin's lymphoma, but accounts for 30- 40% of extranodal cases of non-Hodgkin's lymphoma.

Gastric lymphomas

- Lymphoma accounts for 5% of gastric neoplasms (see also gastric cancer and gastrointestinal stromal tumors (GIST)). Great majority are B-cell lymphomas, either non-Hodgkin's or low-grade mucosa-associated lymphoid tissue (MALT) lymphomas (or MALTomas). The latter account for 40% of primary gastric lymphomas.
- The term MALT lymphoma has come to be used interchangeably with marginal zone B cell lymphoma, which in the stomach is associated with *Helicobacter pylori* infection. *Helicobacter pylori* found in up to 98% of cases of MALT lymphoma, with CagA-positivity particularly linked. Incidence is about 1:50 000 H. pylori-infected people. MALT lymphomas usually found in antrum, but may be multifocal, and tend to metastasize late.

- About 50% of gastric lymphomas are diffuse large cell B lymphomas. Relationship to *H. pylori* infection is uncertain but these tumors are of high grade and do not respond to antibiotics alone. Treatment of this condition now involves combined chemotherapy and radiotherapy, because surgery is no longer needed for diagnosis or staging.
- Early gastric lymphoma may be asymptomatic, but later clinical presentation is similar to gastric cancer, but night sweats and fever may be prominent. Polypoid, fungating mass may be seen, and be difficult to distinguish endoscopically from adenocarcinoma. Endoscopy and biopsy provides 95% sensitivity, and <u>endoscopic ultrasound</u> allows assessment of stage of disease. CT used to assess distant spread.
- Eradication of *H. pylori* may lead to complete remission of MALT lymphoma in > 80% of cases, but for *H. pylori*-negative MALT lymphomas, or where eradication has not induced remission, chemotherapy is still often effective. Newer agents including monoclonal antibodies against B-cell antigen CD20 (e.g., rituximab) show promise.

Small-bowel lymphomas

- B-cell lymphomas encompass immunoproliferative small-intestinal disease (IPSID) and non-IPSID subtypes including marginal zone B-cell lymphoma (MALT type, but not associated with *H. pylori*), large B-cell lymphoma, mantle cell lymphoma, follicular lymphoma, and Burkitt's lymphoma. T-cell lymphomas are usually associated with <u>celiac disease</u>.
- Of the B-cell small-bowel lymphomas, marginal zone and follicular lymphomas are regarded as indolent processes, incurable but controllable by chemotherapy. Diffuse large-cell lymphomas and mantle-cell lymphomas are more aggressive and require chemotherapy.

Enteropathy-associated T-cell lymphoma occurs as a complication of <u>celiac disease</u>. Intraepithelial T cells in celiac are CD3$^+$CD8$^+$ and are polyclonal. Monoclonal proliferation of T cells in celiac can result in a spectrum of processes from refractory sprue, where response to gluten-free diet is lost, through ulcerative jejunitis to enteropathy-associated intestinal T-cell lymphoma. Clinical features include diarrhea, abdominal pain, weight loss, and vomiting. A minority present with intestinal perforation or obstruction. Anemia is common, albumin usually low, LDH is elevated in 25%. Treatment is usually combined surgery and chemotherapy, but prognosis is poor (response rate 60%, remission rate 40%, but relapse in six months 80% with one- and five-year survival rates of 30–40% and 10–20%, respectively).

Immunodeficiency-related lymphoma

- Posttransplant immunoproliferative disorders (PTLD) occur in 1–20% of solid organ transplants (e.g., <u>liver transplantation</u>) and bone marrow transplants and usually result from proliferation of Epstein–Barr virus transformed cells. Treatments include antiviral agents, B cell antibodies (rituximab), and donor leucocyte infusions.
- B-cell NHL can develop in HIV positive patients. EBV is implicated in about 50%.

Meckel's diverticulum

- Arises from persistence of the omphalo-mesenteric or vitelline duct, which connects the embryonic gut tube with the yolk sac but normally disappears early in fetal life. It occurs in 2% of people and is the commonest congenital GI tract abnormality. Can be as proximal as ligament of Treitz but most are within 100 cm of ileocecal valve. Associated with other congential anomalies (cleft palate, annular pancreas).
- **Clinical features.** Painless <u>lower GI bleeding</u> in the young (mean age 5 years); obstruction (commonest presentation in adults). Diverticulitis, perforation, and carcinoma are much less common.
- **Diagnosis** is with technetium pertechnate scan(Meckel's scan): this assumes uptake by heterotopic gastric mucosa, but nearly all bleeding diverticula contain gastric mucosa. False positives may occur with <u>intussusception</u> and <u>Crohn's disease</u>.
- **Surgical resection** is the treatment of choice.

Mesenteric venous thrombosis

Accounts for perhaps 10% of cases of acute mesenteric ischemia: intestinal infarction is rare unless the branches of peripheral arcades and vasa recta are involved. Causes are similar to those for <u>portal vein thrombosis</u> and include hypercoagulable states, portal hypertension, abdominal infections, blunt abdominal trauma, pancreatitis, and malignancy in the portal area.

Clinical features. **Acute mesenteric venous thrombosis** presents with pain in 90%; lower GI bleeding or hematemesis occurs in 15% and suggests bowel infarction. Most patients are febrile and 25% show signs of septic shock. Patients with **chronic mesenteric venous thrombosis** are usually asymptomatic at time of diagnosis but may develop GI bleeding from varices secondary to <u>portal vein thrombosis</u>.

Diagnosis. Selective angiography can establish a definite diagnosis and can differentiate arterial from venous ischemia but is not always available in an emergency. CT angiography is very useful and probably the investigation of choice.

Treatment. Most patients with acute mesenteric venous thrombosis are treated as for <u>intestinal ischemia</u>. If surgery is required, postoperative heparinization reduces recurrence and progression. Treatment of chronic mesenteric venous thrombosis centers on controlling bleeding from varices.

Peutz–Jeghers syndrome

Peutz 1921; Jeghers 1949.

- Hamartomas represent a type of <u>polyp</u> characterized by glandular epithelium supported by a framework of smooth muscle continuous with muscularis mucosa. Usually multiple.
- The syndrome is autosomal dominant and involves germ-line mutation of a serine–threonine kinase gene of chromosome 19.
- There is characteristic mucocutaneous pigmentation that resembles freckles (see Color Plate 23). Polyps can be anywhere in the GI tract but are commonly small intestinal.
- Diagnosis made in person with histologically confirmed hamartoma and two of the following: family history of autosomal dominant inheritance, mucocutaneous hyperpigmentation, small-bowel polyposis. Genetic testing available, but not 100%.
- There is a high overall risk of cancer (90% by age 65). Risk of colon cancer is 40%, with similar risks of stomach and pancreatic cancer. Also elevated risk of small-bowel carcinoma. There is an increased risk of breast cancer, uterine cancer, and testicular cancer.
- Guidelines for screening include colonoscopy from late teens every two to three years; upper GI endoscopy every two years; annual Hb and surveillance of small bowel (SBFT, ? CE); annual EUS of pancreas every one to two years; annual breast exam or mammogram; and annual pelvic examination and Pap smear; transvaginal ultrasound and serum CA-125 annually. Males under age 12 should have yearly testicular exams.

Protein-losing enteropathy

Excess protein loss from the gut (which is nonselective and not limited to low-molecular-weight proteins as in the nephritic syndrome) can be due to:

- Increased mucosal permeability.
- Mucosal ulceration.
- Lymphatic obstruction.

Clinical features

- Edema, diarrhea, fat or carbohydrate malabsorption, signs of fat soluble <u>vitamin</u> deficiency, and consequences of reduced cellular immunity.
- **Laboratory abnormalities** may include ↓ serum albumin, Igs, proteins (e.g., ceruloplasmin, alpha-1 antitrypsin, transferrin, hormone binding proteins), and lymphocytopenia if there is lymphatic obstruction.

Diagnosis

The gold standard is measuring the loss of intravenously labeled albumin; this has disadvantages in terms of radioactive exposure and expense, so fecal measurement of alpha-1 antitrypsin is the preferred method. Note that because alpha-1 antitrypsin is degraded at pH < 3, it cannot be used to measure gastric protein loss and interpretation is difficult in patients with positive <u>fecal occult blood</u>.

Differential diagnosis includes:
- Increased mucosal permeability: i.e., Celiac disease, tropical sprue, Menetrier's disease
- Mucosal ulceration: i.e., IBD, malignancy, NSAID enteropathy
- **Lymphatic obstruction:** i.e., intestinal lymphangiectasia, CHF, cirrhosis, intestinal lymphoma

Work up of etiology of protein losing enteropathy includes EGD +/– small-bowel imaging +/– colonoscopy

Treatment

Based on underlying etiology. Also, maintenance of nutritional status.

Roux-en-Y anastomosis

- Procedure involves dividing jejunum approximately 15 cm from ligament of Trietze, and mobilizing a loop of jejunum. Proximal limb is anastomosed to the appropriate anatomic site (see Figure 3.3.1). Divided end of jejunum is anastomosed to jejunal loop along its course.
- Indications for Roux-en-Y anastomosis include <u>biliary reflux</u> following partial <u>gastrectomy</u>, biliary reconstruction following bile duct injury (hepaticojejunostomy between jejunal loop and common hepatic duct); as anti-obesity (bariatri) surgical intervention (jejunal anstomosis on to proximal stomach); and treatment of <u>postgastrectomy syndromes</u>. See also <u>biliary bypass procedures</u>.

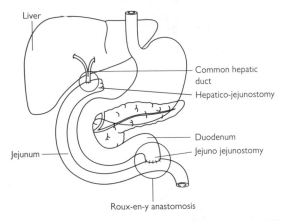

Figure 3.3.1 Roux-en-Y anastomosis and hepatico-jejunostomy as part of <u>biliary bypass procedure</u>.

Short bowel syndrome

- A malabsorption syndrome resulting from extensive intestinal resection. Major causes in adults are <u>Crohn's disease</u>, mesenteric infarction, and <u>radiation</u> injury. Degree of malabsorption is related to remaining length of small and large bowel. Nutrient absorptive capacity is higher in proximal small intestine than distal small bowel; intestinal failure can be avoided if there is 100 cm of jejunum with no colon or if there is 50 cm of jejunum with colon in continuity.
- **Water and electrolyte malabsorption**. Net sodium and fluid balance is related to jejunal length. Patients with <100 cm jejunum are often net secretors, whereas those with >100 cm are net absorbers. In these patients, use of <u>oral rehydration solutions</u> can decrease stoma output and convert some patients from net secretors to net absorbers: sodium concentration should be in the range 90–120 mM. Importantly, sport drinks and commercially made liquid formula feeds contain too little sodium for maximal fluid absorption in patients with short bowel and a jejunostomy.
- **Site-specific transport processes.** Calcium and magnesium are absorbed in the duodenum and proximal jejunum but the malabsorption is potentiated by fat malabsorption because the mineral are precipitated intraluminally by long chain fatty acids. Ileal resection of more than 50 cm frequently impairs vitamin B12 absorption and resection of more than 100 cm cause bile acid malabsorption.

Box 3.3.4 Complications of short bowel

- **Cholesterol <u>gallstones</u>**. Reduced hepatic-bile-acid secretion leads to cholesterol supersaturation
- <u>Oxalate kidney stones</u>.
- **D-lactic acidosis.** If the colon is *in situ*, carbohydrate overfeeding can result in excess short chain fatty acids. This lowers colonic pH, which promotes Gram-positive anerobes that produce D-lactate. Humans lack D-lactate dehydrogenase. Absorbed D-lactate may produce nystagmus, ataxia, and confusion. Patients look drunk but blood alcohol is normal; D-lactate levels are high (>3 mM/l)

Tropical sprue

Initially described by Hilary in 1759 who wrote observations of chronic diarrhea in Barbados. Characterized by chronic diarrhea and malabsorption in residents or visitors to the tropics. Recently redefined as **malabsorption of at least two different substances in people in the tropics when other causes have been excluded.**

Epidemiology

Restricted to Southern and Southeast Asia, the Caribbean, and Central South America. Usually occurs in long-term visitors or residents of over six months, but epidemics have occurred in India and Burma. The prevalence may be decreasing due to increasing self-medication with antibiotics.

Clinical features

Chronic diarrhea with steatorrhea, anorexia, cramps, and bloating. There may be lactose intolerance, vitamin B12 or vitamin A deficiency, hypocalcaemia, anemia, stomatitis, glossitis, and edema.

Pathological features

Includes atrophic gastritis (although this may relate to co-infection with *Helicobacter*) and mild changes in colonic epithelial cells, but the major changes are in the small intestine. There is reduced disaccharidase activity and reduced fat absorption: the latter may account in part for altered transit time through the small bowel. Etiology still uncertain but likely to involve chronic infection with enteropathogens.

Diagnosis

Requires demonstration of partial villous atrophy, exclusion of specific cause of diarrhea and malabsorption, and presence of fat and B12 malabsorption.

- Search carefully for intestinal pathogens; three stool specimens for microscopy, with particular attention to looking for microsporidia and *Isospora* in the immunocompromised. Fecal microscopy is insensitive for <u>Giardia</u> and <u>Stronglyoides</u>.
- Duodenal biopsy or serological ELISAs may be helpful to diagnose giardiasis and *Stronglyoides*.
- <u>Celiac</u> serology is important to exclude gluten-sensitive enteropathy.
- Contrast examination or capsule endoscopy of the small bowel may be needed to exclude <u>lymphoma</u>.

Treatment

"Simple" general measures (restoring water and electrolytes, replacing nutritional deficiencies of iron, folate, B12) have reduced mortality of epidemic tropical sprue. The use of antibiotics is controversial, but overland travelers improve on tetracycline 250 mg qid, usually given for several months.

Prognosis is good, particularly in expatriates returning from the tropics. There is some evidence of recurrence in indigenous populations of the tropics.

VIPoma

See <u>Pancreatic Endocrine Tumors</u>.

Liver

Acetaminophen overdose

Background
- Drug very safe at therapeutic levels (< 4 g/day), but in overdose (particularly > 10 g), depletion of hepatic glutathione leads to accumulation of toxic metabolites (para-amino benzo quinonamaine), and liver injury.
- Increased toxicity associated with chronic alcohol excess, fasting, late presentation (> 16 hours since ingestion), and concomitant use of certain drugs (phenobarbitone, phenytoin, isoniazid, zidovudine) that promote acetaminophen metabolism to toxic metabolites.

Clinical features
- Patients may be well, or have nausea/vomiting for first 24 hours.
- Liver failure, with progressive jaundice, hypoglycemia, hepatic encephalopathy (often associated with cerebral edema), and multiorgan failure develops from approximately 48 hours postoverdose.
- Acute renal failure may occur independent of liver failure.

Investigation
- Plasma acetaminophen levels (see nomogram) taken > 4 hours postingestion predict toxicity (and need for treatment).
- Baseline Chem 7, LFTs, Glu, CBC, PT/INR. Abnormalities at presentation suggest overdose > 18 hours previously, or pre-existing liver disease.

Specific management
- N-ACETYLCYSTEINE (NAC) replenishes hepatic glutathione stores, virtually abolishes severe hepatotoxicity if given < 12 hours postingestion, and may provide benefit even if started up to 36 hours after overdose.
- Indications for NAC include:
  - Serum acetaminophen levels above cut off > 4 hours postingestion.
  - Patients presenting > 12 hours postoverdose.
  - History of staggered overdose, or history unreliable.
  - Serum acetaminophen levels below treatment line, but risk of increased toxicity (as earlier).

General management
- See acute liver failure.
- Daily bloods: Urea & Electrolytes, LFTs, Glu, CBC, PT/INR.
- AST/ALT may rise massively (10,000 U/l not uncommon) at day 2–3, but patient's clotting (INR/PT), and overall clinical state (e.g., hepatic encephalopathy) much more important prognostic markers. If INR normal at 48 hours, significant liver damage will not occur.
- Contact specialist liver unit early, especially if any of following: arterial pH < 7.3; INR > 3; creatinine > 2.0 mg/dL, hypoglycemia, or any degree of encephalopathy 48 hours after ingestion.
- Acetaminophen overdose remains important indication for urgent liver transplantation.

Acquired immune deficiency syndrome

See: <u>HIV and the liver</u>

Acute fatty liver of pregnancy (AFLP)

Background

- Rare disease, characterized by mitochondrial cytopathy, with incidence 1:14,,000 pregnancies in the United States.
- Unlike other liver conditions specifically related to pregnancy (<u>HELLP syndrome</u> and <u>obstetric cholestasis</u>), AFLP frequently associated with <u>acute liver failure.</u>
- Pathogenesis unclear, but associated with inherited long chain 3-hydroxyacyl coenzyme A dehydrogenase (LCHAD) deficiency, first pregnancies, and in those carrying male fetuses or twins.

Clinical features

- Usual presentation at 34–37 weeks of pregnancy, only rarely before 20 wecks or after delivery.
- Characteristic presentation with nausea, vomiting, abdominal pain, and confusion, with pre-eclampsia (thirst, headache, blurred vision, proteinuria, hypertension, peripheral edema).
- Jaundice common (in contrast to <u>HELLP syndrome</u>), with additional features of <u>acute liver failure</u> (hypoglycemia, bleeding, <u>hepatic encephalopathy</u>). Pruritus may be an initial symptom and clinical overlap with <u>obstetric cholestasis</u> rarely seen. Diabetes insipidus reported.

Investigations

- Blood results may show ↑ WCC, ↑ AST/ALT (but usually < 750 U/l), ↑ bilirubin x 6–8 ULN. ↑ PT suggests significant liver impairment, and ↑ uric acid, urea, and creatinine also common.
- Imaging with <u>ultrasound</u> should be performed, in part to exclude other conditions (e.g., biliary obstruction, subcapsular hematoma, Budd Chiari syndrome), but no diagnostic features of AFLP.
- <u>Liver biopsy</u> classically shows microvesicular fat. Rarely performed during pregnancy if delivery to be expedited. May be performed by transjugular route, if coagulopathy present.

Management

- Intensive care setting, with specialist hepatology and obstetric input essential. Prompt delivery is cornerstone of treatment, with management of <u>acute liver failure</u> and <u>hepatic encephalopathy</u> as necessary.
- DDAVP may be required for diabetes insipidus.
- <u>Liver transplantation</u> has been successful, but is rarely required unless delivery is delayed.
- Maternal mortality < 1% with specialist care, and perinatal mortality 7%.
- Mother, infant, and father should be tested for the G1528C mutation in LCHAD.

Albumin (use in liver disease)

- Few issues cause greater disagreement in hepatology than use of human albumin solutions (e.g., 25% HAS) in patients with cirrhosis, ascites, and hypoalbuminemia. Problem arises due to absence of well-designed randomized controlled studies.
- Supporters (usually hepatologists) argue that HAS has been used for years with few problems, helps to maintain intravascular volume and, thus, renal perfusion. Recent studies have demonstrated additional benefits in hepato-renal syndrome when combined with Terlipressin[1] and in prevention of HRS in the setting of spontaneous bacterial peritonitis.
- Opponents point to data[2] suggesting no benefit of albumin over saline in critically ill patients (but this study included a hugely variable patient group, and not liver patients); only transient improvement in plasma oncotic pressure with HAS; and argue that adequate volume expansion, rather than HAS *per se*, is the key.
- Albumin is about 10 times more expensive than 4% Gelofusin® solution).

Alcoholic liver disease

Epidemiology and pathogenesis

- Alcohol accounts for 40–80% of cases of cirrhosis in the developed world. United States Health and Human Services recommend consumption of alcohol in moderation—defined as the consumption of up to one drink per day for women and up to two drinks per day for men. In individuals drinking > 40 units/week, 6–8% will develop cirrhosis within 12 years, with 20–30% of long-term heavy drinkers developing significant liver disease.
- Alcohol excess very strongly linked to antisocial behavior and domestic violence, and risks of binge drinking among young people are increasingly recognized. See also <u>alcohol dependency</u>.
- Number of clinical patterns of disease may occur.

Alcohol-induced fatty liver

Results from heavy alcohol intake over months. Usually asymptomatic, but associated with hepatomegaly, mildly elevated transaminases, and increased liver echogenicity on <u>ultrasound</u>. History should allow differentiation from <u>nonalcoholic fatty liver disease (NAFLD)</u>. Although usually resolves after several weeks of abstinence, progression to cirrhosis in 20% who continue to drink, and very rarely may present with <u>acute alcoholic hepatitis with liver failure</u>.

Alcoholic hepatitis

Usually develops in those drinking very large amounts over a long period. An undefined trigger (usually develops in absence of recent increased intake) initiates severe proinflammatory response, associated with oxidant

1 Gastroenterology. 2008 May;134(5):1352–1359
2 SAFE Study Investigators (2004). N. Engl. J. Med. 350: 2247

injury and neutrophilic liver infiltration. In those who recover from alcoholic hepatitis, cirrhosis develops in >10% per year.

Clinical features: Acute onset of malaise, jaundice, anorexia, diarrhea, and nausea. Tender hepatomegaly and signs of decompensated liver disease (e.g., ascites, <u>hepatic encephalopathy</u>), which may worsen after hospital admission, despite stopping alcohol. Malnutrition is common, correlates with poor prognosis, and >50% of total energy intake in these patients comes from alcohol. Mortality 60% in alcoholic hepatitis relates to the sequelae of liver failure—sepsis, renal failure, and variceal bleeding.

Investigations

- CBC may show ↑WCC (50% cases), ↓platelets (direct toxic alcohol effect, or due to hypersplensim), ↑MCV.
- Electrolytes may show ↓Na⁺, K⁺, Ca²⁺, Mg²⁺. Renal failure may be due to sepsis, dehydration, or <u>hepatorenal syndrome</u>.
- <u>Liver function tests</u>: AST/ALT characteristically < × 3 ULN, with AST > ALT in > 70%. ↑bilirubin and PT incorporated into discriminant function (DF) test (see Box 4.1) predicts mortality (DF > 32 correlates with >35% 4 week mortality), but does not differentiate alcoholic hepatitis from end-stage liver failure/cirrhosis.
- ↑Acute phase markers (CRP, ferritin).
- <u>Liver biopsy</u> establishes diagnosis (and excludes/identifies underlying cirrhosis), with features of hepatocyte ballooning and necrosis, Mallory bodies, and neutrophil infiltrate.

Management

- General supportive measures are paramount, with diligent care of IV lines and prevention of sepsis. No role for antibiotic prophylaxis (fever and ↑WCC, ↑CRP may be feature of alcoholic hepatitis *per se*), but culture of blood, urine, ascites, and use of broad spectrum antibiotics essential in setting of clinical sepsis (e.g., third-generation <u>CEPHALOSPORIN + METRONIDAZOLE, PIPERACILLIN/ TAZOBACTAM</u>), ideally guided by culture results. If sepsis continues, consider systemic antifungal treatment (e.g., fluconazole, amphotericin). See <u>ANTIBIOTICS</u> and <u>ANTIFUNGALS</u>.
- Insert urinary catheter and monitor output if impaired renal function/ poor urine output.
- Insert CVP line if patient shocked, bleeding, or in renal failure.
- Vitamin K 10 mg IV for three days.
- Thiamine 100 mg od (prophylaxis against <u>Wernicke's encephalopathy</u>)
- Protein supplements (> 1.2 g/kg/day) speed nutritional recovery and liver function tests, and do not appear to precipitate or worsen encephalopathy. Parenteral feeding should be avoided if at all possible, because of risks (sepsis, bleeding). Nasogastric feeding can be safely given (and probably reduces bacterial translocation).
- Role of <u>CORTICOSTEROIDS</u> remains controversial, but consensus for use (e.g., commencing prednisolone 40 mg od) in severe disease (DF > 32) with encephalopathy. Variceal bleeding and sepsis are contraindications. Patients who do not exhibit response within a week unlikely to benefit from longer therapy.

- Specific management of complications may be necessary—see:
  - Ascites.
  - Hepatorenal syndrome.
  - Variceal bleeding—See acute upper GI bleeding.
  - Hepatic encephalopathy.
  - Alcohol withdrawal syndrome.
- N–ACETYLCYSTEINE, pentoxifylline 400 mg tds PO (nonselective phosphodiesterase inhibitor), and liver support devices have shown some promise, but their exact role is still to be defined.

Box 4.1 Discriminant function (DF) in alcoholic hepatitis

DF = 4.6 (prolongation of PT in sec) + (bilirubin in µmol/l/17.1).

Consider corticosteroids if DF > 32 (see text).

Alcoholic cirrhosis

Clinical features of cirrhosis due to alcohol are similar to those of other causes, ranging from entirely asymptomatic disease to severely decompensated liver failure (see Approaches: well patients with abnormal liver tests; recent-onset jaundice; cirrhosis; and chronic liver disease). Histology may show micronodular cirrhosis. In alcoholic cirrhotics with ascites, five-year survival is 16–25%. Mortality at five years is reduced by 50% through abstinence, irrespective of degree of liver dysfunction. Death occurs due to complications of cirrhosis, including hepatocellular carcinoma.

Management

includes patient education about the effect of abstinence on prognosis, and management of complications of cirrhosis— see:
- Portal hypertension.
- Emergencies—Acute upper GI bleeding.
- Hepatic encephalopathy.
- Hepatorenal syndrome.
- Ascites.
- Cirrhosis and chronic liver disease.

Many centers require patients to be abstinent for at least 6 months prior to liver transplantation, although five-year survival posttransplantation is equivalent between those with alcoholic and nonalcoholic indications.

"Long quaffing maketh a short lyfe." John Lyly (1554–1606)

"Alcohol is the cause and the solution to many of life's problems." Homer Simpson (1956–)

Alpha-1-antitrypsin deficiency

Epidemiology + pathology

Autosomal recessive condition, commonest in Caucasians (1:1800 homozygous deficient (PiZZ)). Impaired cellular transport of α_1-antitrypsin with intrahepatic accumulation appears to underlie liver injury, but mechanism unclear.

Clinical features

Neonatal cholestasis and jaundice develop in 10% of homozygotes, with subsequent hepatomegaly and portal hypertension. Liver function tests show raised cholestatic enzymes and transaminases. Presentation in adulthood occurs in 10% of homozygotes, with cirrhosis or emphysema (rarely both in the same patient). High rates of portal hypertension and hepatocellular carcinoma reported.

Investigations

Diagnosis made by finding: serum α_1-antitrypsin level < 75% of lower limit of normal (80 mg/dl); ↓α_1-globulin level on protein electrophoresis; genetic phenotyping by immunofixation; periodic-acid Schiff positive globules in periportal hepatocytes on histology.

Management

Prevention of hepatic insults (e.g., alcohol), adequate nutrition, avoidance of smoking (with respect to chest). **Ursodeoxycholic acid** may help with neonatal cholestasis. Liver transplantation remains only treatment for advanced disease, with 80% five-year survival in children. Inhaled α_1-antitrypsin has been used to treat pulmonary disease.

Alpha-fetoprotein (AFP)

Protein normally produced by the liver and fetal yolk. Serum levels elevated (> 10 ng/ml) in a range of cancers, including hepatocellular carcinoma (HCC), germline tumors (e.g., testicular seminoma, teratoma, ovarian tumors), and metastasic liver deposits, but also in active liver disease, and in mothers pregnant with babies carrying neural tube defects or Down's syndrome.

AFP and liver disease. Although level of AFP may correlate with size of HCC, it is not elevated in 30% of HCCs. It is, therefore, not of use alone as a screening or surveillance test. It may also be elevated in 5% of patients with chronic liver disease (particularly during flare of disease, as indicated by raised ALT/AST). However, AFP > 100 ng/ml always necessitates the exclusion of HCC, by means of U/S, contrast-enhanced CT scan, and occasionally angiography.

Ascites

See: Top 10 Clinical Problems: Ascites.

Autoimmune hepatitis (AIH)

Etiology + epidemiology

Necroinflammatory liver disease of unknown etiology. Estimated prevalence of 50–100 cases per million population (F:M ratio 4:1). Strongly associated with HLA alleles DR3 (often younger at onset, more severe course) and DR4 (older, more benign course).

Clinical features

- Bimodal age distribution at disease onset—10–30 years and > 40 years. Young women commonly affected, but found in all other groups.
- Presentation with acute hepatitis in up to 40%, but acute liver failure very rare. Many present with gradual onset of jaundice, fatigue, abdominal pain, and fever, and 30–80% have cirrhosis at presentation.
- Associated with other autoimmune diseases in 48% of cases—thyroid disease, arthritis, vitiligo, ulcerative colitis, diabetes mellitus, lichen planus, alopecia, mixed connective tissue disease.
- Prior to immunosuppression, 50% 3–5- year mortality reported. When disease remission is induced, 90% 10-year survival, even with cirrhosis at outset.
- Overlap syndromes may occur. In the presence of clinical features of AIH, antimitochondrial Abs (AMA) and cholangitis are seen in 8%, suggesting overlap with primary biliary cirrhosis (PBC), and biliary disease suggestive of primary sclerosing cholangitis (PSC) occurs in 6%. Anti-LKM1 Abs shown in 2–5% of patients with HCV infection.

Investigations

Definitive diagnosis requires: circulating autoantibodies >1:80 titre; IgG > × 1 ULN; all other causes of chronic liver disease excluded.

Incorporation of clinical, laboratory, and histological parameters into standardized scoring systems may aid diagnosis where classical features are absent.[1]

Characteristic elevation of transaminases (ALT/AST) by > 1.5 x Ul N for > 6 months. ALT > 1000 U/l rarely seen (note: ALT > 1,000 U/l usually due to drugs, viral hepatitis, or ischemia).

Two subtypes of AIH categorized, according to serological results:

- **Type 1.** 80% of cases of AIH, 70% female < 40 years. Antinuclear Ab (ANA) ± smooth muscle Ab (ASM) +ve. Elevated IgG in 97% of cases. Good response to immunosuppression in 80% of patients, but 25% have cirrhosis at presentation.
- **Type 2.** Very rare in United States; may account for 20% of AIH cases in Europe. Usually diagnosed in children. Associated with antiliver–kidney microsomal Abs (anti-LKM1) and anti-LC-1 Abs, but ANA/ASM usually negative. Rapidly progressive, and poor response to immunosuppression.

Liver biopsy. Periportal/lobular hepatitis characteristic, but no pathognomonic features in AIH (Color plate 8). Histological grade (inflammation) and stage (fibrosis) predict prognosis (bridging necrosis/multilobular necrosis/cirrhosis probably predicts worse outcome). Repeat biopsy on treatment predicts likelihood of maintained remission off treatment.

1 Johnson, PJ and McFarlane, IG. *Hepatology* 1993; 18: 998

Management

Treatment indicated when ALT/AST > 1.5 × ULN, IgG > 2 × ULN, and moderate to severe periportal hepatitis on biopsy. Absolute indication if ALT/AST > 10 × ULN, severe hepatitis and necrosis, or disease progression.

- CORTICOSTEROIDS. Mainstay of treatment, with 80% biochemical and histological remission within two to four years. Initiated alone or with AZATHIOPRINE. Usual starting dose prednisolone 30–50 mg od PO for 2/52, with aim of reduction of 5 mg every 10 days, to maintenance at 5–15 mg/day or less. Drug withdrawal should not be attempted <2 years after starting treatment, and then should be guided by histology (100% relapse if on-treatment progression to cirrhosis, 20% if histological resolution). Disease flares may occur, whatever the response. Progression in 10% despite steroids.
- AZATHIOPRINE. No role as monotherapy for inducing remission. Very useful in combination with steroids, allowing steroid reduction, and as maintenance therapy after steroid withdrawal (maintains remission in > 80% over 1–10 year follow-up). Usual dose 1–1.5 mg/kg/day in combination, increasing to 2–2.5 mg/kg/day as monotherapy after remission achieved. Important side effects and checking TPMT levels prior to commencing treatment is recommended.
- New immunosuppressants. Effectiveness of tacrolimus, cyclosporin, mycophenolate, and others reported, and may be considered for treatment failures, but no established role yet.
- Liver transplantation. Consider in patients with progressive disease, especially if no response after four years of treatment, or early hepatic decompensation. The 5- and 10-year survival posttransplant of 90% and 75%, respectively. AIH may recur in graft, but rarely leads to graft loss.

Bilirubin metabolism

- Bilirubin is an end product of heme degradation, derived from red blood cells (70–80% of total) and extrahematopoietic tissues (mainly liver). Approximately 4 mg/kg of bilirubin produced/day.
- Bilirubin produced by initial conversion of heme to biliverdin (via heme oxygenase), and then biliverdin to bilirubin (via bilverdin reductase).
- Unconjugated bilirubin circulates in plasma bound to albumin. After uptake into hepatocytes (? by organic anion transporting polypeptide (OATP)) it undergoes conjugation in endoplasmic reticulum by bilirubin glucuronyltransferase (UGT-1) (defective enzyme activity associated with Gilbert's syndrome). Conjugation converts hydrophobic bilirubin into water-soluble form (80% as bilirubin diglucuronides), which is excreted into bile via an ATP-dependent export pump (site of defect in Dubin–Johnson syndrome).
- Resorption of conjugated bilirubin from the gut is minimal, but it may be hydrolyzed by bacterial β-glucuronidase interminal ileum/colon, with this unconjugated bilirubin subsequently converted to colorless urobilinogen. Approximately 20% of urobilinogen is resorbed, and excreted in the urine.

Budd–Chiari syndrome (BCS)

Definition and pathogenesis

BCS refers to obstruction of main hepatic veins (HVs) by thrombus, and is viewed as separate from veno-occlusive disease, which involves hepatic venules. Causes of BCS include generalized thrombophilia in > 40% (e.g., myeloproliferative disorders, factor V Leiden deficiency), hepatocellular carcinoma, and anomalies of inferior vena cava. In clinical practice the diagnosis is rarely made unless it's considered.

Clinical features

Usual pattern involves abdominal pain, ascites, and hepatomegaly developing over several months, but acute liver failure may rarely occur. Jaundice is variable. Features of portal hypertension, including splenomegaly and bleeding varices, may develop. Clinical course varies considerably, but three-year survival in chronic BCS of 50% has been reported.

Investigation

Diagnosis usually made with Doppler ultrasound or contrast CT scan (but alert radiologists to clinical possibility!) Venography and venous pressure measurement allow the site of obstruction to be defined. Caudate lobe hypertrophy (due to separate drainage into inferior vena cava) on imaging is a characteristic, but only seen in 50% of cases. Unlike most cases of portal hypertension, the ascitic fluid in acute Budd–Chiari syndrome is often an exudate (i.e., SAAG < 11 g/dl. See ascites). Perform thrombophilia screen to identify underlying cause (see portal vein thrombosis).

Management

In acute BCS, thrombolysis and subsequent anticoagulation has been used, to attempt recannulation of HVs, and in the rare cases of acute liver failure (see emergencies) liver transplantation may be required. In chronic BCS anticoagulation should also be considered, but management of complications is central, including ascites and portal hypertension. Ascites is diuretic-resistant in 30% from presentation. Liver transplantation probably carries better prognosis than surgical portocaval shunting, but TIPSS has been used to good effect.

Caroli's disease

Congenital segmental cystic dilatation of intrahepatic bile ducts, thought to relate to a ductal plate malformation, and associated with autosomal recessive polycystic kidney disease. Sometimes classified as type 5 choledochal cyst. Hepatic fibrosis may occur, but the extrahepatic tree is unaffected. Often presents in early 20s, and clinical features include jaundice, cholangitis, and intraductal stones. Cholangiocarcinoma (reported in 7%) and portal hypertension may develop. Diagnosis often made with non-invasive imaging (e.g., U/S, CT, MRCP). Endoscopic biliary drainage may be attempted, but is of limited use in draining intrahepatic ducts. Hepatectomy is effective if disease confined to one lobe, but liver transplantation may be indicated for recurrent cholangitis and extensive disease.

Child–Pugh score

Widely used grading system in patients with chronic liver disease, because it is easy to calculate and uses straightforward clinical and biochemical/hematological parameters (see Table 4.1).

This grading system is of prognostic use, and is widely used as the basis for assessing patients with cirrhosis for <u>liver transplantation</u> (e.g., Child–Pugh score > 7 as indication for referral).

Table 4.1 Child's grading (with Pugh's modifications)

Criteria	Points		
	1	**2**	**3**
<u>Hepatic encephalopathy</u> grade	None	1–2	3–4
Serum bilirubin (mg/dl)	<2	2–3	3
Serum albumin (g/dl.)	>35	3.5–2.8	<2.8
Prothrombin time prolongation (sec)	<4	4–10	>10
Total score	5–6	7–9	10–15
Child's grade equivalent	A	B	C

Table 4.2 Percentage survival in chronic liver disease

Child's grade	1 year	5 years	10 years
A	84	44	27
B	62	20	10
C	42	21	0

Drug-induced hepatotoxicity

Background

Accounts for < 5% of cases of jaundice, but 30–50% of cases of <u>acute liver failure</u>. Incidence approximately 1:10,000 to 1:100,000 persons exposed to drug. Risk factors for drug reaction include: female sex; old age (may relate to reduced hepatic blood flow and renal clearance); obesity (e.g., methotrexate-induced hepatic fibrosis); fasting (e.g., acetaminophen); multiple drug use (induction of cytochrome P450 may be important); alcohol (especially acetaminophen, isoniazid, methotrexate); chronic liver disease (increased risk of anti-TB and HAART-related liver reactions in patients with chronic viral hepatitis).

The injury caused can be considered in terms of the mechanism of toxicity, and the site of injury within the liver.

Table 4.3 Common causes of drug-induced liver injury

Injury	Common examples	Comments
Hepatocellular	Acetaminophen	Hepatic necrosis
	Methotrexate, tetracycline, valproate, herbal remedies, HAART, amiodarone	Steatosis
	Isoniazid, sulfonamides, disulfuram, aspirin, ketoconazole, terbinafine, minocycline	Acute or chronic hepatitis
Cholestasis	Amoxicillin–clavulanate acid, flucloxacillin, erythromycin, amitryptiline, phenytoin, chlorpromazine, trimethoprim–sulfamethoxazole	Cholestatic hepatitis (hepatocanalicular)
	Anabolic steroids, estrogens	Canalicular
Granulomas	Diltiazem, allopurinol, hydralazine, carbamazepine, quinidine, quinine	Varying degrees of cholestasis/hepatitis
Fibrosis	Methotrexate	-
Vascular	Azathioprine, busulphan	Veno-occlusive disease
	Vitamin A, methotrexate	Noncirrhotic portal hypertension

Mechanism of toxicity

Drugs may induce liver injury through two broad types of reaction.
- Dose-dependent, direct hepatotoxic effects. Toxic effects may relate to "increased dose'\" (e.g., acetaminophen) or "cumulative dose."
- Idiosyncratic effects. Reaction unpredictable, not dose related. Likely to occur due to "multi-hit" process involving genetic and immune mechanisms. Onset 5–90 days after ingestion, and usually damages hepatocytes, leading to hepatitis (i.e., ↑ AST/ALT). Continued use or re-exposure to drug may be fatal.

Site of injury

Clues to the causative agent may be gained by the morphological pattern of liver injury (Table 4.3). Hepatocellular injury may manifest as steatosis, hepatic necrosis, or acute/chronic hepatitis.

Clinical features

- No pathognomonic features of drug-induced liver injury.
- Fever, rash, lymphadenopathy may be present in allergic idiosyncratic reactions, and jaundice may be preceded by prodrome of nausea, vomiting, and anorexia (as with viral hepatitis).
- Cholestatic patterns of injury may mimic biliary obstruction (i.e., pruritis and jaundice).

Diagnosis/investigation

- Usually no specific diagnostic tests (except in <u>acetaminophen overdose</u>), so diagnosis relies on clinical suspicion, careful drug history (including all prescribed, complementary, and recreational drugs/preparations), consideration of the temporal relationships between drug ingestion and liver disease, and exclusion of other disorders.
- "Liver screen" of blood tests necessary to define pattern and severity of liver injury, and other causes (see <u>Approaches to recent-onset jaundice</u> and <u>well patient with abnormal liver tests</u>). Serum ALT > 1,000 U/l strongly suggests drug injury, acute viral hepatitis, or hepatic ischemia.
- Peripheral eosinophilia may point toward an allergic drug reaction.
- Liver U/S excludes biliary obstruction in patient with cholestasis.
- <u>Liver biopsy</u> findings are rarely specific for a drug reaction (although eosinophils and granulomas may suggest an allergic reaction).

Avoid diagnostic rechallenge with the suspected drug in almost all cases (risk of even more severe reaction), unless drug toxicity is highly questionable, or no alternative to suspected drug for a serious condition.

Management

- Stopping causative drug is fundamental intervention (failure to do so is associated with high mortality). In patients on combination of drugs, the one started most recently may be the likeliest culprit. Nevertheless, stopping all drugs is the wisest maneuver, if clinically possible. If patient improves, drugs least likely to be responsible may be carefully reintroduced.
- <u>CORTICOSTEROIDS</u> may be used for severe allergic-type reactions, and <u>URSODEOXYCHOLIC ACID (UDCA)</u> for cholestatic reactions, but no clear trial evidence of benefit.
- Patients with evidence of liver failure (e.g., INR >1.5, or <u>hepatic encephalopathy</u>) require transfer to a <u>liver transplant</u> center (also see <u>acute liver failure</u>).

Dubin–Johnson syndrome

- Rare, autosomal recessive cause of conjugated hyperbilirubinemia (see <u>recent-onset jaundice</u> and <u>bilirubin metabolism</u>). Impaired excretion of bilirubin, leading to mild jaundice (Bn < 120 µmol/l, 50% conjugated), but normal liver function. No specific treatment, but good prognosis.

Fatty liver

- A spectrum characterized by the presence of fat deposits within hepatocytes. May range from fatty liver alone (steatosis) to fatty liver associated with inflammation (steatohepatitis). It can occur with the use of alcohol (see <u>alcoholic liver disease</u>) or in its absence (<u>nonalcoholic fatty liver disease</u>—NAFLD). Nonalcoholic steatohepatitis (NASH) increasingly considered as part of the spectrum of NAFLD, but associated heptatocyte inflammation and cell death in NASH may lead to fibrosis and cirrhosis.
- Steatosis affects > 20% of US adult population, with most common associations including alcohol, obesity, and diabetes mellitus. Steatosis also found on <u>liver biopsy</u> in 50% of patients with chronic <u>hepatitis C</u>. Prognostic factors in developing fibrosis include age > 45 years, diabetes mellitus, and high <u>body mass index</u> (BMI).
- Most patients asymptomatic. Hepatomegaly is common, but splenomegaly and ascites suggests cirrhosis.
- In <u>liver function tests</u>, AST-to-ALT ratio of > 2 suggests alcohol use, whereas ratio < 1 more consistent with NAFLD.
- On U/S liver is hyperechogenic, or bright. Steatosis is detected only when > 30% fatty change present.
- Diagnosis of fatty liver only definitively established with <u>liver biopsy</u>. Histologic findings include steatosis, which is usually macrovesicular, and neutrophil/mononuclear cell infiltrate. Fibrosis or cirrhosis may be present in advanced cases.
- Management depends on addressing the cause (e.g., weight reduction, diabetic control, abstinence from alcohol, drug cessation), but specific treatments for <u>nonalcoholic fatty liver disease</u> show promise. Fatty liver may completely resolve, with no residual architectural damage.

Focal nodular hyperplasia (FNH)

- Most commonly found in women < 40 years, and incidental finding in majority.
- Nonspecific abdominal pain in 15%, and spontaneous hemorrhage is rare. No clear link with oral contraceptive, in contrast with hepatic adenomas. FNH is thought to arise as hyperplastic response to pre-existing vascular malformation (and condition linked to cavernous <u>haemangiomas</u> elsewhere.
- On CT, central hypodense scar, and vascular enhancement with IV contrast, is characteristic. Most lesions < 5 cm, with histology resembling cirrhosis (but with surrounding normal parenchyma), and central stellate scar often containing thick-walled blood vessels.
- Surgical resection may be indicated if significant symptoms are clearly attributable to FNH, if complication has occurred (e.g., hemorrhage), or if there is doubt about the diagnosis.

Gilbert's syndrome

Described by Nicolas Augustin Gilbert, 1858–1927, French physician, so "soft" G in pronunciation.

Gilbert's syndrome is the commonest of the disorders of hyperbilirubinemia (see <u>bilirubin metabolism</u>), and is found in 5–10% of Caucasian populations. Diagnosis often made on routine blood testing (raised bilirubin (usually < 4 mg/dl), with all other liver tests entirely normal; or occasionally when intercurrent illness leads to transient clinical jaundice (see <u>recent-onset jaundice</u>). Prolonged fast may downregulate bilirubin uridine diphosphate glucuronosyltransferase (UGT)-1 enzyme, so precipitating jaundice, but test has low sensitivity in making diagnosis. <u>Liver biopsy</u> is rarely needed, or the risks justified. Life expectancy normal, and no specific treatment.

HELLP syndrome

Background

- HELLP syndrome (hemolysis, elevated liver enzymes, low platelets) is a microangiopathic disease, and one of the liver conditions specifically related to pregnancy (see also <u>acute fatty liver of pregnancy</u>, <u>obstetric cholestasis</u>).
- Occurs in 20% of patients with pre-eclampsia, and associated with significant fetal and maternal morbidity/mortality.

Clinical features

- Presentation usually weeks 27–36 of pregnancy, but after delivery in 30%.
- Classic features include malaise, right upper quadrant pain, nausea, vomiting, and symptoms/signs of pre-eclampsia (thirst, headache, blurred vision, proteinuria, hypertension, peripheral edema). May develop in absence of pre-eclampsia. Clinical jaundice in only 5%.
- Maternal complications include disseminated intravascular coagulation (in 20%), placental abruption, subcapsular hematoma.
- Maternal mortality 1%; perinatal mortality up to 30%.

Investigations

- ↓Hb (usually < 9 g/dl), fragmented cells on film, ↑and serum lactate dehydrogenase (LDH) level > 600 IU/l suggest hemolysis. Platelets < 100 x 10⁹/l.
- Serum aminotransferase (AST, ALT) levels x 2–15 ULN (mean approx 250 U/l), and bilirubin x2 ULN (i.e., approx 2 mg/dl). Massive elevation of AST/ALT (e.g., > 2000 U/l) suggests liver infarction/haematoma.
- ↑D-dimers may predict severity.
- <u>Liver biopsy</u> demonstrates periportal hemorrhage/necrosis and fibrin deposition, but rarely warranted, as findings correlate poorly with laboratory tests and outcome, and there are increased risks of procedure.
- <u>U/S</u> or <u>CT scan</u> may show subcapsular hematoma/infarction.

Management

- Delivery as soon as possible (ideally beyond 32 weeks, by vaginal delivery), usually leads to prompt resolution. CORTICOSTEROIDS are often given prior to delivery (largely for speeding fetal lung maturity), but no clear evidence of improvement in outcome of HELLP.
- Liver transplantation has been successful in those with acute liver failure.
- Recurrence of HELLP in future pregnancies of < 5%.

Hemangioma

- Benign vascular liver lesion, with reported prevalence of 1–20% of adult population. More common in women (may get larger in pregnancy), and usually identified at age 30–50 years. Range from < 1 cm to > 20 cm (most < 5 cm), and usually asymptomatic (rarely present with pain, hemorrhage, or rupture).
- Diagnosis on transabdominal ultrasound suggested by subliver capsule, well-defined hyperechoic lesion. CT scan classically shows low density lesion with delayed filling with contrast. Appearance on MRI of hyperintensity on T2-weighted images. Angiography occasionally necessary.
- Surgery indicated if hemangioma very large, getting larger (e.g., on 6–12 monthly U/S), or diagnosis uncertain (misdiagnosis of malignant liver tumors as hemangiomas is well recognized).

Hemochromatosis

Epidemiology + pathogenesis

- Hemochromatosis denotes iron overload, and may be "primary" (genetic hemochromatosis (GH)), or "secondary" (repeated transfusions, excess dietary iron). Usual total body iron is 3–4 g; in GH it may be > 20 g.
- 90% of GH cases are due to substitution of tyrosine for cysteine at position 282 of the HFE gene located on chromosome 6 (C282Y mutation). It shows autosomal recessive inheritance, with 10% of northern European populations heterozygous (+/−) and 1% homozygous (+/+) for C282Y mutation. There is low penetrance of clinical disease, partly due to menstruating iron loss in pre-menopausal women.
- Understanding of mechanism of iron overload is incomplete, but may involve reduced expression of HFE gene product at cell surface, increasing affinity of transferrin receptor for transferrin. Cellular iron may induce tissue injury through oxidant injury.
- Relationship between alcohol and iron overload is complex. In patients with GH (C282Y +/+), cirrhosis is nine times more common in those drinking > 60 g of alcohol/day than in those taking less. Reasons for this are unclear, but likely due to cofactor effect of alcohol and GH on oxidative stress, hepatic stellate cell activation, and hepatic fibrogenesis. Hepatic iron overload may also occur in alcoholic liver disease per se, independent of GH (but C282Y mutation should be excluded in alcoholic patients with any evidence of iron overload—see later).
- C282Y+/− has been linked with a number of clinical scenarios (porphyria cutanea tarda, increased fibrosis in hepatitis C, alcoholic

liver disease, nonalcoholic steatohepatitis (see nonalcoholic fatty liver disease), but evidence for clinical iron overload in compound heterozygotes (C282Y+/−, H63D+/−) is more convincing.

Clinical features

- Abdominal: hepatomegaly, cirrhosis, hepatocellular carcinoma (15% of untreated cases), splenomegaly.
- Cardiovascular: cardiomyopathy.
- Endocrine: diabetes mellitus, hypogonadism, panhypopituitarism, testicular atrophy.
- Skin: pigmentation ("bronze diabetes"), porphyria cutanea tarda (vesicular rash, back of hands), loss of axillary/pubic hair (secondary to hypopituitarism).
- Skeletal: chondrocalcinosis (often affecting knees), arthritis in second and third metacarpophalangeal joints.

Investigations

- Serum ferritin (upper normal limit males: > 300 µg/l, females: > 200 µg/l). In absence of other causes of elevated ferritin (e.g., inflammatory disease), serum ferritin > 1000 µg/l strongly suggests GH.
- Transferrin saturation: > 45% suggestive of iron overload.
- Liver Biopsy (Color plate 7). Gold standard for diagnosis, with assessment of severity and pattern of Perl's haemosiderin stain (grade I–IV siderosis), and measurement of hepatic iron index (HII; µmol iron per g dry weight of liver/age in years). HII > 1.9 suggests GH.
- C282Y gene analysis useful, but incomplete penetrance of C282Y+/+ and fact that GH also occurs in C282−/− patients necessitate full biochemical tests in those with features suggestive of GH.
- MRI scanning has high specificity for demonstrating liver iron overload, but poor sensitivity, and has not replaced need for biopsy in most cases.
- Liver function tests. Often normal or minimally deranged.
- Fasting glucose.
- LH/FSH. May be reduced, with impaired response to gonadotrophin-releasing hormone.

Management

- Venesect one unit of blood (450 ml; 0.25 g of iron) every one to three weeks, with measurement of ferritin and Hb every four to six sections. Aim for Hb lower end of normal range, and ferritin < 50 µg/l. May take two years, but when achieved can reduce venesection rate to every three to six months.
- Iron chelation (desferrioxamine infusion 2 g x 3/week) occasionally needed when venesection not tolerated (e.g., patients with heart failure), but less effective, and rarely first-line treatment.
- Excluded hepatocellular carcinoma, especially if cirrhotic, with alpha fetoprotein + ultrasound every three to six months.
- Refer to endocrinologist for management of hypogonadotrophic hypogonadism. Hormone replacement often required.
- Strongly advise stopping/minimizing alcohol (no clear safe lower limit defined).
- Screening of relatives for GH is vital. If index case has C282Y+/+, screen using genetic analysis, transferrin saturation, and serum ferritin. If index case does not have genetic mutation demonstrated, screen biochemically.

Hepatic drug metabolism

- Phase 1 metabolism usually involves oxidation reaction, with insertion of a hydroxyl group, catalysed by the cytochrome p450 family of enzymes. There are 20 cytochrome p450 members falling into three groups. Some are inducible and some not.
- Phase 2 metabolism involves conjugation to polar ligands (glucuronide, sulphate, glutathione, amino), which generally enhances water solubility.
- Effects on drug metabolism (e.g., induction of cytochrome p450) underlie some types of drug-induced hepatotoxicity.

Hepatic encephalopathy

Background

- Hepatic encephalopathy (HE) encompasses a spectrum of neuropsychiatric disturbances observed in patients with significant liver dysfunction. It may also occasionally occur in patients with large portosystemic shunts in the absence of intrinsic liver disease.
- May develop in Acute liver failure or in patients with chronic liver disease and portal hypertension. In the latter, HE may be acute and episodic, related to a precipitant, or chronic and persistent, due to the combination of portosystemic shunting and liver dysfunction (see cirrhosis and chronic liver disease).
- Debate remains about the most important toxins contributing to HE, but there is consensus that it develops due to reduced hepatic metabolism of gut-derived metabolites, as a result of impaired liver synthetic function and portosystemic shunting. Ammonia appears to be important, but hypotheses have also implicated the role of opiates, manganese, false neurotransmitters, and tryptophan.

Clinical features

- HE is a clinical diagnosis that should be considered in any patient with liver disease and confusion or altered consciousness.
- Subclinical HE may be difficult to diagnose, but may have a significant effect on the lives of > 30% of patients with cirrhosis. Diagnosis may require electroencephalography or psychometric testing. A clinical grading system is applied to overt HE (Table 4.1). Overt HE in chronic liver disease carries a poor prognosis, with a 1 year survival of < 50%.

Assessment

In the history, ask about increased sleepiness and reversal of normal sleep pattern. Has patient or friends/family noted any change in personality or intellect?

Investigations

- In the patient with suspected HE, in whom a diagnosis of liver disease has not previously been made, the extent and cause of liver injury need to be established (see recent-onset jaundice).

Table 4.4 Grade of hepatic encephalopathy

Grade	Features	Liver flap (asterixis)
1	Impaired higher functions (e.g., arithmetic), but no effect on consciousness	Usually absent
2	Disorientation and personality change with inappropriate behavior	Usually present
3	Confusion and gross disorientation with increased somnolence	Present
4	Coma	Usually absent

Table 4.5 Precipitants of HE and hepatic decompensation

Progressive liver injury	Dehydration (may be secondary to diuretics)
Additional liver insult (e.g., alcohol, hepatitis A)	Constipation
Upper GI bleeding	Renal failure
Hepatocellular carcinoma	Drugs (e.g., opiates)
Infection (e.g., spontaneous bacterial peritonitis)	Noncompliance with treatment
Increased portosystemic shunt (e.g., new TIPSS formation)	Large protein meal
Zinc deficiency	

- Laboratory findings that suggest underlying liver disease include ↑prothrombin time, ↑bilirubin, ↓albumin (the three tests most indicative of poor liver function), ↑liver enzymes (AST/ALT/ALP/GGT), ↓platelets (?splenomegaly/hypersplensim in portal hypertension), ↓serum Na⁺.
- In patients with known cirrhosis, HE in association with worse liver function requires a search for an additional liver insult (e.g., alcohol binge, acute viral hepatitis, ischemia.
- Abdominal U/S or CT scan may show evidence of portal hypertension.
- Tests for HE *per se* are relatively nonspecific. Raised serum ammonia levels are elevated in patients with portal hypertension, but correlation with HE is poor. Sensory evoked potentials remain a research tool. On EEG, normal waveform may be replaced in HE by slower, higher amplitude delta waves. Although similar changes seen in renal or respiratory failure, their appearance may predate overt HE, and so EEG has a role.
- Seek a precipitant, including septic screen (culture of blood, urine, sputum, acites), exclusion of GI bleed (? ↓Hb, melena on examination, serum urea disproportionately elevated with respect to creatinine), or renal impairment.

Management

- **Supportive care** for the patient in coma is essential. ICU assessment and admission is necessary for patients with grade 3/4 HE, with consideration of endotracheal intubation if safe airway not maintained.
- **Treatment** of precipitants alone leads to resolution of HE in > 60% of cases. Give antibiotics for overt sepsis, as well as for patients with variceal bleeding, in view of an association of sepsis with bleeding (see acute upper GI bleeding), and the potentially additive effects of sepsis and high protein gut load leading to HE. Obsessive care of potential new sites of sepsis, such as IV cannulae, pressure areas, is vital. Precipitant drugs should be stopped. Renal impairment should be treated by controlling sepsis and ensuring adequate plasma expansion (also see hepatorenal syndrome).
- **Diet.** There is little evidence for the time-honored role of protein restriction in patients with HE and, as these patients are often malnourished, it may exacerbate problems. Protein intake should be maintained at 1–1.5 g/kg/day, with a transient reduction to 0.5 g/kg/day only if overall treatment fails. Vegetable-based protein diets may be more effective than animal-based ones.
- **Bowel cleansing** helps to reduce ammoniagenic substrates from the gut. Give lactulose 30–50 ml four times per day orally or via NG (no evidence that fine-bore NG tubes precipitate bleeding in patients with varices), aiming to ensure two to four soft stools passed daily. Improvement in HE is expected in 24–48 hours.
- **Antibiotics** against urease-producing gut bacteria are rarely used as first-line treatment, but may have a role in patients unresponsive to standard therapy e.g., neomycin 1–2 mg/day; metronidazole 250 mg tds PO; Rifaximin 550 mg twice a day. Antibiotics should not be given long term in view of toxicity.
- **Newer treatments** may gain an established role. Sodium benzoate 10 g/day PO improves ammonia clearance by increasing nitrogen excretion, and may be used with lactulose. Metabolic substrates for the conversion of ammonia to urea (e.g., ornithine aspartate 9 g/day PO) have been shown to reduce period of clinical HE. Conversion of ammonia to urea is zinc-dependent, and zinc acetate 600 mg daily has been shown to improve HE, compared to placebo.

Hepatic granulomas

- Granulomas are found in 4–10% of liver biopsies, and there is a wide range of causes, although autoimmune liver disease, sarcoidosis, and TB probably account for most (see Box 4. 2). They are frequently found in patients with HIV, often related to underlying infection (*M. tuberculosis*, *M. avium intracellulare*, *Cytomegalovirus*, *Toxoplasma*), lymphomatous infiltration, or drug reaction. Hepatic granulomas may develop as part of a lupus-like drug reaction.
- The classical presentation is varied (reflecting the wide range of underlying causes), but hepatomegaly is found in only 20% of cases. Granulomatous hepatitis presents with fever of unknown origin in

50% of cases, and there is debate as to whether it is a variant of sarcoidosis.
- LFTs often show ↑ALP/GGT. Range of diagnostic tests may be needed to identify cause (e.g., CXR and serum angiotensin-converting enzyme (SACE) for sarcoidosis).
- Treatment depends on the cause. Corticosteroids may improve fever and LFTs in hepatic sarcoid/idiopathic granulomatous hepatitis. Drug-related granulomatous reaction usually responds to cessation.

Box 4.2 Causes of hepatic granulomas

Drugs
- Sulphonamides
- Hydralazine
- Procainamide
- Allopurinol
- Isoniazid
- Carbamazepine
- Chlorpropramide
- Phenylbutazone
- Quinidine
- Tolbutamide

Infection
- Mycobacterium <u>Tuberculosis</u>
- M. avium intracellulare
- Brucella
- Syphilis
- Leprosy
- <u>Schistosomiasis</u>
- <u>Whipple's disease</u>
- Q fever
- Coxiella burnetii
- <u>HIV</u>/AIDS

Industrial
- Berylliosis

Neoplasia
- Hodgkin's lymphoma
- NonHodgkin's lymphoma

Immunological disease
- <u>Inflammatory bowel disease</u>
- <u>Sarcoidosis</u>
- Systemic lupus erythematosis
- Granulomatous hepatitis
- <u>Primary biliary cirrhosis</u> (PBC)
- PBC/autoimmune hepatitis <u>overlap syndrome</u>
- <u>Polyarteritis nodosum</u>
- Wegener's granulomatosis

Hepatitis A

Epidemiology

Hepatitis A virus (HAV) infection remains the cause of a large number of reported cases of acute viral hepatitis in the United States. Transmission is through fecal–oral route, infected water supply, and ingestion of uncooked shellfish. It is the most common vaccine-preventable infection in travelers to areas of high endemicity (e.g., N. Africa, S. America, where > 95% of children by 10 years have been exposed).

Clinical features

- HAV only causes acute, never chronic, hepatitis. Likelihood of developing jaundice increases with age (79% in patients > 15 years), and this occurs three to five weeks after infection, often preceded by a prodrome of malaise, anorexia. Adults often feel unwell for six weeks.
- Prolonged cholestasis may occur in 5% of cases. Acute liver failure reported in < 0.1% of cases, but may be more common in conjunction with chronic hepatitis C.

Investigation

Liver function tests demonstrate markedly ↑ALT (often > 1000 U/l) during acute icteric phase. Diagnosis usually confirmed by HAV IgM Ab in serum, which appears five to eight weeks after onset of symptoms. Liver biopsy rarely indicated.

Management

- No specific treatment of acute hepatitis A is necessary.
- Prednisolone 40 mg PO daily, and tapering off over two to four weeks, may speed resolution of prolonged cholestasis. See acute liver failure for very rare severe hepatitis A.
- "Prevention is better than cure." HAV vaccine is very effective, and should be offered to: travelers to areas of increased risk; IV drug users; men who have sex with men; patients with hemophilia or chronic liver disease (including hepatitis C, who may have increased risk of acute liver failure); those at occupational risk (e.g., child care centre workers). 1 ml of vaccine given initially, and then at six to twelve months, provides 95% protection for > five years.
- Passive immunization, with human normal immunoglobulin (HNIG) has few indications, due to the rapid efficacy of HAV vaccine (even postexposure), and worries about transmission of prion disease (HNIG manufactured from pooled serum).

Hepatitis B

Epidemiology

- More than 300 million people worldwide are infected with hepatitis B virus (HBV), with chronic infection in 0.1–2% in Western Europe and United States, and up to 20% in areas of Southeast Asia.

- Most common route of transmission is perinatally (90% infection rate in infants born to HBeAg+ve mothers), but blood inoculation through unclean needles remains important. Sexual transmission accounts for 30% of infections in developed countries.

Clinical features

Acute hepatitis B. Jaundice, malaise, and right upper quadrant pain may develop one to four months after infection. Although <u>acute liver failure</u> may develop in 2% of cases, acute hepatitis results in viral clearance in > 95% of infected adults.

Chronic hepatitis B. Defined by HBsAg+ve in serum > 6/12. Age at infection strongly determines chronicity, reflecting host immunity (> 90% in neonates, 20–50% age 1–5 years, < 5% in adults). Different patterns of chronic infection correlate with serological markers (see Table 4.6). Highest rate of complications in highly replicating disease (i.e., HBeAg+ve, or precore mutant infection). Spontaneous clearance of infection (i.e., becoming HBsAg–ve) occurs in 1% of chronically infected patients/year. **Complications** include:

- **Cirrhosis**. Once develops (usually 30–40 years after perinatal infection, but very variable), five-year survival of approximately 80%, but this falls to 35% after episode of decompensation (see <u>cirrhosis and chronic liver disease</u>).
- <u>Hepatocellular carcinoma</u>. Nearly 100-fold increased risk in chronic hepatitis B. Annual incidence 2–6% in those with cirrhosis, 0.4–0.6% in noncirrhotics.
- Membranous glomerulonephritis.
- <u>Polyarteritis nodosum</u>.

Investigations

- HBV serology: HBsAg (indicates ongoing infection); HBeAg (presence confirms high viral replication, but may be negative in HBeAg–ve chronic hepatitis B ('pre-core mutant'); anti-HBe (reciprocal of HBeAg); anti-HBc IgM (acute infection); anti-HBc IgG (previous or ongoing infection); anti-HBs (resolved infection or vaccinated).
- HBV DNA by PCR: Essential if HBsAg+ve, HBeAg–ve, in order to exclude precore infection (HBeAg+ve, HBV DNA > 10^5 copies/ml, ↑ALT).
- <u>Liver function tests</u>. AST/ALT usually > 1,000 U/l in acute hepatitis. LFTs may fluctuate in chronic infection, but ALT < 80 U/l strongly predicts lack of HBeAg seroconversion (loss of HBeAg, development of serum anti-HBe) in response to antiviral therapy (i.e., a lack of sustained treatment response).
- <u>Alpha fetoprotein</u>. Perform every six months with liver <u>ultrasound</u>, especially in cirrhotics, in view of <u>hepatocellular carcinoma</u> risk.
- <u>Liver biopsy</u>. Rarely needed in acute hepatitis B. Indicated in chronic infection, when treatment is considered (see management algorithm).
- HIV testing should be considered in all with chronic hepatitis B, especially if lamivudine planned for HBV infection (as lamivudine monotherapy for undiagnosed HIV infection may promote HIV treatment-escape mutants).

Table 4.6 Patterns of HBV infection and serology

Clinical state	HBsAg	HBeAg	Anti-HBc IgM	Anti-HBc IgG	Anti-HBs	Anti-HBe	HBV DNA	Serum ALT	Comments
Acute infection	+	+/−	+	+/−	−	+/−	+/−	↑↑	HBsAg may be −ve at presentation
Chronic low replication	+	−	−	+	−	+	+	N	
Chronic high replication	+	+	−	+	−	−	+++	N/i	ALT may be > 1,000 U/l, and anti-HBcIgM+ve in flare of disease
HbeAg−ve chronic hepatitis B ('pre-core mutant')	+	−	−	+	−	+	++	↑	Common in S Europe
Vaccinated	−	−	−	−	+	−	−	N	
Resolved infection	−	−	−	+/−	+	+/−	−	N	Anti-HBc IgM+ve if recently resolved

Box 4.3 Practice points in interpreting HBV serology

- HBsAg may rarely be negative at presentation in acute hepatitis B (and particularly in severe/fulminant disease, due to profound immune-mediated response to infection, and associated liver damage). However, anti-HBc IgM will be positive.
- HBeAg positive confirms high level of HBV DNA (measurement of absolute level of virus rarely changes management in this setting). In contrast HBV DNA quantification is essential in all cases of HBeAg-negative chronic infection, to exclude "pre-core mutant" infection.
- Anti-HBc IgM may occasionally be positive in acute flares of chronic infection. Differentiation from acute primary infection often difficult, but chronic infection may be suggested by knowledge of prior positive serology, and subsequent lack of HBsAg seroconversion (as occurs in > 95% of cases of acute infection). Liver biopsy may be needed to confirm chronic disease.

Management

- *Acute hepatitis B*. No definitive evidence that antiviral therapy effects disease course, but lamivudine has been given for fulminant hepatitis B.
- *Chronic hepatitis B*. Usual goal of treatment is to suppress HBV replication, induce HBeAg seroconversion (clearance of HBeAg, appearance of anti-HBe), and reduce liver injury. Ultimate goal is to clear HBsAg and prevent cirrhosis and HCC. Treatment is indicated for those with replicative disease (i.e., HBeAg+ve, or pre-core infection) and liver injury. Rate of HBeAg seroconversion with present antivirals closely related to pre-treatment ALT (<10% if ALT < x2 ULN, >50% if ALT > x5 ULN).
  - <u>INTERFERON ALPHA</u> (IFN-α) (e.g., 6 MU x3/week for six months) induces HBeAg seroconversion in 30% at one year, and HBsAg loss in 5–10%. Standard IFN increasingly being replaced (in trials and clinical practice) by pegylated (PEG) IFN, with recent trials showing 30–36% HBeAg seroconversion following one-year course of treatment.[1] Range of important side effects of IFN (see <u>hepatitis C</u>), and contraindicated in decompensated cirrhosis.

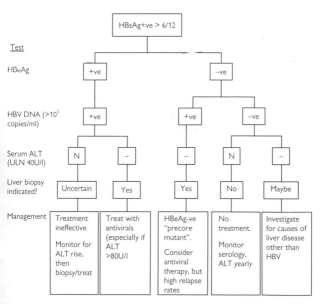

Figure 4.1 Management algorithm for chronic hepatitis B. *Note*. Consider surveillance for hepatocellular carcinoma in all chronically infected patients (e.g., every six months AFP and U/S).

1 Lau, GKK et al. (2005). *N. Engl. J. Med.* 352: 2682; Janssen, HL et al. (2005) Lancet 365: 123

- LAMIVUDINE has few side effects and is easy to take. Induces HBeAg seroconversion in 25% after 1 year of use, 56% after three years, but treatment-resistant YMDD variants may develop in > 40% after three years of use. Conflicting trial results on merit of combination LAMIVUDINE + PEG IFN therapy, but recent large trials of HBeAg+ve infection (see above) suggest no additional benefit of adding LAMIVUDINE to PEG IFN. Lamivudine remains drug of choice in patients with decompensated cirrhosis, and prior to liver transplantation to control replication.
  - ADEFOVIR depixol. Main indication at present as additional therapy in patients on maintenance LAMIVUDINE who develop YMDD variants, especially posttransplantation.
  - ENTECAVIR AND TENOFAVIR ARE NOW APPROVED. BOTH AGENTS ARE POTENT WITH HIGH RATES OF HBV DNA SUPPRESSION AND MINIMAL RATES OF DRUG INDUCED RESISTANCE.
- HBeAg-ve chronic infection ("precore mutant"). Need for effective treatment, as disease is often more progressive than HBeAg+ve disease. However, although antivirals may control HBV DNA during treatment (e.g., LAMIVUDINE, IFN, PEG IFN, combination), viral replication increases again after cessation.
- Other disease groups. LAMIVUDINE indicated in patients co-infected with HIV, in combination with other antiretroviral therapy. Antiviral therapy leading to control of replication may improve membranous glomerulonephritis and polyarteritis nodosum. LAMIVUDINE given to control replication prior to transplantation, and (± hepatitis B immunoglobulin (HBIG) peritransplant) may reduce infection of new graft.
- Hepatitis B vaccination. In USA vaccination of new born infants is universal. Passive immunization with hepatitis B immunoglobulin (HBIG) (Table 4.7) given at 0.1 ml/kg body weight after exposure (or birth to chronically infected mother) with immunization are recommended.

Table 4.7 Indications for HBV immunization

Active (hepatitis B vaccine)	Passive (HBIG)
Family contacts of individual with HBV infection	Postexposure prophylaxis
Babies born to infected mothers (± HBIG if mother HBsAg+ve, HBeAg+ve)	Newborns of mothers who are HBsAg+ve, HBeAg+ve (with vaccine)
IV drug users	
Regular receivers of blood (e.g., hemophilia)	Newborns of mothers with acute hepatitis B in 3rd trimester
Patients with chronic renal failure	
Health care workers	
Sexual contacts of infected individual	
Travelers to areas of high endemicity	

Hepatitis C

Epidemiology

- More than 150 million people worldwide are infected with hepatitis C virus (HCV), an RNA virus of the flavivirus family. Up to 2% of people have been exposed to HCV, with higher rates in Asia and Africa.
- Transmission mainly through injection-drug use or blood-product transfusion (virtually eliminated in developed countries now due to screening of donated blood). Use of nondisposable needles during treatment of <u>schistosomiasis</u> may have contributed to the high prevalence of HCV in Egypt (15% of population). Skin piercing procedures of proven risk. Rate of HCV transmission in monogamous heterosexual relationships appears low (< 6%). Transmission from mother to infant occurs in about 5% of cases, but increased to 18% if mother co-infected with HIV. Breastfeeding transmission not reported. No risk factors reported in 10–20% of cases.
- Six main HCV genotypes (1–6), with subtypes (a–c). Geographical variation in predominant genotype: e.g., 1, 2, 3 in Europe, United States; genotype 4 in Egypt, Middle East.

Clinical features

- Less than 15% of patients develop acute icteric hepatitis (although spontaneous viral clearance may then occur in up to 50%).
- Chronic infection follows infection in 50–85% of cases, as defined by persistence of HCV RNA in the serum. Infection usually clinically silent, with liver damage occurring over many years. Studies suggest that 20% of patients will develop severe fibrosis/cirrhosis after 20 years of infection, but recent data suggest a lower rate in the absence of cofactors (e.g., alcohol). Risk factors for disease progression include high circulating virus level, long duration of disease, male sex, older age at acquisition, alcohol excess, and co-infection with HIV/<u>hepatitis B</u>.
- Up to 4% of patients per year with HCV cirrhosis develop <u>hepatocellular carcinoma</u>.
- Nonspecific complaints, including fatigue, headache, and poor concentration, are commonly reported. HCV may have direct CNS effects.
- Extraintestinal manifestations have been associated with chronic HCV (See Box 4.4), the pathogenesis of which remains uncertain.

Investigation

- Anti-HCV antibody. Positive ELISA test (and particularly RIBA test) confirms exposure to HCV, but not persistence of infection. May be negative in early phase of acute infection.
- HCV RNA by PCR. HCV RNA positivity confirms ongoing infection, with cut-off variable, but usually 10–1000 viral copies/ml.
- HCV genotype. Essential to determine this in patients considered for treatment, as influences regimen/treatment response.
- <u>Liver function tests</u>. ALT/AST ↑ approximately x1.5–2.5 ULN in chronic hepatitis C, but fluctuations throughout the course of disease

Box 4.4 Extrahepatic associations of hepatitis C

- Cryoglobulinemia
  - Detectable in 36–54% of chronic patients
  - Most patients asymptomatic
  - Arthralgia and pruritis in 18%
  - Neuropathy and glomerulonephritis in 2%
- Membranous glomerulonephritis
- Sjögren's syndrome
- Lichen planus
- Autoimmune hepatitis
- Thyroiditis
- Polyarteritis nodosum
- Polymyositis
- Porphyria cutanea tarda

are common, and there is a poor correlation between the level of ALT and either level of viremia or severity of histological disease. Other liver disease may also need to be excluded.

- Liver biopsy. Only definitive method of assessing the degree of inflammation (grade) and fibrosis (stage), and may guide a decision concerning need for treatment. Should be considered in all HCV RNA+ve patients, especially if AST/ALT persistently abnormal.
- Additional blood tests. Antismooth muscle antibodies because, although they may be an epiphenomenon in chronic HCV, true autoimmune hepatitis is a disease association, which can be exacerbated by antiviral therapy. Thyroid function tests and antithyroid autoantibodies, as abnormalities more common in hepatitis C, and thyroid abnormalities may occur with interferon therapy, particularly in the presence of antithyroid antibodies. HBsAg should be tested for as chronic hepatitis B is associated with more progressive histological disease in those with HCV. HIV testing should also be considered, in view of shared modes of acquisition.
- Abdominal U/S prior to liver biopsy, and to identify features of cirrhosis and portal hypertension. Repeat every six months (with alpha fetoprotein) in patients with proven cirrhosis, in view of risk of hepatocellular carcinoma.

Management

- Crucial to ensure that patient is aware of natural history of the disease, as many believe that progression to end-stage liver disease is inevitable, and that treatment is ineffective. Progression usually seen in those who drink excess alcohol, and no safe lower limit of alcohol known.
- Patients should be advised not to donate blood, and the risks of shared needles by drug users should be reiterated. Avoid sharing razors and toothbrushes. Sexual transmission is unusual, but condoms should be used during casual sexual contacts, to lower the risk of a range of

transmitted infections (e.g., HIV). It is prudent to test regular sexual partners of patients, but to advise that the risk of transmission is low.
- Vaccinate against <u>hepatitis A</u> and <u>hepatitis B</u>, as co-infection may lead to disease progression (hepatitis B), or fulminant liver failure.

Antiviral therapy
- Treatment has advanced significantly over last 10 years.
- NIH consensus statement declared that treatment is indicated in a patient with positive anti-HCV antibody, positive HCV-RNA, raised liver enzymes (AST, ALT), and moderate–severe hepatitis on liver biopsy, but studies may confirm that treatment benefits all viremic patients, even if minimal liver injury. Interferon is contraindicated in decompensated cirrhosis.
- Long-acting pegylated-α<u>INTERFERON</u> (PEG-IFN) + <u>RIBAVIRIN</u> has replaced standard α<u>IFN</u> alone as treatment of choice.
- "Gold standard" for assessing treatment response is sustained virological response (SVR), defined as negative HCV RNA 6 months after completing treatment. Contraindications and side-effects of treatment should be discussed (see Table 4.8).

Acute hepatitis C. Rare clinical diagnosis, but > 95% SVR with 6 months of <u>INTERFERON ALPHA</u> (IFN-α) monotherapy has been shown.[1] In practice, most experts would use PEG-IFN + <u>RIBAVIRIN</u> in this setting, in view of superior efficacy of this combination in chronic infection (although not as yet proven to be better than standard IFN for acute infection).

Chronic hepatitis C
- Standard <u>IFN-α</u> + <u>RIBAVIRIN</u> for 12 months leads to overall SVR of 38%, with a number of factors influencing treatment response (see Table 4.9).
- For HCV-genotype 2/3, PEG-IFN/<u>RIBAVIRIN</u> gives SVR of 80% on 6-month course (can even reduce to 4 four months if HCV RNA negative at 6 weeks). Genotype 1 is less responsive, with 45–55% SVR after 12-month course (discontinue drug if HCV RNA has not decreased x 2 logs at 3 months or positive at 6 months, as response unlikely).
- Special clinical scenarios in which treatment may be effective, but which require expert involvement include:
  - Patients with HIV/HCV co-infection.
  - Adults who have relapsed following a previous response to treatment.
  - Children with chronic hepatitis C.
- End-stage liver disease due to chronic hepatitis C is now the commonest indication for orthotopic <u>liver transplantation</u>. Recurrence of HCV in the grafted liver is almost universal, with cirrhosis sometimes occurring at an accelerated rate in these immunocompromised patients (up to 10% of patients within five years of transplantation).

1 Jaeckel, E. et al. (2001). *N. Engl. J. Med.* 345: 1452

Table 4.8 Side effects of hepatitis C treatment

Alpha interferon	
Influenza-like symptoms	Depression (even suicidal ideation)
Nausea	Myelosuppression
Lethargy	Hypersensitivity
Weight loss	Hypo/hyperthyroidism
Autoimmune reactions	Hair loss
Ribavirin	
Hemolysis (2 g fall in Hb usual)	Teratogenicity

Table 4.9 Predictors of long-term response to IFN

Nonviral genotype 1	Absence of cirrhosis on biopsy
Low pretreatment viremia	Low hepatic iron stores
Loss of detectable virus (negative HCV-RNA) after 1 month of treatment	ALT normalized in first 12 weeks of treatment
Younger age	Female
Nonblack racial origin	

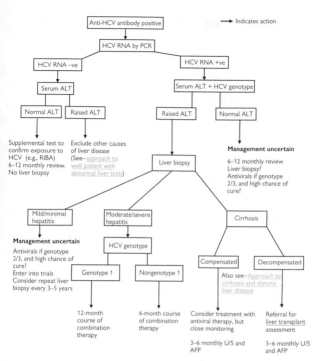

Figure 4.2 Management of hepatitis C.

Hepatitis D virus (HDV)

- RNA virus that requires <u>hepatitis B</u> virus (HBV) for complete virion assembly (5% of HBV carriers co-infected with HDV).
- As with HBV infection, HDV may cause acute hepatitis (even <u>acute liver failure</u>), asymptomatic viral carriage, or progressive chronic liver disease with cirrhosis and <u>portal hypertension</u> (more aggressive course of HDV/HBV co-infection than HBV alone). For uncertain reasons, HDV infection associated with lower risk of <u>hepatocellular carcinoma</u> than HBV infection alone.
- Presence of HBsAg necessary for diagnosis of hepatitis D. Anti-HDV IgM present in acute infection, and IgG antibodies appear in resolved or chronic infection. In contrast to hepatitis B, IgM antibodies persist at high titre in chronic infection. Serum HDV RNA detectable by PCR in acute infection and chronic disease, but test not widely available.
- Vaccination against <u>hepatitis B</u> protects against hepatitis D.
- Treatment with standard IFN (9 MU x 3/week) for 48 weeks has been associated with reduced HDV RNA, but most studies show increased viral replication following cessation of a range of treatments, and antiviral therapy remains disappointing.
- <u>Liver transplantation</u> may be required in decompensated HDV/HBV cirrhosis (again, posttransplant survival better for HDV/HBV co-infection than for HBV alone, possibly related to inhibitory effects of HDV on HBV).

Hepatitis E virus (HEV)

- RNA virus that is endemic in India, Pakistan, Middle East, and Southeast Asia (accounts for > 90% of major hepatitis outbreaks in India).
- Virus spread by fecal–oral route, in association with poor sanitation (with epidemics often during monsoon season, on 10-year cycle).
- Incubation period 15–65 days, followed by acute icteric hepatitis (jaundice, malaise, nausea, anorexia). Cholestatic hepatitis more common than for <u>hepatitis A</u> or <u>hepatitis B</u>. Chronic hepatitis rarely occurs, and usually settles clinically within 6 weeks. Chronic infection has been described in immunocompromised organ transplant recipients.
- <u>Acute liver failure</u> may occur, with a reported maternal mortality in those infected in third trimester of > 20%.
- Diagnosis made by excluding other causes of acute hepatitis (see <u>recent-onset jaundice</u>), and IgM anti-HEV in the serum confirms recent infection (may be performed in specialist laboratories).
- Treatment is supportive, with <u>liver transplantation</u> considered for those with acute liver failure.

Hepatitis G virus (HGV)

HGV, and closely related GB virus, appear to be parenterally transmitted viruses, and were originally thought to be cause, in some cases, of nonA–E hepatitis. However, no clear evidence that they cause liver disease.

Hepatocellular carcinoma (HCC)

Epidemiology

- Sixth commonest cancer worldwide.
- 75–90% of patients with HCC have cirrhosis, and this complication develops in 4% of cirrhotics per year (less common if cirrhosis due to autoimmune hepatitis, primary biliary cirrhosis). Chronic hepatitis B increases risk of HCC 100-fold. Rare in hepatitis C in the absence of cirrhosis. Other risks include aflatoxins produced by fungi on nuts stored in damp conditions (e.g., common etiology of HCC in North Africa, China).

Clinical features

- Pain, weight loss, anorexia, malaise are common symptoms.
- Hepatomegaly common; hepatic bruit sometimes found.
- HCC may be the precipitating cause of hepatic decompensation and hepatic encephalopathy.
- 10% of patients present with variceal bleeding, which may be linked to portal vein thrombosis.

Investigations

- Alpha fetoprotein (AFP) elevated in 70% of cases, with levels > 400 ng/ ml strongly suggestive of HCC (normal range < 20 ng/ml). However, high levels also seen during hepatitis flares (i.e., in association with ↑↑ALT). > 60% HCCs < 4 cm have AFP < 200 ng/ml.
- Ultrasound widely used in screening/surveillance, and first modality if ↑AFP (sensitivity 95% for 1.5–3 cm HCCs). See Box 4.5 for differential diagnosis.
- CT or MRI may be necessary, particularly for multifocal HCC in cirrhotic liver.
- Angiography (± lipiodol) indicated if clinical suspicion (e.g., ↑↑AFP), but no mass on U/S, CT, MRI.
- Liver biopsy confirms histological diagnosis, but avoided if resection an option, because of risk (albeit < 2%) of needle track seeding.

Management

- Range of options for HCCs confined to the liver, determined by number, size, distribution of tumors, and underlying liver histology/ function, but ongoing debate on optimal treatment. Without treatment, three-year survival for small HCC in noncirhotic liver 45%.
- Hepatic resection if HCC confined to single lobe of noncirrhotic liver (liver biopsy of nontumorous lobe indicated prior to surgery), with 45–60% five-year survival. Resection also indicated

in well-compensated cirrhosis (<u>Child–Pugh score</u> A), but risk of decompensation.

- <u>Liver transplantation</u> effective for decompensated cirrhotic with solitary HCC < 5 cm, or no more than three lesions all < 3 cm.
- In nonsurgical candidates with localized HCCs, local ablation (e.g., percutaneous alcohol injection or radiofrequency ablation) may provide good palliation and survival comparable with hepatic resection, with mortality largely correlated with underlying liver function.
- Transcatheter chemoembolization (TACE) relies on engendering ischaemia in HCC, and targeting chemotherapy, but is contraindicated in decompensated cirrhosis and multifocal HCC.
- Systemic chemotherapy regimes disappointing to date.

Surveillance for HCC (probably with U/S every six months and AFP) indicated for all patients with cirrhosis (although rate of HCC appears lower for autoimmune aetiologies, such as <u>primary biliary cirrhosis</u>); <u>haemochromatosis</u>; and chronic <u>hepatitis B</u> (irrespective of presence of cirrhosis).

Box 4.5 Causes of mass lesions in liver

- <u>Hepatocellular carcinoma</u>
- Fibrolamellar carcinoma
- Metastases (commonest cause, due to e.g., <u>colon</u>, <u>pancreas</u>, <u>gastric cancer</u>, <u>neuroendocrine tumor</u>)
- Intrahepatic <u>cholangiocarcinoma</u>
- <u>Gallbladder carcinoma</u>
- <u>Focal nodular hyperplasia</u>
- <u>Nodular regenerative hyperplasia</u>
- Hepatic adenoma
- <u>Hemangioma</u>
- <u>Liver abscess</u>*
- <u>Hydatid disease</u>*
- <u>Lymphoma</u>
- Angiosarcoma
- Benign regenerative nodule
- Simple cyst*

*Cystic lesions.

Hepatorenal syndrome (HRS)

Background

- HRS is defined as development of renal failure in patients with severe liver disease (acute or chronic), in absence of other cause of renal pathology.
  - **Type 1 HRS** occurs acutely, often in conjunction with acute liver disease or decompensation of cirrhosis. Often in association with marked jaundice and coagulopathy.
  - **Type 2 HRS** is more chronic, usually in patients with refractory ascites and relatively mild jaundice.
- Common clinical mistake is to assume that any liver patient with renal impairment has hepatorenal syndrome. Wide range of other causes (see Table 4.10).
- Pathological process in HRS is that of profound renal arteriolar vasoconstriction leading to renal hypoperfusion in setting of hemodynamic changes of decompensated liver disease (↑ heart rate, ↑cardiac output, ↓systemic vascular resistance, ↓ mean arterial pressure).

Diagnosis

- Clinical diagnosis based around major diagnostic criteria:
  - Acute or chronic liver disease with advanced hepatic failure and ascites.
  - Serum creatinine > 1.5 mg/dl, or creatinine clearance < 40 ml/min.
  - Other causes of renal impairment excluded (hypovolaemia, bacterial sepsis, nephrotoxic drugs).
  - No sustained improvement with plasma expansion (Albumin 1 g/kg, (max 100 g) per day for 2 days).
  - Proteinuria < 0.5 g/day.
  - Normal renal tract U/S.
- Note that low urinary Na⁺ no longer major criterion for diagnosis.

Management

- Stop all potentially nephrotoxic drugs (e.g., diuretics).
- Correct hypovolemia (see also <u>albumin (use in liver disease)</u>).
- Search for and treat sepsis (common precipitant of liver decompensation). Send blood, sputum, urine, ascitic fluid.
- Drain ascites if tense (see <u>paracentesis</u>).
- Consider octreotide and midodrine
- Consider renal support (usually hemofiltration) if likely improvement in liver function/liver transplantation. (HRS rarely resolves unless liver function improves. HRS has 50–95% mortality dependent on etiology.)

Table 4.10 Causes of renal dysfunction in patient with liver disease

Hepatorenal syndrome	<u>Leptospirosis</u>
Hypovolemia (e.g., over diuresis)	<u>Amyloidosis</u>
Nephrotoxic drugs (e.g., NSAIDs, aminoglycosides, acetaminophen)	Membranous glomerulonephritis (e.g., due to <u>hepatitis B</u>)
Sepsis	Renal tubular abnormalities
Polycystic disease	<u>Acute fatty liver of pregnancy</u>

HIV and the liver

Background and etiology

Liver test abnormalities occur in 80% of patients with HIV, due to:

- Coexistent liver disease. Hepatitis B and hepatitis C common, due to similar modes of acquisition, and run more aggressive course than in nonHIV patient. Acute exacerbation of liver disease may occur following start of anti-HIV treatment due to enhanced immunity against hepatitis B.
- Immunosuppression-related infection (e.g., CD4 < 50 μl): e.g., *Mycobacterium avium intercellulare* (MAI), *M. tuberculosis* (MTB), fungal infection (e.g., *Histoplasma capsulatum*), *Pneumocystis carinii*.
- Treatment. Highly active retroviral therapy (HAART) frequently associated with LFT derangement (see Table 4.11). Acute liver failure may occur, with syndrome of hepatomegaly, steatosis, lactic acidosis, and liver failure probably related to mitochondrial toxicity. Severe toxicity in 10% taking nonnucleoside reverse transcriptase inhibitor nevirapine.
- Tumors, including nonHodgkin's lymphoma, Kaposi's sarcoma.
- Biliary disease. HIV-cholangiopathy associated with low CD4 count, with diffuse biliary strictures similar to primary sclerosing cholangitis, or distal biliary stricture/papillitis.

Clinical features Variable, dependent on type of liver injury.
Hepatomegaly common.

Investigations

- In view of high frequency of LFT derangement, clinical balance needed between not missing important/reversible liver disease, and exposing otherwise well patient to invasive investigations.
- See recent-onset jaundice and well patient with abnormal liver tests. Viral serology should be performed in all cases.
- U/S or CT may exclude biliary dilatation or liver masses.
- ERCP may be necessary to diagnose HIV cholangiopathy.
- Liver biopsy abnormalities in 90% (e.g., hepatic granulomas, steatosis), but new diagnoses only made in 8% of biopsies in HIV patients (e.g., Kaposi's sarcoma, mycobacterium).

Management

- Depends on making a specific diagnosis.
- Hepatitis B coinfection usually treated with lamivudine or tenofavir, which is also active against HIV, as part of combination HAART.
- Standard treatment for hepatitis C appears to be less effective in patients with, than without, HIV, but sustained responses possible.
- LFTs should be regularly monitored during HAART (especially first eight weeks and with reverse transcriptase inhibitors), and stopped if signs of significant hepatotoxocity (e.g., serum ALT > x5 ULN).
- Mitochondrial toxicity and liver failure have been successfully treated with liver transplantation.

Table 4.11 Common drug causes of liver derangement in HIV patients

Drug	Type/use
Indinavir	Anti-HIV protease inhibitor
Saquinivir	
Ritonovir	
Stavudine	Anti-HIV reverse transcriptase inhibitor
Didanosine	
Nevirapine	
Trimethoprim–sulfamethoxazole	*Pneumocystis* prophylaxis/treatment
Ketoconazole	Antifungal
Isoniazid	Anti-TB
Rifampicin	

Hydatid disease

Epidemiology + pathogenesis

Caused by tapeworm *Echinococcus*. Most commonly seen in farming or rural communities, where man is an accidental host for *E. granulosum*, whose life cycle usually involves the ingestion of eggs by a definite host (carnivore, e.g., dog), from an infected intermediate host (e.g., sheep).

Clinical features

Cystic echinococcosis affects the liver (63% of cases), lungs (25%), and more rarely bones, kidneys, brain.

Many cysts asymptomatic, but may cause symptoms due to mass effect (e.g., obstructive jaundice, abdominal pain) or cyst complications (rupture with anaphylaxis, secondary infection).

Investigations

- Echinococcus ELISA has 90% sensitivity for hepatic echinococcosis.
- Eosinophilia in 25%; LFTs may be elevated in patients with hepatic disease.
- CT is 98% accurate, and highly sensitive at demonstrating characteristic daughter cysts.

Management

- Surgery is optimal approach, as only 30% are cured with medical therapy alone. Surgery includes cystectomy alone, or partial affected organ resection. During surgery, sterilization of the cyst, and prevention of spillage, with risk of anaphylaxis, is essential. Chemotherapy with benzimidazoles (e.g., albendazole, mebendazole) is given for at least one month over perioperative period to prevent secondary infection.
- If surgery is not an option, "PAIR" technique of aspiration of cyst contents and injection of a scolicidal agent, followed by isotonic saline, in conjunction with oral benimidazole treatment, may be effective.

Intrahepatic cholestasis of pregnancy

Background
- Form of intrahepatic cholestasis that is responsible for 20% of cases of jaundice in pregnancy.
- Prevalence reported as 0.5–1% of pregnancies. In those women who developed cholestasis on high estrogen oral contraceptive pill, 50% developed obstetric cholestasis in subsequent pregnancies.

Clinical features
- Usual onset in second or third trimester, but may develop earlier.
- Pruritis predominates, but jaundice in 20–60% develops two to three weeks later.
- Right upper quadrant pain unusual.

Investigation
- Vital to exclude other causes of symptomatic cholestasis (e.g., choledo-cholithiasis).
- ↑Bilirubin (largely conjugated), but usually <6 mg/dl, ↑ALP (usually <1,000 U/l), ↑AST/ALT (sometimes >1,000 U/l). Curiously, GGT often normal. ↑PT may be due to deficiency of vitamin K-dependent clotting factors, rather than liver failure.
- Imaging with ultrasound essential to exclude biliary obstruction.
- Liver biopsy rarely necessary, but shows intrahepatic cholestasis, bile plugging, and minimal inflammation.

Management
- Symptoms most reliably controlled by delivery.
- URSODEOXYCHOLIC ACID 15–20 mg/kg/day usually very effective at controlling itch. CHOLESTYRAMINE is alternative, but may exacerbate vitamin K-deficiency, necessitating parenteral vitamin K in latter stages of pregnancy.
- Antihistamines, phenobarbitol, S-adenosylmethionine (SAMe), and steroids have also been tried.
- Pregnancy should not continue beyond term. Maternal outcome is good. However, there is risk to the fetus. Higher rates of fetal prematurity, meconium stained amniotic fluid, intrauterine demise and an increased risk for neonatal respiratory distress syndrome. Recurrence of cholestasis in future pregnancies in 60% of mothers.

Liver abscess

Epidemiology/etiology
- In pre-antibiotic era most pyogenic liver abscesses occurred following appendicitis. Abscess formation may occur in pre-existing liver lesions, including hepatocellular carcinoma, especially in those with prior instrumentation, or in setting of significant tumor necrosis (e.g., following chemoembolization/radiofrequency ablation). May also arise from biliary tract, in association with cholangitis, choledocholithiasis,

and <u>Clonorchis</u> infection, and following ERCP. Intraabdominal disease (e.g., <u>colon cancer</u>, <u>diverticular disease, Crohn's disease</u>) may give rise to portal bacteremia and liver abscess.

- Infections usually polymicrobial, involving gut-derived Gram-negative (e.g., *E. coli, Klebsiella*), Gram-positive (e.g., *Enterococci, Streptococcus milleri*), and anerobic organisms (e.g., *Bacteroides* spp). Rarer causes include <u>hydatid disease</u>, TB, and *Candida albicans*. *Entamoeba histolytica* is an important cause in developing countries (see <u>amebiasis</u>). In patients who present with <u>cholangitis</u>, but who remain septic despite relief of biliary obstruction, it is vital to exclude liver abscess.

Clinical features

- Significant variability in severity and duration of symptoms. May present acutely with right upper quadrant pain, high fever, and septic shock, or more indolently (> 1 month) with fever of unknown origin (FUO), malaise, anorexia, weight loss, and dull abdominal discomfort.
- Examination may reveal tender hepatomegaly, and occasionally jaundice.

Investigation

- Bloods show mildly abnormal LFTs (often ↑ALP/GGT, even in absence of large duct obstruction), ↑ WBC (neutrophilia), ↑ ESR/CRP.
- Blood cultures positive in 50–80%.
- Imaging. Abscesses may be single or multiple. <u>Ultrasound</u> is usually first modality, and is highly specific. <u>CT scanning</u> is nearly 100% sensitive for liver abscess, often showing hypodense lesion with "rim enhancement" with contrast. Vital to exclude biliary obstruction.
- Differential diagnoses of liver abscess on imaging include amebic liver abscess (<u>amebiasis</u>), <u>hydatid disease</u>, simple cysts, necrotic tumor.
- Abscess aspiration needed if blood cultures negative, and failure to respond to initial treatment (but organism isolated in 90% of cases if abscess aspirated prior to antibiotics).
- Look hard for a reason for liver abscess (e.g., colonoscopy to exclude <u>colon cancer</u> in *Streptococcus milleri* abscess).

Management

- If abscess associated with biliary obstruction, biliary drainage (preferably endoscopically by <u>ERCP</u>) is essential.
- Antibiotics tailored to culture sensitivities but, until available, broad-spectrum empirical cover (e.g., third generation <u>CEPHALOSPORIN</u> and <u>METRONIDAZOLE</u>, or <u>PIPERICILIN/TAZOBACTAM.</u> Antibiotics usually given for two weeks IV, then further six weeks orally. May take weeks/months for resolution of abscess—be guided primarily by clinical progress, not radiological change.
- Percutaneous aspiration/drainage of abscesses used in combination with antibiotics (important to give metronidazole prior to aspiration if amebiasis suspected).
- Surgery for abscess drainage rarely required, but may be necessary if: multiple abscesses, loculated abscesses, abscesses with viscous contents obstructing the drainage catheter, underlying disease requiring primary surgical management, inadequate response to percutaneous drainage within seven days.

Liver function tests (LFTs)

Conventional liver function tests (AST, ALT, ALP, GGT) provide little information as to synthetic function of the liver. This is best indicated by serum albumin, clotting (prothrombin time, INR) and bilirubin.

Bilirubin (normal serum range < 1.5 mg/dl)

↑ levels may reflect ↑ production (e.g., hemolysis), ↓ hepatic uptake/conjugation (e.g., Gilbert's syndrome), ↓ biliary excretion (e.g., choledocholithiasis). See bilirubin metabolism and recent-onset jaundice.

Prothrombin time (PT; normal range 10–14 s)

In absence of vitamin K deficiency (excluded by giving vitamin K 10 mg PO/IV/day for three days), PT provides good indicator of liver synthetic function. Strong prognostic indicator of poor outcome and need for liver transplantation in acute liver failure and after acetaminophen overdose (and so do not correct PT in this setting (e.g., with fresh frozen plasma), unless bleeding. International Normalized Ratio (INR) standardizes PT measurement to eliminate variability. Commonly used.

Albumin (normal serum range 3.5–5.0 g/dl)

Reasonable indicator of liver synthetic function. In chronic liver disease, serum albumin reflects disease severity and prognosis (see Child–Pugh score). Always consider other causes of low albumin (malnutrition, severe intercurrent illness, renal losses (e.g., nephrotic syndrome), and gut losses (protein-losing enteropathy).

Aspartate aminotransferase (AST; normal range 5–45 IU/l)

Intracellular enzyme present in a number of tissues other than hepatocytes (e.g., striated muscle). As with ALT, ↑ levels in many types of liver disease, but levels > 1,000 IU/l suggest acute hepatocyte injury due to drugs (e.g., acetaminophen overdose), viruses (e.g., hepatitis A, hepatitis B), or ischemia (e.g., hypotensive episode). AST > ×2 higher than ALT characteristic of alcoholic liver disease; also in cirrhosis.

Alanine aminotransferase (ALT; normal range 5–45 IU/l)

Also intracellular enzyme, but more specific than AST for hepatocyte injury. ALT > AST often found in viral hepatitis and nonalcoholic fatty liver disease.

Alkaline phosphatase (ALP; normal range 40–165 IU/l)

Present in biliary epithelial cells, bone, and intestine. Isoenzyme may identify source, but associated ↑ GGT in setting of ↑ ALP rarely makes measuring this necessary. ↑ ALP seen in intrahepatic cholestasis (e.g., primary biliary cirrhosis) or extrahepatic biliary obstruction (e.g., pancreatic cancer).

Gammaglutamyl transpeptidase (GGT; normal range 10–60 IU/l)

Marker of cholestasis, but may be ↑ due to alcohol and other drugs through enzyme induction. Extensive investigation of ↑ GGT, in absence of other LFT derangement, rarely identifies significant pathology.

Liver support devices

- Liver transplantation as the only therapeutic option for the patient with end-stage acute or chronic liver failure is unsatisfactory for many reasons (e.g., lack of donors; life-long immunosuppression; ethical issues).
- Artificial liver support systems remain a "holy grail" in hepatology, and could have particular role as a bridge to transplant in those with acute liver failure awaiting a donor liver, and to allow time for spontaneous recovery of native liver (e.g., post acetaminophen overdose).
- Two broad types of devices:
  - **Nonbiological**. These devices use noncellular technologies to mimic some aspects of liver function. Molecular absorbance recirculation system (MARS) is an extracorporeal device attached to a conventional hemodialysis machine. Patient's blood circulates through a special hollow-fiber filter with a membrane, and protein (albumin)-bound toxins pass through membrane and attach to albumin in the dialysate compartment. The dialysate albumin is cleaned of toxins by continuously passing over charcoal and anion exchange resin columns, and then recirculates. MARS reduces hyperbilirubinemia and may improve hepatic encephalopathy and intractable pruritis, but definite effects on the outcome in liver failure are not yet established. Available in Europe. The HemoTherapies Liver Dialysis Unit is a charcoal-based, blood detoxification product that has been approved by the FDA for the treatment of drug toxicity and liver failure. This system has demonstrated safety; however, small controlled trials have not demonstrated a survival benefit in either acute or chronic liver disease. Not commonly utilized.
  - **Biological**. These devices employ isolated liver cells to mimic liver function, often in conjunction with charcoal and resin columns. Advantage of providing some synthetic activity and toxin clearance that is comparable to native liver function. In trial of commercial system, overall 30-day survival not improved, but survival benefit shown in small subgroups. Devices appear to be safe, but more expensive than nonbiological systems.
- Other methods of liver support under development include hepatocyte transplantation, stem-cell transplantation, and transgenic xenografts.

Liver transplantation

Background
- Management of chronic liver disease has been transformed by orthotopic liver transplantation (OLT) over the last 20 years.
- Alternatives to human livers for transplantation (e.g., xenotransplantation from other mammals such as pigs, or large-scale production of functioning hepatocytes) remain an elusive goal (also see liver support devices).

- End-stage liver disease due to cirrhosis accounts for 60% of OLT, malignancy 10% (see hepatocellular carcinoma), acute liver failure 5–10%, cholestasis 10–15%.
- Overall patient survival post-OLT at one and three years are 86% and 76%, respectively.

Technique

Pretransplant assessment, surgical approach, and postoperative care, are beyond the scope of this text.

Types of transplant

- Whole cadaveric graft—represents great majority of transplants. Totally reliant on limited supply of organs.

Box 4.6 When to refer for OLT consideration?

This is not an exact science, but simple answer is 'sooner rather than later'. Liver units don't want to first hear of the patient with acute liver failure when in grade III hepatic encephalopathy, or of the decompensated cirrhotic when they have become cachectic and malnourished. Broadly, consider OLT when anticipated survival < two years.

Acute liver failure (see emergencies and Table 4.12). Note that progression of liver synthetic dysfunction determines timing/need for OLT. Prothrombin time (PT) is an ideal marker of this (and so do not correct elevated PT (e.g., with fresh frozen plasma) unless actively bleeding).

Chronic liver disease

Indications

- Refractory ascites (see ascites), hepatic encephalopathy, and variceal bleeding (not effectively controlled with medical/endoscopic therapy—see portal hypertension).
- After first episode of spontaneous bacterial peritonitis (SBP), as predicts 50% two-year mortality.
- Poor quality of life (e.g., pruritis, severe fatigue) in cholestatic liver disease (e.g., primary biliary cirrhosis).
- Child–Pugh score >7, and more recently MELD score (see Box 4.7) have been used as indicators of need for referral.

Contraindications

- HIV positivity [although some transplant programs are reviewing this in view of efficacy of highly active antiretroviral therapy (HAART)].
- Active sepsis
- Advanced cardiopulmonary disease
- Extrahepatic/extensive intrahepatic malignancy (also see hepatocellular carcinoma and cholangiocarcinoma)
- Active alcohol dependency or substance abuse (most programs require six-month abstinence prior to transplantation for alcoholic cirrhosis)
- Psychosocial factors that may impair ability to comply with immunosuppression

---

- Split-liver graft—also cadaveric, but splitting liver may allow two recipients to be transplanted.
- Auxiliary liver transplantation—donor liver is implanted next to part, or whole, of recipient liver. May be used for acute liver failure (when regeneration of native liver might occur) or metabolic liver disease.
- Live-related transplantation—hemi-hepatectomy and liver lobe donation from family member. Likely good immunological match, but huge ethical considerations (e.g., small but definite risk of donor mortality).

Posttransplant complications

Myriad complications, related to immunological rejection, technical problems, drug effects, infection, and recurrence of underlying disease. All may contribute to early or late graft dysfunction.

- **Rejection**. Three types:
  - **Hyperacute**—antibody and complement-mediated reaction, with massive hepatic necrosis < 10 days after OLT. Only treatment is urgent retransplantation.
  - **Acute**—occurs in 30–70% of patients, often clinically silent, diagnosed on liver biopsy, usually day 7–9 post-OLT. Often rapid response to high dose immunosuppression.
  - **Chronic**—progressive bile duct loss, with fibrosis and cholestasis. Associated with previous recurrent acute rejection, cytomegalovirus (CMV), and hepatitis C infection. Adjustment of immunosuppression may help, but graft failure is usual.
- **Technical problems**. Hepatic artery, portal vein, vena cava thrombosis (may necessitate urgent retransplantation if occurs acutely), or anastomotic leak and hemorrhage. Biliary anastomotic leaks in 10%, with anastomotic strictures in 3–20% (treatment with endoscopic stenting ± surgical revision).
- **Drug effects**. As well as predisposing to infective complications, immunosuppressives may have hepatotoxic, and extrahepatic, effects (see CORTICOSTEROIDS, AZATHIOPRINE, CYCLOSPORINE, TACROLIMUS).
- **Infection** may relate to immunosuppression. Bacterial infection accounts for most infective episodes (35–70% of patients), but viral infection may be linked to early or late graft dysfunction (e.g., HSV, CMV). See Table 4.12. Epstein–Barr virus (EBV) reactivation occurs two to six months post-OLT, and is linked with posttransplant lymphoproliferative disorder (PTLD).
- **Disease recurrence**. Reinfection of graft with hepatitis C is universal, and may lead to accelerated cirrhosis and graft loss. Hepatitis B reinfection may be prevented/limited with hepatitis B immunoglobulin (HBIg) and LAMIVUDINE ± ADEFOVIR DEPIXOL. 20–30% of patients transplanted for alcoholic liver disease return to drinking. Recurrence of autoimmune hepatitis, primary biliary cirrhoisis, and primary sclerosing cholangitis posttransplantation has been reported.

Table 4.12 Selection criteria for liver transplantation in acute liver failure: King's College criteria

Acetaminophen	Nonacetaminophen
Arterial pH < 7.3 (should be interpreted with caution—may improve with N-Acetylcysteine and aggressive rehydration)	PT > 100 s, INR > 6.7
Or all 3 of:	Or any 3 of:
• PT > 100 s	• Etiology: halothane hepatitis, drug reaction, seronegative hepatitis
• Cr > 300 μmol/l	• Age <10, > 40 years
• Grade III or IV encephalopathy	• PT > 50, INR > 4.0
	• Serum bilirubin > 18 mg/dl

Reproduced with permission from O'Grady JR (1997) Acute liver failure. *J Coll. Physicians* Lond. 31(6):603–7.

Box 4.7 MELD score

Model for end-stage liver disease (MELD) score based on retrospective study of prognosis with chronic liver disease in absence of OLT.

$$3.8 \times \log(e) \text{ (bilirubin mg/dl)} + 11.2 \times \log(e) \text{ (INR)} + 9.6 \log(e) \text{ (creatinine mg/dl)}$$

- MELD scores range from 6 to 40. (< 9 = 4% three-month mortality, > 30 = 83% three-month mortality.)
- Advantage of MELD over <u>Child–Pugh score</u> in having no subjective components (e.g., clinical ascites).
- In 2002, MELD adopted in United States as means of determining OLT candidate's priority for organ allocation.

Table 4.13 Infectious agents postliver transplantation

Bacterial	Gram-positive, Gram-negative, anerobes
Viral	Epstein–Barr virus, *cytomegalovirus, herpes simplex virus, varicella zoster* virus
Mycobacteria	*M. tuberculosis, M. avium intracellulare*
Fungal	*Aspergillus* spp, *Pneumocystis carinii, Candida* spp, *Cryptococcus*

MELD score

See: liver transplantation.

Mirizzi's syndrome

Refers to the impaction of a gallstone in the cystic duct, with obstruction of common bile duct/common hepatic duct, and gallbladder. Patients present with jaundice, right upper quadrant pain, and fever, and may mimic choledocholithiasis or cholangitis. Distended gallbladder may be palpable and tender (see cholecystitis), and gallbladder empyema may develop. Ultrasound or CT scan reveals biliary dilatation above the cystic duct. ERCP may demonstrate the obstructing stone, and a biliary stricture in region of common hepatic duct with obstructed cystic duct (features may mimic cholangiocarcinoma).

Endoscopic stone removal is often not possible, and definitive treatment is usually surgical, with open cholecystectomy and surgical repair of bile duct if necessary.

Nodular regenerative hyperplasia (NRH)

- Most common cause of noncirrhotic portal hypertension in the West. May be associated with other multisystem diseases (e.g., rheumatoid, polyarteritis nodosum) or medications. Usually asymptomatic. May present with malaise, fever, abdominal discomfort, ascites, or variceal bleeding. Liver function is usually well preserved.
- **Diagnosis** may be difficult. Histology shows nodule formation, but without fibrous septae (in contrast to cirrhosis). These nodules are usually 0.2–2 cm, and may be seen on imaging. Finding on vascular studies of presinusoidal portal hypertension in presence of patent portal vein supports diagnosis of NRH.
- **Treatment** is based on removing offending agent (if known), treating the underlying medical condition, and treating the complications of portal hypertension.

Nonalcoholic fatty liver disease (NAFLD)

Background and etiology
- NAFLD is gaining acceptance as the term for a chronic liver disease with histological features similar to those of alcohol-related liver disease, but without significant alcohol intake. Nonalcoholic steatohepatitis (NASH) constitutes 20% of NAFLD, and is part of spectrum of disease.
- Increasing prevalence of NAFLD closely parallels rate of obesity in population, and 25% of patients have fatty liver on U/S in study in United States.
- Mechanism of steatosis and liver injury uncertain, but may involve hyperinsulinemia, endotoxemia, oxidative stress. Wide range of conditions is associated with NAFLD (see Box 4.8).

Box 4.8 **Risk factors for NAFLD**

- Middle age female
- Obesity
- Diabetes mellitus/glucose intolerance
- Hyperlipidemia
- Total parenteral nutrition
- Jejuno-ileal bypass
- Starvation
- Drugs (e.g., amiodarone, methotrexate, tetracycline)
- Metabolic disease (e.g., abetalipoproteinemia, glycogen storage disease, Wilson disease)

Clinical features
- Many patients asymptomatic, with diagnostic suspicion raised by incidentally raised serum aminotransferases (e.g., ALT) or "fatty liver" on U/S. Fatigue, malaise, right upper quadrant discomfort may be reported.
- Hepatomegaly common.
- Can progress to end-stage liver disease and portal hypertension, but natural history remains poorly defined, and many patients run indolent course.
- As with other etiologies of chronic liver disease, patients with cirrhosis related to NAFLD are at risk of hepatocellular carcinoma (HCC).

Investigation
- Important to exclude other causes of chronic liver disease, including careful alcohol history.
- Characteristic pattern of LFTs showing ↑ALT/AST, ↑GGT (ALP usually normal) with ↑fasting cholesterol, lipids, glucose. Elevated serum ferritin may be seen, and role of heterozygosity for HFE hemochromatosis gene in accelerated fibrosis in NAFLD remains controversial.
- U/S, CT, and MRI are all accurate at showing fatty liver.
- Liver biopsy is the only definitive way to define liver injury, as LFT derangement poorly predicts fibrosis, and approximately 20% of patients with persistent ↑ALT have advanced fibrosis/cirrhosis. Histology may show steatosis (fatty liver), steatohepatitis (fatty liver plus inflammation, which may progress to fibrosis/cirrhosis), or established fibrosis. Role of liver biopsy remains controversial, as carries definite risk, and many hepatologists advise initial identification and treatment of risk factors prior to biopsy in otherwise uncomplicated case.

Management
- Cornerstone is control of risk factors (weight loss, treatment of hyperlipidemia and hyperglycemia, and discontinuation of possible drug causes). However, these measures effective in only minority.
- Control of hyperinsulinemia shows promise, even in nondiabetics, with preliminary trials of metformin, and also rosiglitazone (a ligand for the peroxisome proliferator-activated receptor-γ, which promotes insulin responsiveness), showing improved liver biochemistry and histology in NASH. However, NASH returns on stopping rosiglitazone, and there are concerns about liver toxicity. Routine use of these agents awaits clarification, but evidence supports consideration of metformin in diabetic patients with NASH.

Overlap syndromes

Refers to clinical scenario in which two chronic liver diseases are simultaneously present. Found in 10% of patients with autoimmune liver disease.

- <u>Autoimmune hepatitis</u> (AIH)/<u>primary biliary cirrhosis</u> (PBC) overlap occurs as two variants: one with predominant cholestatic LFTs, antimitochondrial Ab (AMA) positive, but histological evidence of AIH; the other (also known as autoimmune cholangitis or AMA-negative PBC) with histological criteria for PBC, but AMA-negative, but often antinuclear Ab (ANA) and anti-smooth muscle Ab (SMA) positive. <u>URSODEOXYCHOLIC ACID</u> (UDCA) is usually given (12–15 mg/kg/day) in addition to steroids ± <u>AZATHIOPRINE</u> in those with prominent AIH features.
- AIH/<u>primary sclerosing cholangitis</u> (PSC) overlap mainly reported in children/young adults, with cholangiogram (MRCP/ERCP) and histological features consistent with PSC, but biochemical and serological markers of AIH. UDCA ± immunosuppressants used, but response unpredictable.
- AIH/<u>hepatitis C</u> characterized by chronic HCV infection with anti-LKM-1, ANA, SMA Abs, and ↑serum IgG. Treatment difficult, as <u>INTERFERON</u> may worsen liver disease if AIH predominant (e.g., Ab titres > 1:320), yet immunosuppression for AIH may increase HCV replication.

Portal hypertension

Background

- If pressure gradient between hepatic and portal venous systems (hepatic venous pressure gradient (HVPG)) increases to > 10–12 mmHg (normal 4 mmHg), portosystemic collaterals (varices) may develop.
- Most commonly due to intrahepatic disease at the site of liver sinusoid (e.g., cirrhosis), but presinusoidal, and postsinusoidal causes also important (see Table 4.14).
- Increased intrahepatic vascular resistance important, due to fibrosis and disruption of microcirculation at sinusoid, but resistance may be dynamic, with likely role for myofibroblasts, derived from hepatic stellate cells. Increased portal blood flow also contributes.
- Bleeding due to varices occurs in 30–40% of patients with cirrhosis, with risk factors including variceal size and <u>Child–Pugh score</u>.
- Gastro-esophageal region commonest site for varices, but stomach, rectum, duodenum, and surgical anastomoses (e.g., stomas) also affected.

Table 4.14 Causes of portal hypertension

Pre-sinusoidal	Sinusoidal	Postsinusoidal
Extrahepatic		*Extrahepatic*
Portal vein thrombosis	Cirrhosis	Right heart failure/valve disease
	Alcoholic hepatitis	
Splenic vein thrombosis	Nodular regenerative hyperplasia	Constrictive pericarditis
Arterio-venous fistula	Primary biliary cirrhosis	
Portal vein stenosis	Primary sclerosing cholangitis	
Intrahepatic		*Intrahepatic*
Schistosomiasis		Budd–Chiari syndrome
Sarcoidosis		Veno-occlusive disease
Early–primary biliary cirrhosis		
Early–primary sclerosing cholangitis		
Idiopathic noncirrhotic portal hypertension		

Clinical features

- Bleeding from gastro-esophageal varices usually presents with hematemesis > melena, with first bleeds carrying 25–50% mortality. Chronic blood loss and anemia may occur due to portal hypertensive gastropathy (PHG).
- Left upper quadrant discomfort due to splenomegaly occasionally reported.
- Signs of chronic liver disease may be present, including ascites, splenomegaly, dilated superficial veins, and rectal hemorrhoids.

Investigation

- Aimed at defining type of portal hypertension, and underlying etiology.
- Upper GI endoscopy showing varices confirms portal hypertension, and should be considered in all patients after diagnosing cirrhosis. Various grading systems for variceal size used (broadly: small=grade 1 = < 25% lumen occluded on endoscopy; medium = grade 2 = 25–50% lumen occluded; large = grade 3 = >50% lumen occluded) (Color plate 15).

- Doppler <u>ultrasound</u> informs abnormalities of hepatic and portal vein flow, <u>portal vein thrombosis</u>, and liver architecture. <u>CT scanning</u> with contrast and <u>MRI</u> also highly effective.
- Measurement of HPVG is invasive and rarely necessary to make diagnosis, but allows clarification of whether cause is presinusoidal, postsinusoidal, or sinusoidal. Transjugular <u>liver biopsy</u> and portal venography can be performed at same time.
- Other tests will depend on site of obstruction causing portal hypertension (e.g., see <u>Budd–Chiari syndrome</u>, <u>schistosomiasis</u>), and whether patient known to have liver disease. Liver function is usually excellent in presinusoidal portal hypertension. Portal hypertension *per se* may cause ↓WBC, ↓ platelets, due to hypersplenism.

Management
- Acute variceal bleeding is an emergency (see <u>acute upper GI bleeding</u>).
- Treat underlying cause of chronic liver disease (see <u>cirrhosis and chronic liver disease</u>).
- Prophylaxis—important, and often overlooked.
- **Primary prophylaxis** (to prevent first bleed) indicated when moderate–large varices found on screening endoscopy. Nonselective β-blockers (e.g., propanolol 40–80 mg bd PO) lower portal pressure, reduce risk of bleed (from 30% to 14% over two years in patients with large varices), and most hepatologists use these as first line therapy (but compliance may be poor, and side effects preclude long-term use in 30%). Adjust dose to maintain heart rate 60 bpm. Exact role of variceal band ligation (VBL) uncertain, as may effectively eradicate varices (e.g., with endoscopies every two to four weeks until eradicated), but invasive, may precipitate bleeding in a few (e.g., postbanding ulcers), and no benefit for gastric variceal/PHG bleeding.
- **Secondary prophylaxis** (to prevent re-bleed) is essential, as 60% of patients re-bleed < 1 year. β-blockers and VBL both effective.
- Ongoing areas of debate: role of invasive HPVG measurement to assess response to β-blockers; role of adding nitrates (e.g., isosorbide mononitrate) to β-blockers in nonresponders; and relative merits of VBL versus β-blockers as prophylaxis. Eradication of varices with VBL in combination with β-blockers appears most effective.
- Recurrent variceal bleeding that is difficult to control medically is an indication for transjugular intrahepatic portosystemic shunt (<u>TIPSS</u>) and consideration of <u>liver transplantation</u>.
- The AASLD has made recommendations regarding the treatment of varices:
- After an episode of variceal bleeding, cirrhotics should receive therapy to prevent recurrence (secondary prophylaxis).
- Combination of nonselective ß-blockers plus EVL is recommended as secondary prophylaxis.
- Nonselective ß-blocker should be adjusted to the maximal tolerated dose.

- EVL every one to two weeks until obliteration of varices. First surveillance EGD performed 1 to 3 months after obliteration and subsequently every 6 to 12 months to check for recurrence of varices.
- Consider TIPS in Child A or B who experience recurrent variceal bleeding despite nonselective beta blockers plus EVL. Surgical shunt can be considered in Child A patients.
- Refer to transplant center if patient is a candidate.

Table 4.15 Endoscopy and primary prophylaxis in compensated cirrhosis

Endoscopic finding	Action
No varices	Repeat endoscopy 2–3 years
Small varices	Repeat endoscopy 1 year
Medium–large varices	Life-long β-blockersVariceal band ligation if intolerant of β-blockers

Garcia-Tsao G, Sanyal AJ, Grace ND et al. (2007). Prevention and management of gastroesophageal varices and variceal hemorrhage in cirrhosis. Hepatology, 43(3):922.

Portal vein thrombosis (PVT)

Background

Thrombosis may involve only PV, or extend into splenic vein and splanchnic venous bed. Combination of local cause and systemic thrombotic predisposition important in development (see Table 4.16).

Clinical features
- Acute PVT (usually defined as presentation within two months of thrombosis) may present with abdominal pain, fever, and signs of mesenteric infarction.
- Chronic PVT presents with complications of <u>portal hypertension</u>. Splenomegaly and hypersplenism common, but ascites rare (unless associated liver disease). Variceal bleeding occurs in 30%, but excellent prognosis, due to preserved liver function (the latter may also explain low rate of <u>hepatic encephalopathy</u>). Ten-year survival > 80% in absence of cirrhosis.
- Biliary abnormalities (due to compression by varices or variceal mass around portal vein—"cavernoma") seen in 80%, but obstructive jaundice due to <u>biliary stricture</u> is rare.

Investigation

Aimed at defining cause (can be found in 80%) and extent of thrombosis.
- PVT accurately diagnosed with Doppler <u>U/S</u>, contrast <u>CT</u>, <u>endoscopic ultrasound</u>, and MRI. Formal angiography rarely required.
- Bloods may show signs of hypersplenism (↓WCC, ↓platelets).
- Tests for prothrombotic tendency essential if no clear cause identified (see Table 4.16).

Management

- No randomized trials to guide management.
- See <u>acute upper GI bleeding</u> for management of variceal bleeding.
- Small studies suggest resolution of acute PVT in 80% of cases with prompt formal anticoagulation (heparin followed by warfarin) ± prior thrombolytic therapy. Duration of anticoagulation uncertain, but may be needed lifelong if thrombotic tendency persists (as for pulmonary embolism).
- In chronic PVT no clear consensus on variceal bleeding prophylaxis, as RCTs performed in patients with chronic liver disease, and low rate and severity of bleeding in isolated PVT, but primary and secondary prophylaxis probably indicated (see <u>portal hypertension</u>). Recent large case series suggest that oral anticoagulation leads to no increase in frequency or severity of variceal bleeding, and may reduce mortality due to mesenteric infarction. Pragmatic approach may be consideration of warfarinization after eradication of gastro-esophageal varices with endoscopic band ligation.
- Surgical portosystemic shunt and <u>TIPSS</u> considered for recurrent bleeding. Low rate of hepatic encephalopathy.

Table 4.16 Causes of portal vein thrombosis

<u>Cirrhosis</u>	Postsurgical (e.g., <u>liver transplantation</u>)
<u>Portal hypertension</u> (any cause)	Umbilical vein catheterization
Prothrombotic tendency (see below)	PV compression by nodes (e.g., TB, lymphoma)
Malignancy (local/ distant)	Drugs (e.g., <u>oral contraceptive pill</u>)
Sepsis (local/ systemic)	Pregnancy/postpartum
<u>Schistosomiasis</u>	<u>Pancreatitis</u> (acute and chronic)

Table 4.17 Prothrombotic factors associated with portal vein thrombosis

Myeloproliferative disorders (e.g., polycythemia rubra vera, essential thrombocytosis, myelofibrosis)	G20210A prothrombin gene mutation
Anticardiolipin antibody	Hyperhomocysteinemia
Protein C, S, antithrombin III deficiency	Paroxysmal nocturnal hemoglobinuria
Antiphospholipid syndrome	Factor V Leiden deficiency

Primary biliary cirrhosis (PBC)

Epidemiology + pathogenesis

Chronic, progressive cholestatic disorder, predominantly of middle-age women (90%). Prevalence 20–400/million. Etiology unclear, but environmental trigger in genetically susceptible individuals likely leads to t-cell mediated auto-immune response against bile duct epithelial cells.

Clinical features

- Pruritis and lethargy classical presenting features, but 50% identified in asymptomatic stage. Associated autoimmune diseases (sicca syndrome (80%), thyroid disease, Raynaud's, Addison's disease). Osteoporosis is common. Hypercholesterolemia. Malabsorption. Increased risk of hepatocellular carcinoma (although lower than for chronic viral hepatitis, hemochromatosis, and alcoholic liver disease).
- Clinical signs include xanthelasma around eyes, skin hyperpigmentation, excoriations due to pruritis, clubbing, and signs of chronic liver disease.
- Median survival from presentation of 10–16 years for asymptomatic; 7–10 years for symptomatic patients.

Investigations

- ↑ALP, ↑GGT, with transaminases raised only mildly. Bilirubin ↑occurs late, and rise then usually inexorable. ↑PT may be due to impaired synthetic function or vitamin K malabsorption. ↑serum IgM.
- Ultrasound performed in all cases to exclude biliary obstruction.
- Antimitochondrial antibodies (AMA) in 95% of cases of PBC. If negative, but histological features of PBC, and ↑antinuclear antibody titers, likely "autoimmune cholangitis," variant of PBC (see overlap syndromes).
- Role of liver biopsy debated, because little need when diagnosis is clear (↑ALP, ↑IgM, AMA strongly +ve), as histology rarely changes management and of little prognostic value. Biopsy indicated where there is diagnostic uncertainty. Four histological stages (Color plate 9):
  1. Florid bile duct lesion, portal hepatitis, granulomas.
  2. Periportal fibrosis and hepatitis, portal tract enlargement, ductular proliferation.
  3. Bridging necrosis, septal fibrosis, scarring.
  4. Cirrhosis; but staging again limited by the patchy distribution of lesions.
- DEXA scan (see bone densitometry), calcium, and parathyroid hormone levels to investigate bone disease. Measure fat soluble vitamins (vitamins A, D, E, K). Lipid panel.

Management

- Complications of cirrhosis are managed along established lines (see cirrhosis and chronic liver disease).
- Wide range of immunomodulators tried in PBC (e.g., steroids, methotrexate, colchicine), without significant benefit shown to date.

- URSODEOXYCHOLIC ACID (UDCA) 10–15 mg/kg/day is safe and
  well tolerated, and improves liver biochemistry, but its effect on
  disease progression and transplant-free survival is much debated.
- For pruritis, give CHOLESTYRAMINE 4 g four times per day PO, and
  alternatives include UDCA, rifampin, naloxone, phenobarbitol, and even
  extracorporeal liver support (e.g., MARS—see liver support devices).
- Treat osteoporosis and osteopenia if present (low threshold for giving
  calcium/vitamin D supplements, even without DEXA scan). Measure
  vitamin D level.
- If vitamin deficient, give orally vitamin A 10,000 IU/day, vitamin D +
  calcium (see above), vitamin E 400 IU/day, vitamin K 5–10 mg/day.
- Liver transplantation is highly effective (> 80% five-year survival),
  and may be indicated for intractable pruritis and fatigue, as well as
  progressive liver failure.

Primary sclerosing cholangitis (PSC)

Epidemiology + pathogenesis

Cholestatic liver disease characterized by biliary stricturing and dilatation.
Prevalence 60–80/million, and associated with inflammatory bowel disease
(IBD) in 80% of cases (3–10% of patients with IBD, mainly ulcerative colitis,
will get PSC). Immunogenetic factors (e.g., association with HLA A1, B8,
DR3) and environmental factors (e.g., portal venous entotoxins/ bacteria)
likely to be important, but exact etiology remains unclear.

Clinical features

Common presentation with fatigue, pruritis, intermittent jaundice, and
right upper quadrant discomfort. Usually asymptomatic at diagnosis.
- Jaundice may result from intrahepatic stricturing, impaired liver
  function, "dominant" extrahepatic biliary stricture (in 20%), biliary
  stone disease, or cholangiocarcinoma (lifetime risk 20–30%).
- Features of cholangitis (fever, pain, jaundice) usually occur following
  instrumentation (e.g., ERCP), rather than de novo.
- Signs of chronic liver disease and portal hypertension may be present.
- Osteoporosis and metabolic bone disease and steatorrhea may occur.
- Time from symptomatic presentation to death or liver transplant
  12–21 years.

Investigation

- LFTs show cholestatic pattern (↑ALP, GGT), but with AST/ALT ↑ <
  x5 ULN. Bilirubin often fluctuates (unlike in primary biliary cirrhosis),
  with increases related to cholangitis/biliary stones/strictures.
- ERCP remains "gold standard" for diagnosis, but MRCP may also show
  cholangiographic changes of multifocal intrahepatic ± extrahepatic
  stricturing and beading.
- Liver biopsy (Color plate 10) often not diagnostic, but histological
  features include bile duct proliferation, ductopenia, and concentric
  peribiliary fibrosis ("onion skin").
- p-ANCA is elevated in 65–85% of PSC patients.

- Diagnosis of <u>cholangiocarcinoma</u> in PSC always difficult at early stage, but combination of CT, biliary brush cytology at ERCP, and serum tumor markers CEA and CA19–9 used (although CA19–9 >180 U/ml reported to be > 95% specific, > 66% sensitive, high levels also seen in biliary obstruction). Lifetime risk 10–15%.
- Yearly surveillance colonoscopy program in PSC patients with colitis is indicated in view of markedly increased <u>colonic cancer</u> risk. Surveillance starts at the time of diagnosis (unlike other IBD patients where surveillance is not indication until 8-10 years of colitis).

Management

- <u>URSODEOXYCHOLIC ACID</u> (<u>UCDA</u>) improves LFTs, but no effect on symptoms, histology, or survival at conventional doses (10–15 mg/ kg/day). However, it may protect against colonic neoplasia, and at > 20 mg/kg/day improve liver histology. > 30 mg/kg are not recommended.
- "Dominant" extrahepatic biliary strictures endoscopically dilated ± stented.
- <u>ANTIBIOTICS</u> (e.g., <u>CIPROFLOXACIN</u>) for proven cholangitis, but no role for prophylaxis (except prior to ERCP).
- Pruritis managed initially with <u>CHOLESTYRAMINE</u> 4 g/day, with other options including rifampicin 150 mg bid (see PBC above).
- Correct <u>vitamin A</u>, <u>D</u>, <u>E</u>, <u>K</u> deficiencies, if present.
- <u>Liver transplantation</u> provides 80–90% five-year survival, but 20% recurrence at five years. <u>Cholangiocarcinoma</u> is absolute contraindication in most centers.

Box 4.9 Differential diagnosis of PSC

- Biliary stone disease
- Postcholecystectomy <u>biliary strictures</u>
- <u>Caroli's disease</u>
- HIV cholangiopathy
- <u>Cholangiocarcinoma</u>
- Ischemic strictures
- Exposure to biliary toxins (e.g., formalin)
- <u>Autoimmune pancreatitis</u> with biliary involvement
- *Clonorchis* infection

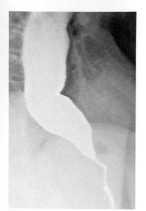

Plate 1 Fluoroscopic spot film from upper GI series. "Bird's Beak" appearance (tapered high-grade narrowing) at the esophagogastric junction with esophageal dilation and redundancy is classic for achalasia.

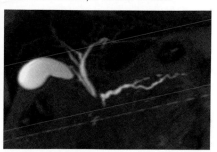

Plate 2 Maximum Intensity Projection (MIP) from a respiratory-triggered 3-D T2-weighted MRCP sequence shows a classic "Double Duct" sign from pancreatic adenocarcinoma in the head and neck of the pancreas obstructing both the main pancreatic duct and the common bile duct.

(a)

(b)

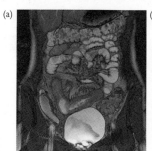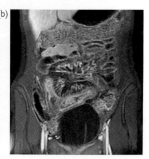

Plate 3 Balanced Steady State Free Precession image (a) and gadolinium-enhanced fat-saturated 3D T1-weighed gradient echo image (b) in a patient with Crohn's disease showing irregular thickened mucosa with increased enhancement, mural thickening and edema, serosal irregularity and increased enhancement, and mesenteric vascular engorgement ("comb sign").

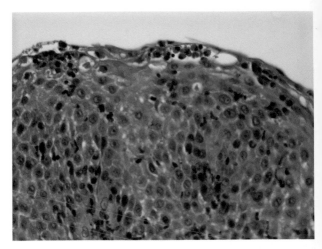

Plate 4 Eosinophillic esophagitis: esophageal squamous epithelium showing numerous intraepithelial eosinophils, increased density of eosinophils in the superficial epithelium, eosinophilic microabscesses, and degranulation (H&E, 400x).

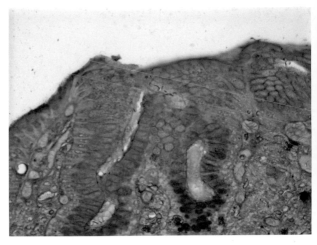

Plate 5 H.pylori gastritis: view of the superficial gastric epithelium with numerous V-shaped bacterial organisms consistent with Helicobacter pylori present at the luminal aspect of the epithelium (Steiner stain, 400x).

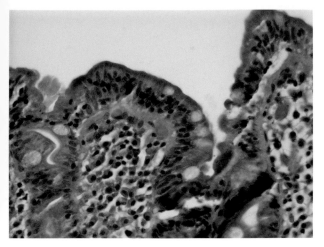

Plate 6 Celiac disease: small intestinal biopsy shows marked villous shortening, crypt hyperplasia, and numerous intraepithelial lymphocytes (H&E, 400x).

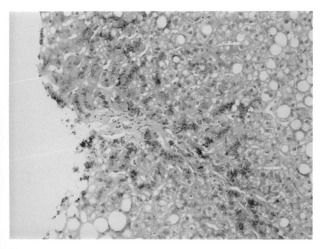

Plate 7 Hemochromatosis: view of a portal area with surrounding periportal hepatocytes having diffuse deposition of blue, granular cytoplasmic pigment consistent with iron deposition (Prussian Blue Iron stain, 200x).

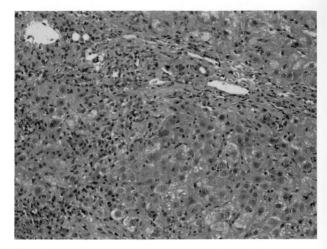

Plate 8 Auto-immune hepatitis: medium-power view of a portal and periportal mixed inflammatory infiltrate with prominent plasma cells with scattered apoptotic hepatocytes at the interface (H&E, 200x).

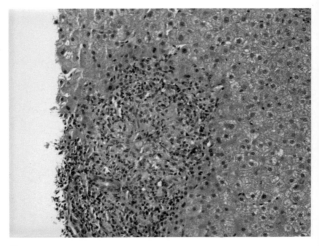

Plate 9 Primary Biliary Cirrhosis: portal area expanded by a mixed inflammatory infiltrate, mainly comprised of lymphocytes, histiocytes, and plasma cells, which surrounds a damaged small interlobular bile duct (H&E, 200x).

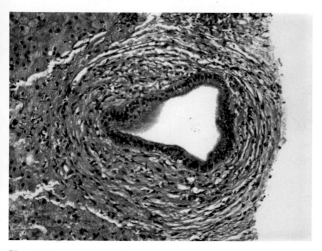

Plate 10 Primary Sclerosing Cholangitis: prominent concentric fibrosis surrounds this medium-to-large interlobular bile duct (Masson's Trichrome stain, 200x).

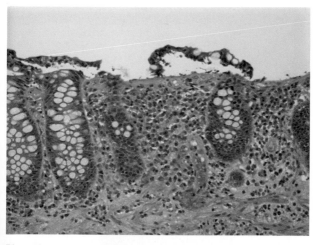

Plate 11 Collagenous Colitis: colonic mucosal biopsy showing expansion of the lamina propria by chronic inflammation, a striking increase in the subepithelial collagen layer with embedded capillaries, and epithelial denudation (H&E, 400x).

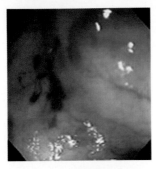

Plate 12 Angiodysplasia in the caecum. Courtesy of William B. Silverman.

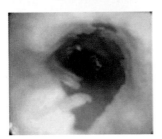

Plate 13 This figure shows an irregular and abnormal junction between esophageal squamous (white) mucosa and gastric (pink) mucosa. This is Barrett's esophagus but it is impossible to accurately define the extent from this picture because the gastro-esophageal junction (point of disappearance of the gastric rugal folds) is not clearly seen.

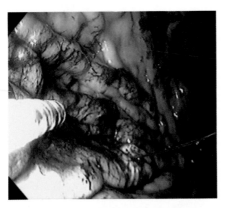

Plate 14 Endoscopic image of spurting Dieulafoy lesion. Courtesy of Klaus Mönkemüller and Walter Curioso.

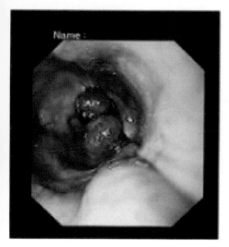

Plate 15 Variceal band ligation. 2 rubber bands are seen applied to a varix in the 5 o'clock position. Reproduced with permission from Yamada T, et al. Handbook of Gastroenterology. 2005 Lippincott Williams and Wilkins.

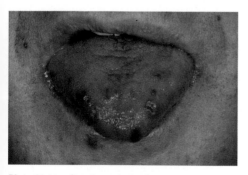

Plate 16 Hereditary hemorrhagic telengectasia.

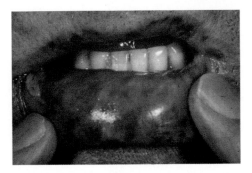

Plate 17 Brown macules on lips in patient with Peutz-Jeghers syndrome.

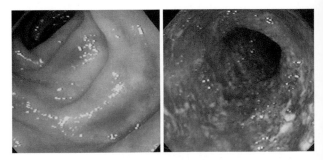

Plate 18 Mild (left) and severe (right) ulcerative colitis. This figure was published in Feldman M, et al. Sleisenger and Fordtran's gastrointestinal and liver disease, 7th ed. Copyright Elsevier 1998.

Spontaneous bacterial peritonitis (SBP)

Background
- SBP is present in 10–30% of hospitalized cirrhotic patients with ascites.
- Increased risk related to gastrointestinal bleeding, ascitic protein: <1.0 g/dL, advanced liver disease, and previous episodes.
- Bacterial translocation, bacteremia, and impaired antimicrobial activity of ascitic fluid contributes to its development. Gram-negative bacilli (especially *Escherichia coli*) cause 80% of infections.

Clinical features
Majority present with fever, systemic signs of sepsis, but few abdominal features. Abdominal pain and rebound tenderness occur in minority. Asymptomatic in 10%. Liver decompensation, with worsening hepatic encephalopathy, and renal failure are important associations.

Investigation
Diagnostic ascitic tap mandatory in all patients admitted to hospital with ascites, because of high rate of SBP (see ascites).
- Ascitic white count: WCC > 500 cells/µl, neutrophils > 250 /µl strongly suggestive of SBP, unless intra-abdominal source of infection.
- Ascitic protein: < 1.0 g/dL merits consideration of antibiotic prophylaxis.
- Microscopy and culture: 5–10 ml of fluid should be inoculated into blood culture bottles with media for aerobes and anaerobes (not just into specimen bottles). Despite this, 20–40% of presumed SBP (i.e., ↑WCC) are culture negative. Isolation of multiple organisms raises possibility of contamination or intra-abdominal source (e.g., diverticular perforation).

Management
- Treat on finding ascitic neutrophils > 250 cells/µl, without waiting for microbiological confirmation. Give third-generation CEPHALOSPORIN (e.g., cefotaxime 2 g bid IV). In nonseverely ill, oral quinolones (e.g., CIPROFLOXACIN 500 mg bid) may be considered.
- Continue antibiotic until clinical sepsis resolved, and ascitic neutrophils < 250 cells/µl.
- Routine infusion of human albumin (1.5 g/kg at time of diagnosis and 1 g/kg at 48 hours) advised by some (may ameliorate renal failure), but controversial (see albumin (use in liver disease)).
- Resolution of infection in 75–90%, but hospital mortality remains at 20–40% (predicted by degree of renal failure (also see hepatorenal syndrome), and largely due to hepatic decompensation).
- Antibiotic prophylaxis with a quinolone (e.g., norfloxacin 400 mg od PO, ciprofloxacin 750 mg/week PO) reduces risk of SBP over next year from 70% to 20%.
- Episode of SBP predicts 50% two-year mortality. Its occurrence requires consideration of suitability for liver transplantation.

TPMT (thiopurine methyltransferase)

Plays a key role in metabolic pathway of <u>AZATHIOPRINE</u>/6 mercaptopurine (6-MP). Variations in TPMT (largely determined genetically) allow for shunting of 6-MP into 6-methylmercaptopurine when levels are normal or high. Patients homozygous for a recessive mutation resulting in inactivation of TPMT (1 in 300 people) produce very high levels of 6-thioguanine nucleotides that make them unlikely to tolerate thiopurines at all (with high risk of side effects, such as significant neutropenia). People heterozygous for the TPMT mutation (10% of people) require lower doses of thiopurines.

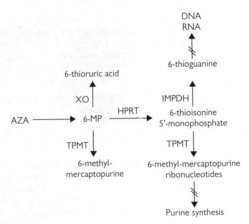

Figure 4.3 Metabolism of <u>AZATHIOPRINE</u>/6-MP. Azathioprine is converted to 6-MP nonenzymatically. AZA, azathioprine; 6-MP,6-mercaptopurine; XO, xanthine oxidase; HPRT, hypoxanthine phosphoribosyltransferase; TPMT, thiopurine methyltransferase; IMPDH, inosine monophosphate dehydrogenase.

Varices

See: <u>portal hypertension</u>.

Wilson disease

Background

- Autosomal recessive disorder, incidence 1:30 000.
- In normal individuals, approximately 10% of the 1–2 mg/day of ingested copper is absorbed, and bound to albumin in serum. After transport to the hepatocyte, copper is either incorporated into ceruloplasmin and excreted into plasma (90% of circulating copper in this form), or bound to ATPase Wilson disease protein (WDP) and excreted in bile.
- The *ATP7A* gene encodes for WDP, with mutations resulting in retention of copper in the liver and impaired incorporation of copper into ceruloplasmin.

Clinical features

- Disease may present at age 3–40 years, with range of features (see Table 4.18).
- Liver disease most common presentation in childhood. Chronic hepatitis may be similar to autoimmune hepatitis, and acute liver failure often associated with hemolysis. First presentation may be with complications of cirrhosis. Gallstones occur due to recurrent hemolysis.
- Neuropsychiatric presentation usual in adolescence/early adulthood.
- Kayser–Fleischer rings are rarely absent in patients with neurological disease (brown-green discoloration around periphery of cornea).

Investigations

Diagnosis rarely made unless considered, and biochemical parameters may be inconsistent particularly in patients with liver disease (see caveats in Table 4.19). No test result should be viewed in isolation, and diagnosis usually made through combination of clinical picture and highly suggestive results. **Unexplained liver disease in young person with Coomb's negative hemolytic anemia should raise suspicion.**

- LFTs nonspecific, but ALT usually < 1,500 U/l, even in acute liver failure.
- Slit lamp examination to exclude Kayser–Fleischer rings.
- Plasma ceruloplasmin < 20 mg/dL in 85% of cases.
- Serum copper < 11 µmol/l.
- 24-hour urinary copper > 100 µg (found in 65% of Wilson, but penicillamine challenge (500 mg 12 hourly x 2) leads to diagnostic elevation of > 1600 µg 24 hours).
- Liver biopsy. Hepatic copper > 250 µg/g dry weight (normal < 50 µg/g). Liver histology may show necrosis, chronic hepatitis, or cirrhosis, depending on clinical presentation. Suggestive features include fatty change, Mallory hyaline, copper staining, and vacuolated nuclei.
- Genetic analysis.

Management
- Acute liver failure:
  - Manage as for <u>acute liver failure</u> and transfer to specialist liver unit for <u>liver transplantation</u>.
- Liver disease without liver failure:
  - Avoid high copper-containing foods (e.g., chocolate, shellfish).
  - Penicillamine 250–500 mg/day increasing incrementally to 1,000 mg/day with pyridoxine 25 mg/day leads to urinary copper excretion and good prognosis. Trientine (750–1500 mg/day in divided doses) is an alternative. Zinc (150–300 mg/day) may be used for maintenance.

Table 4.18 Clinical features of Wilson disease

System	Features
Liver	Acute hepatitis
	<u>Acute liver failure</u>
	Decompensated cirrhosis
	<u>Portal hypertension</u>
	<u>Gallstones</u>
Neurological	Behavioral change
	Parkinsonism/tremor
	Cognitive impairment
	Dysarthria, dystonia, dysphagia
Renal	Renal tubular acidosis
	Renal calculi
Musculoskeletal	Arthropathy
	<u>Osteoporosis</u>
	Osteomalacia
Hematological	Hemolytic anemia
Ophthalmic	<u>Kayser–Fleischer rings</u>

Table 4.19 Caveats in diagnosing Wilson disease

Kayser–Fleischer rings	Copper deposition in other cholestatic liver diseases (e.g., <u>primary biliary cirrhosis</u>, <u>primary sclerosing cholangitis</u>)
↓ Ceruloplasmin	Acute phase reactant, so may be falsely ↑ in Wilson with active liver inflammation. Falsely ↓ in chronic liver disease due to ↓ synthesis
↓ Serum copper	May ↑ due to leakage of nonceruloplasmin bound copper from necrotic liver in acute Wilson
Liver histology	Copper staining may be negative, despite raised liver copper concentrations
Genetic analysis	Mutation analysis is not commercially available in the United States.

Zieve's syndrome

(Also see Piccini, J et al. (2003) *Am. J. Med.* **115**: 729.)

First described in 1957 by Leslie Zieve, who reported a triad of jaundice, hyperlipidemia, and transient hemolytic anemia in a cohort of 20 male patients with alcoholic steatohepatitis. Most patients have upper abdominal/right upper quadrant pain and macrocytic anemia. The hypercholesterolemia and jaundice both resolve within three weeks if the patient stops drinking. The exact mechanism of hemolysis is not known, but may involve several acquired intracellular defects (unstable pyruvate kinase, membrane alterations).

Pancreas

Acute pancreatitis (AP)

Background

Incidence varies (5–25 per 100,000). Alcohol dependency and gallstones account for most cases (see Table 5.1.1). Evidence of acute pancreatic inflammation (sometimes with other organ involvement) differentiates AP from chronic pancreatitis, but clinical distinction may be difficult. Activation of trypsinogen, leading to pancreatic autodigestion, occurs early, but role of primary pancreatic duct obstruction remains uncertain.

Clinical features

Severe, unremitting epigastric pain radiating to the back, with nausea and vomiting. Signs of shock may be present. Bruising in flanks ("Grey–Turner sign") or umbilical area ("Cullen's sign") seen in 1%, and indicates hemorrhagic pancreatitis with poor prognosis. Ileus is common.

Complications

Local complications: inflammatory mass, infected necrosis, pancreatic pseudocyst formation, pseudoaneurysm, obstructive jaundice, gastric outflow obstruction, portal vein thrombosis.

Systemic complications: sepsis, acute respiratory distress syndrome, acute renal failure, disseminated intravascular coagulation.
- Severe AP usually associated with pancreatic necrosis, which occurs in 20–30% of cases of AP. Infected necrosis occurs in 30–70% of cases of pancreatic necrosis, and accounts for > 80% of deaths.
- 5–10% overall mortality, with first episode of AP ×10 more likely to lead to organ failure than recurrent episodes. Obesity is linked with more severe course. Half of deaths occur in first 14 days.

Investigation and assessment of severity
- Serum amylase makes the diagnosis (> 1,000 U/l in appropriate clinical setting), but poor correlation with disease severity.
- CBC, Urea & Electrolytes, LFT, Glu, Ca, CRP, Bicarb essential in all (see Table 5.1.2). Serum ALT/AST > 150 U/l is > 95% specific for gallstones as cause of AP, rather than alcohol.
- Difficult to predict course/prognosis at onset, but various scoring systems have been verified (e.g., Ransom/Glasgow/APACHE II). No criteria 100% reliable, and may be hampered by need for assessment at 48 hours. Best at predicting patients with mild disease, rather than those at risk of severe attack. High serum CRP (e.g., > 210 mg/l at 48–72 hours) appears highly sensitive for necrotizing pancreatitis. Other indicators of poor prognosis include clinical impression of severe disease at 24 hours, obesity (body mass index > 30), > 2 Glasgow criteria (see Table 5.1.2), and organ failure.
- Abdominal ultrasound excludes stones in gallbladder and biliary dilatation, but often poor views of pancreas.
- Plain AXR may show "sentinel loop" due to local small bowel ileus. Pleural effusion on CXR correlated with severe disease.
- Contrast-enhanced CT scan should be performed 48 hours after clinical onset, unless pancreatitis clinically mild, as necrosis predicts

prolonged course and potential mortality (see Table 5.1.3). CT and MRI also define peripancreatic inflammation, and evidence of chronic pancreatitis (e.g., calcification). MRI/MRCP may also define pancreatic duct disruption.

Table 5.1.1 Causes of acute pancreatitis

Gallstones/sludge (35%)	Drugs (e.g., HAART for HIV, azathioprine, NSAIDs, valproate)
Alcohol (30%)	Pancreas divisum
Hypertriglyceridemia	Hereditary pancreatitis
PostERCP	
Ampullary disease (e.g., stenosis, sphincter of Oddi dysfunction)	Infection (e.g., mumps, coxsackie, Ascaris, Chlonorchis, scorpion bites)
Hypercalcemia	TraumaCause unknown/idiopathic (30%)
Pancreatic cancer	

Table 5.1.2 Modified Glasgow criteria

WBC > 15 × 10⁹/l	Urea > 45 mg/dl
Glucose >180 g/dl	Ca^{2+}< 8 mg/dl
LDH > 600 IU/l	Albumin < 3.2 g/dl
AST > 200 IU/l	PaO_2 < 60 mmHg

More factors, worse the prognosis.

Table 5.1.3 Correlation of pancreatic necrosis with outcome in AP

CT finding	Morbidity	Mortality
Necrosis	82%	23%
No necrosis	6%	0%

Management
- Mortality low with prompt intensive care for those who need it; 20% if specialist referral delayed.
- Expert supportive therapy paramount.
- Intravascular volume expansion (colloid/crystalloid) vital, as large losses due to ileus, "third spacing" in peripancreatic tissue. Consider central line insertion to monitor fluids.
- Analgesia (OPIATES usually required).
- Enteral feeding (naso-jejunal tube) may reduce bacterial translocation, so preferable to TPN (but ensure ileus resolved). Start within 72 hours.

- Prophylactic antibiotics for severe AP remains controversial, but recent evidence suggests no reduction in mortality. If clinical suspicion of sepsis, take cultures urgently (including aspiration of necrotic collections) and give high dose IV antibiotics (e.g., imipenem, third-generation CEPHALOSPORIN + METRONIDAZOLE), guided by microbiology. Surgery in pancreatic necrosis only rarely needed.
- Urgent ERCP + sphincterotomy for presumed gallstone pancreatitis only clearly indicated if elevated bilirubin (and not settling at 48 hours), or definite cholangitis. ERCP in all cases of gallstone pancreatitis not advised, as may worsen pancreatitis further, and stones already passed in 80% of cases. In gallstone pancreatitis, cholecystectomy should be performed as soon as AP settled (prior to discharge).

Amylase

- Pancreas produces 40% of serum amylase; salivary glands the rest. Total serum amylase (pancreatic isoenzymes are highly sensitive and specific, but rarely needed clinically) increases 6–12 hours after onset of acute pancreatitis (AP), and levels > 1,000 U/l are strongly indicative of this diagnosis in the correct clinical setting. Amylase may be elevated, but usually < 1,000 U/l, due to a wide range of abdominal causes, including acute appendicitis, cholecystitis, choledocholithiasis, viscus perforation, and salpingitis. Disease of the salivary glands (e.g., mumps), lung and ovarian tumors, head injury, and diabetic ketoacidosis can all cause elevation. Chronic elevation of serum amylase occurs in macroamylasaemia. Condition is of no clinical relevance (beyond confusing the diagnosis of AP), and can be differentiated from pancreatic amylase by the absence of amylase in urine.
- Diagnosis of AP should not rely solely on the level of amylase, which may not be significantly elevated due to underlying pancreatic insufficiency (i.e., with acinar cell loss, therefore, unable to make amylase), or if AP due to hypertriglyceridemia (an amylase inhibitor may be present). Level of amylase in AP does not predict prognosis. Serum lipase sensitive and specific for AP, and raised levels persist for longer, but less readily available than amylase.
- High levels of amylase within pancreatic pseudocysts help to differentiate them from pancreatic cystic tumors, and high amylase levels in ascitic fluid are diagnostic of pancreatic ascites, related to pseuodocyst or pancreatic duct rupture.

Autoimmune pancreatitis

- Rare condition, mainly reported from Japan. May clinically mimic pancreatic cancer, and is a cause of chronic pancreatitis and pancreatic insufficiency. Also associated with intrahepatic biliary strictures similar to primary sclerosing cholangitis.
- Characterized by:
  - Diffuse pancreatic enlargement ("sausage pancreas").
  - Pancreatic duct abnormality.
  - Low common bile duct stricture.
  - Lymphoplasmacytic infiltrate on biopsy.
  - Raised serum IgG4 levels.
  - Associated autoimmune disease (e.g., Sjögren's, Crohn's disease).

Response to CORTICOSTEROIDS.

Chronic pancreatitis

Definition and etiology

Benign disease characterized by permanent alteration of anatomy and function due to chronic inflammation. Causes include alcohol (> 70% of cases); tropical pancreatitis (onset < 40 years in equatorial regions, and may be linked to protein–energy malnutrition); pancreatic duct obstruction (e.g., tumors, intraductal stones, traumatic strictures); hereditary pancreatitis; idiopathic chronic pancreatitis (20% of cases); intraductal papillary mucinous tumor (IPMT—see pancreatic cystic tumors); cystic fibrosis; and autoimmune pancreatitis. Episodes of acute pancreatitis may occur during course of chronic disease.

Clinical features

- Epigastric pain, often radiating to back, and associated with anorexia and weight loss. Pain resolves in 80% within 10 years of onset, often in parallel with development of endocrine and exocrine pancreatic insufficiency.
- Insulin-dependent diabetes develops in 40–70% of patients.
- Steatorrhoea (pale, loose, foul smelling stools that are difficult to flush).

Complications

- Portal vein thrombosis and portal hypertension in 1%.
- Jaundice due to low biliary stricture.
- Pancreatic pseudocyst formation.
- Pancreatic cancer develops in approximately 3% of patients (eightfold risk over general population).
- Life expectancy in patients with chronic pancreatitis is shortened by 10–20 years.

Investigation. Diagnosis made by assessing pancreatic structure and function.

Structure
- KUB may show pancreatic calcification (25–60% of cases).
- <u>CT, MRCP, ERCP</u>, and <u>endoscopic ultrasound</u> are complementary, and may show anatomical features of chronic pancreatitis: irregular main pancreatic duct, with dilatation and/or strictures; side branch irregularity; pancreatic parenchymal heterogeneity, enlargement, or atrophy.

Function
- Functional abnormalities in chronic pancreatitis include a decrease in stimulated secretory capacity, exocrine insufficiency (maldigestion and steatorrhea), and endocrine insufficiency (diabetes mellitus).
- MRCP with secretin. Reduced secretin output, or obstruction of flow due to pancreatic stricture may be seen.
- Fasting glucose/glucose tolerance test. Serum <u>vitamins A,D,E,K</u>.
- Fecal elastase 1 produced by pancreas, and passed in stool largely unaltered (and unaffected by coadministration of <u>PANCREATIC ENZYME SUPPLEMENTS</u>). Highly sensitive and specific for exocrine function (except for falsely low levels with significant diarrhea), and much easier to perform than urine pancreolauryl test or three-day fecal fat (also see <u>pancreatic function tests</u>).

Management
- Remove precipitant (e.g., alcohol).
- <u>Pain control</u>. Start with simple nonopiates (e.g., paracetamol, NSAIDs), cautiously increasing to mild <u>OPIATES</u> (e.g., coproxamol, tramadol) and then stronger opiates (e.g., Fentanyl patches). Endoscopic removal of stones from pancreatic duct in head of pancreas may occasionally help. Celiac plexus block (percutaneously or via <u>endoscopic ultrasound</u>) may be effective, but occasionally surgical drainage procedures or total pancreatectomy used.
- Treat diabetes (most patients require insulin, although doses may be low, due to associated loss of glucagon-producing α cells).
- In patients with exocrine insufficiency, oral <u>PANCREATIC SUPPLEMENTS</u> with meals (e.g., creon, nutrizym) may help reduce weight loss, malabsorption, and steatorrhea (give with proton pump inhibitor to reduce inactivation of enzymes in stomach).
- Endoscopic stenting of <u>biliary strictures</u> may be required, but if no improvement in 12–18 months, consider surgery (see <u>biliary bypass procedures</u>).
- Nutritional support (± fat soluble vitamins).
- Surgery, including pancreatic resection (e.g., <u>Whipple's procedure</u>) or drainage procedure (e.g., Frey, Puestow) occasionally indicated.

Hereditary pancreatitis

- Hereditary pancreatitis displays autosomal dominant pattern due to specific genetic defect. Familial pancreatitis is more generic term when more members in family affected with pancreatitis than expected, but without obvious cause.
- Range of mutations in hereditary pancreatitis (e.g., in cationic trypsinogen gene (PRSS1), secretory trypsin inhibitor gene (SPINK1)). Trypsinogen converts to trypsin, which then activates pancreatic proenzymes to enzymes (except amylase and lipase). Trypsinogen conversion is tightly controlled; hence trypsinogen gene mutations associated with excess enzyme production, autodigestion, and pancreatitis.
- Genetic testing available, and 80% with PRSS1, R122H, or N29I mutations will develop pancreatitis (80% penetrance). Negative test in family with known mutation eliminates risk.
- Recurrent episodes of pancreatitis begin < 40 years (mean 10 years), with chronic pancreatitis developing in 50%. Standard management for acute and chronic pancreatitis applies.
- Cumulative risk of pancreatic cancer may be > 40% by 70 years. No effective cancer screening program established for gene carriers.

Islet cell tumors

See: pancreatic endocrine tumors.

Pancreas divisum

- In embryonic development, dorsal and ventral pancreatic buds join, so that body and tail of pancreas drain predominantly through major papilla, with common bile duct, via ventral pancreas. In 4% of population ventral duct is not linked to dorsal duct, which then drains through smaller accessory duct (duct of Santorini). The small ventral duct drains through the major papilla and the larger dorsal duct drains through the smaller minor papilla. See Figure 5.1.1.
- Most common congenital pancreatic abnormality.
- Diagnosis made by MRCP or ERCP.
- May be a cause of recurrent acute or chronic pancreatitis, and accessory sphincterotomy may improve symptoms. However, etiological link controversial, as minimal increase in prevalence of pancreatitis in patients with pancreas divisum.

Pancreatic cancer

Epidemiology
- Fourth leading cause of cancer death in United States and Europe (incidence approximately 10 cases per 100,000). Median age at diagnosis 65 years, slightly more common in males and African-Americans.
- Risk factors include chronic pancreatitis, cigarette smoking, diabetes. 8% of patients with pancreatic cancer have first-degree relative with disease, related to both underlying hereditary pancreatitis (40% risk by age 70 years) and familial pancreatic cancer.

Pathogenesis
- Pancreatic cancer usually refers to ductal adenocarcinoma, which accounts for 90% of pancreatic tumors (others include pancreatic cystic and pancreatic endocrine tumors).
- Genetic mutations within KRAS2 and CDKN2A genes in > 90% of cancers.
- 75% of cancers in pancreatic head, 10–15% in body, 5–10% in tail.
- Metastases to regional lymph nodes, liver, and occasionally lung.

Clinical features
- Jaundice (at presentation in 50%), weight loss, anorexia, and upper abdominal pain radiating to back are classical symptoms. Symptoms of chronic pancreatitis (e.g., pancreatic insufficiency) occasionally present.
- Nausea and vomiting may relate to duodenal obstruction.
- Palpable gallbladder in 30% (Courvoisier's sign—see Box 5.1.1).
- Migratory thrombophlebitis (i.e., Trousseau sign) and venous thrombosis (including portal vein thrombosis) occur at increased frequency.
- Differential diagnosis includes distal cholangiocarcinoma, ampullary cancer, focal pancreatitis in head of pancreas, and rarely autoimmune pancreatitis.

Box 5.1.1 Courvoisier's law

Ludwig Georg Courvoisier, Swiss surgeon 1843–1918

"Jaundice in the presence of a palpable gallbladder is not explained by gallstone obstruction of bile duct."

Probably explained by slow onset of biliary dilatation with distal bile duct tumors (e.g., pancreatic cancer, ampullary cancer), and fact that chronically inflamed, thick-walled gallbladders less likely to dilate. Exceptions to this rule include gallbladder empyema with cystic-duct stone obstruction, and Mirizzi's syndrome.

Investigation
- Aimed at making diagnosis and tumor staging.
- LFTs may show cholestatic picture – elevated Bili, ALP/GGT (see Recent onset jaundice).
- Elevated serum CA19–9 elevated in 75–85% of patients, but value > 100 U/ml only highly specific for malignancy in absence of biliary obstruction. Carcinoembryonic antigen (CEA) ↑ in 40% of patients, but of little diagnostic use.

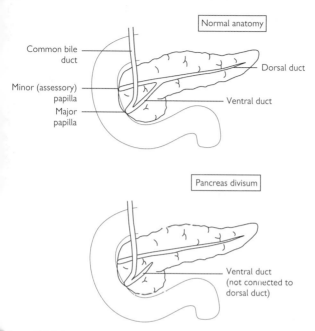

Figure 5.1.1 Anatomic arrangement of pancreatic ducts. (a) The most common arrangement, where most pancreatic secretions empty with the bile through the major duodenal papilla. In about 70% adults, the proximal portion of the dorsal duct remains patent and some pancreatic secretions empty through the accessory papilla. (b) Pancreas divisum: the embryonic dorsal and ventral ducts fail to fuse, with 80–95% of pancreatic secretions emptying from the dorsal duct through the accessory papilla.

- Transabdominal <u>ultrasound</u>: accurately shows biliary dilatation, but views of pancreas often incomplete. Pancreatic-protocol <u>CT</u>: defines tumor and size, demonstrates local vascular involvement (portal vein, superior mesenteric artery/vein), retroperitoneal invasion, and liver metastases. Only imaging modality needed to make diagnosis in > 90 % of cases. Very accurately demonstrates irresectability, but falsely suggests resectability in 25–50% of cases.
- <u>MRI</u> rarely used instead of CT, but has comparable accuracy.
- <u>ERCP</u>: allows endoscopic stenting (with plastic stent until histological confirmation of inoperable cancer), and cytological brushings. "<u>Double duct sign</u>" strongly suggests head of pancreas cancer (Color plate 2).
- <u>Endoscopic ultrasound</u> playing increasing role in staging (as good as <u>CT</u> for defining vascular involvement), allows FNA cytology, and useful for "trouble-shooting" small pancreatic lesions/unexplained strictures.

Management

- Curative resection in <15% of patients (very rare for cancers in body/ tail, as present late), and overall survival at one year and five years is 20% and 4%, respectively. In those undergoing curative resection (Whipple's procedure), five-year survival 10–25%. Histological diagnosis not usually needed or sought prior to attempted curative surgery.
- Palliative chemotherapy with gemcitabine provides improved disease-related symptoms and some survival benefit, but newer combination regimes are awaited. Role of chemo-radiotherapy, including as neoadjuvant therapy (to "downstaging" inoperable tumors to operable), remains uncertain.
- Pain control may be a particular problem, necessitating regular opiates Radiotherapy and celiac plexus block may help.
- ERCP and biliary stenting dependent on presentation (i.e., obstructive jaundice). Metal stents should not be inserted unless histology and clinical assessment/imaging confirm inoperable malignancy. In patients with unresectable tumor and biliary and duodenal obstruction (5% of patients), surgical biliary bypass or enteral and biliary mesh-metal stents are options.

Box 5.1.2 **Differential diagnosis of pancreatic mass**

- Pancreatic cancer (ductal adenocarcinoma)
- Distal cholangiocarcinoma
- Ampullary cancer
- Lymphoma
- TB
- Pancreatic endocrine tumor
- Autoimmune pancreatitis
- Acute and acute-on-chronic pancreatitis
- Von Hippel–Lindau disease
- Pancreatic cystic tumor
- Pancreatic pseudocyst

Pancreatic cystic tumors

Background

- Cystic neoplasms of pancreas account for 10–15% of cystic lesions (pancreatic pseudocysts (80–90%), true cysts, and acute fluid collections after acute pancreatitis account for rest), and represent only 1% of pancreatic neoplasms.
- Mucinous cystic neoplasm (MCN), serous cystadenoma, and intraductal papillary mucinous neoplasm (IPMN) account for > 90% of pancreatic cystic neoplasms (see Table 5.1.4).

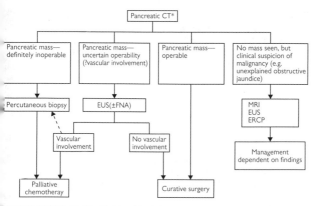

* Includes CT cuts through abdomen and chest, to exclude metastases.

Figure 5.1.2 Staging and management of suspected pancreatic cancer.

Table 5.1.4 Pancreatic cystic tumors

	Mucinous cystic neoplasm (MCN)	Serous cyst—adenoma	Intraductal papillary mucinous neoplasm (IPMN)
Sex	> 80% female	> 80% female	> 50% male
Peak age	50 years	70 years	60–70 years
Presentation	Mass/pain	Mass/pain	Recurrent pancreatitis
Pancreatic site	Body/tail	Head/body	Head
CT findings	Septae, Ca^{2+}	Septae, Ca^{2+}	No septae
	Mactrocysts	Mult. Sm cysts	
ERCP findings			
Pancreatic duct dilatation	No	No	No
Duct–cyst communication	Uncommon	Rare	Yes
Malignant potential	Yes (8–33% of cases)	Very rare	Yes (15–40% cases)

Clinical features

- Increasingly diagnosed incidentally on abdominal imaging.
- IPMN may be misdiagnosed as idiopathic recurrent or <u>chronic pancreatitis</u>, with pancreatic duct abnormalities, and <u>pancreatic insufficiency</u> caused by mucus obstruction of pancreatic duct.
- May occasionally present as for <u>pancreatic cancer</u> (i.e., weight loss, jaundice, pain).

Investigation

- <u>CT</u> and <u>MRI/MRCP</u> may define cyst architecture and relationship with pancreatic duct.
- <u>Endoscopic ultrasound</u> (EUS) has increasing role, and allows cyst fluid aspiration, but may not be necessary where surgery is planned and cross-sectional imaging unequivocal.
- Fluid analysis allows differentiation from <u>pancreatic pseudocyst</u>. Elevated cyst CEA levels suggest malignancy, but CA19–9 does not appear of be of use.
- <u>ERCP</u> may demonstrate mucus, either emanating from wide-open papilla (pathognomonic of IPMN), or within dilated pancreatic duct.

Diagnosis

- Differentiating between pseudocysts, serous cystadenomas, and mucinous cystadenomas can be difficult
- Pseudocyst: suspect with a recent history of pancreatitis, when the lesion contains amylase-rich watery fluid and communicates with the pancreatic duct.
- Serous cystadenoma: suspect when the lesion consists of multiple small cysts (microcysts) and the cyst fluid is thin and watery.
- Mucinous neoplasm: suspect when one or more macrocytic spaces containing mucin are found.
- Unfortunately, these are general guidelines that do not always permit an accurate diagnosis.

Management

No standardized policy. Management in specialist centers. Management depends on diagnosis and certainty of diagnosis. Need to balance potential cure from surgery, against requirement for radical resection (Whipple's procedure or distal pancreatectomy, dependent on site) in asymptomatic patients with cystic tumors of low malignant potential.

The ASGE[1] has issued a guideline on the role of endoscopy in the diagnosis and management of cystic lesions of the pancreas. ACG[2] has also issued a guideline on the diagnosis and management of neoplastic pancreatic cysts. Brief summary:

- Incidentally discovered pancreatic cysts require evaluation.
- EUS finding alone are not sufficient for the evaluation of pancreatic cysts.
- Cyst fluid analysis is most often necessary.

1 Jacobson, BC, Baron, TH, Adler, DG, et al. ASGE guideline: The role of endoscopy in the diagnosis and the management of cystic lesions and inflammatory fluid collections of the pancreas. Gastrointest Endosc 2005; 61:363.
2 Khalid A, Brugge W. (2007). ACG guidelines for the diagnosis and management of neoplastic pancreatic cysts. American Journal of Gastroenterology, 102(1):2339.

Pancreatic endocrine tumors (PET)

- <u>Neuroendocrine tumors</u> of the GI tract classified into two groups—<u>carcinoid</u> tumors and PETs. Latter arise from pancreatic islet cells.
- Primary insulinomas and glucagonomas occur exclusively in pancreas, but 50–70% of <u>gastrinomas</u> arise from extrapancreatic sites. May be associated with other conditions, including <u>multiple endocrine neoplasia (MEN)-1</u>, Von Hippel–Lindau disease, neurofibromatosis type 1 (NF1), and tuberous sclerosis (e.g., >10% NF1 patients develop <u>carcinoid</u> tumor, often duodenal).
- PETs may be functional (associated with clinical syndrome related to hormone release (see Table 5.1.5)) or nonfunctional.

Insulinoma

- Located throughout pancreas (one-third head, one-third body, one-third tail), usually < 5 cm, with multiple lesions in approx 10%. Clinical features relate to symptomatic hypoglycemia, and patients may have weight gain due to overeating to stave off hypoglycemia (18%). Association with MEN-1 in approximately 10%.
- As with other functional PETs, diagnosis depends on localizing tumor, and demonstrating excess hormone. In > 90%, 72-hour fast with three-to-six hourly blood glucose, plasma insulin, and C-peptide levels induces hypoglycemia and demonstrates disproportionately elevated insulin. CT/ MRI localize lesion in < 40% if 1–3 cm, and <u>endoscopic ultrasound</u>, angiography, and selective venous sampling may be required.
- Management includes advice to take small regular meals and diazoxide, a nondiuretic benzothiazide analogue, that inhibits insulin release (this drug and <u>OCTREOTIDE</u> may control symptoms in 60% of cases). Surgery provides complete cure in 70–95%.

Glucagonoma

- Glucagon stimulates glycogenolysis and insulin secretion, and inhibits pancreatic and gastric secretion and gut motility. Association with <u>MEN-1</u> in 20%. Metastases/local invasion in 50–80%. Slow growing.
- Usually > 5 cm, secrete excess glucagons, causing dermatitis (migratory necrolytic erythema), weight loss, glucose intolerance, and anemia. Hyperglycemia in 40–90%.
- Diagnosis made on demonstrating elevated plasma glucagons >500 pg/ml (normal < 200 pg/ml). CT to locate tumor.
- Treatment includes control of diabetes and use of octreotide (may improve weight loss, diarrhea, and rash).
- Surgery performed for local disease, but cure in only 20%.

VIPoma

- Usually solitary tumors in tail of pancreas.
- Characterized by profound watery diarrhea, dehydration, hypokalemia and hypochlorydia.
- Diagnosis made on basis of large-volume diarrhea (> 3 l/day in > 75% of patients), and raised serum VIP levels (>75 pg/ml).

- Medical management includes careful fluid and electrolyte replacement. May need > 5 l fluids, and 350 MEq of potassium/day). <u>OCTREOTIDE</u> controls symptoms, but effect may be short lived. Surgery completely relieves symptoms in approximately 30%.

See: <u>Gastrinoma</u>

Nonfunctional PETs

- One-third of PETs. Usually occur in pancreatic head, are generally larger than functional ones, and 60–90% malignant

Table 5.1.5 Pancreatic endocrine tumors (PET)

Syndrome	Hormone released	Clinical features	Rate of malignancy (%)	Incidence per million
Gastrinoma (Zollinger–Ellison syndrome)	Gastrin	Recurrent upper GI tract ulceration	60–70	1
Insulinoma	Insulin	Hypoglycemic episodes Weight gain	<10	1–2
Glucagonoma	Glucagon	Weight loss Diarrhea, Dermatitis (migratory necrolytic erythema)	60	0.1
VIPoma	Vasoactive intestinal polypeptide	Watery diarrhea↓K, ↓Mg^{2+} Flushing	> 60	0.5
Somato-statinoma	Somatostatin	Diarrhea	> 70	< 0.1

For details on practical aspects of measuring gut hormones, see gut hormone profile.

Pancreatic function tests

- Pancreatic **endocrine** function usually assessed with glucose tolerance test.
- Exocrine function tests used to assess <u>chronic pancreatitis</u> and other causes of exocrine <u>pancreatic insufficiency</u>, and variety of direct and indirect tests available. Malabsorption and steatorrhea only occur when > 90% of **exocrine** pancreas function lost.
- **Direct tests** involve sampling of pancreatic secretions after administration of secretagogue (e.g., secretin, cholecystokinin). Duodenal aspiration and measurement of volume, bicarbonate, and

enzyme concentration (e.g., amylase, trypsin, lipase). Direct tests remain "gold standard," but invasive to perform, and rarely used in clinical practice.

- **Indirect tests** involve measurement of pancreatic enzymes in stool, or of metabolites of pancreatic enzyme breakdown in urine/plasma/stool.
  - **Three-day fecal fat.** Normally < 7% of ingested fat appears in stool, but steatorrhea develops if pancreatic lipase output falls to < 10% of normal, so test poorly sensitive for mild to moderate pancreatic insufficiency. Unpleasant test for patients and laboratory staff, and rarely performed. Qualitative microscopic examination of single stool for oil nearly as sensitive.
  - **Fecal elastase 1 (FE1).** Increasingly used, because it is simple, noninvasive, and accurate (sensitivity/specificity > 90% for significant exocrine insufficiency). Uses monoclonal antibody and ELISA to detect elastase in single spot stool sample. Falsely low FE1 levels (< 200 μg elastase/g of stool) may occur in watery diarrhea, but level < 50 μg elastase/g of stool highly specific for significant exocrine <u>pancreatic insufficiency</u>. Measurement not affected by concomitant use of <u>PANCREATIC SUPPLEMENTS</u>.
  - **Pancreolauryl test.** Fluorescein dilaurate is split by pancreatic enzymes into lauric acid and fluorescein. Fluorescein absorbed in the intestine, partly conjugated in the liver, and excreted in the urine. On day one of test, tablet of fluorescein dilaurate taken and urine collected for 10 hours. On day two, same procedure, but tablet contains free fluorescein (allows for correction of individual variations in intestinal, hepatic, and renal function). Results expressed as the ratio of fluorescein excreted after fluorescein dilaurate (T) and after free fluorescein (K) (T/K ratio < 20% abnormal). Most accurate at diagnosing significant exocrine insufficiency, less sensitive for mild-moderate disease. In clinical practice this test is largely being replaced by FE1 measurement.

Pancreatic insufficiency

- Clinical exocrine insufficiency only occurs when > 90% of exocrine pancreas function lost.
- Causes include <u>chronic pancreatitis</u>, pancreatic resection (see <u>Whipple's procedure</u>), and <u>cystic fibrosis</u>.
- Clinical features relate to malabsorption and include steatorrhea (pale, loose/bulky stools, which may contain visible droplets of oil, float, and be difficult to flush away), weight loss, abdominal bloating and discomfort. Malabsorption of fat soluble vitamins (see <u>vitamins A, D, E, K</u>) may give rise to a range of clinical problems, including metabolic bone disease. In patients with chronic pancreatitis and significant exocrine insufficiency, pain is often absent, reflecting loss of functioning pancreas.
- Diagnosis confirmed using <u>pancreatic function tests</u>, but significant exocrine insufficiency unusual in absence of structural abnormality of pancreas (e.g., pancreatic atrophy, calcification, pancreatic

duct abnormalities). Anatomy usually accurately assessed with pancreatic protocol <u>CT scan</u>, but other complementary modalities include <u>endoscopic ultrasound</u>, <u>ERCP</u>, and <u>MRCP</u>. The latter may be performed before and after secretin injection, providing some indication of volume of pancreatic juice output, and functional hold up at pancreatic sphincter.

- Management includes treating underlying cause, <u>PANCREATIC ENZYME SUPPLEMENTS</u>, treatment/prevention of <u>osteoporosis</u>, and replacement of fat soluble vitamins. Also see <u>Steatorrhea</u>.

Pancreatic pseudocyst

Background

- Localized fluid collection (2–30 cm) with nonepithelialized wall, usually located within lesser sac. Accounts for 80–90% of pancreatic cystic lesions.
- Arises due to pancreatic duct disruption. Complicates 16–50% of cases of <u>acute pancreatitis</u>, 20–40% of <u>chronic pancreatitis</u>, and rarely associated with <u>pancreatic cancer</u> or trauma. By convention, cyst needs to be present for > four weeks after acute pancreatitis to make diagnosis ("acute fluid collection" < 4 weeks).

Clinical features/complications

- May be asymptomatic, or cause symptoms related to:
- Local compression: biliary obstruction; gastric outlet obstruction.
- Vascular involvement: <u>portal vein thrombosis</u> (PVT); pseudoaneurysm: involvement of gastroduodenal/splenic artery. May present with rapidly increasing pain, ↓Hb, or hypovolaemic shock due to rupture.
- Infection: occurs in 10%, usually following instrumentation (e.g., drainage).
- Rupture: may be associated with development of largely asymptomatic pancreatic ascites, or generalized peritonitis.

Investigations

- Diagnosis usually made with transabdominal <u>U/S</u> or contrast <u>CT scan</u>.
- Diagnostic cyst aspiration occasionally needed (via <u>endoscopic ultrasound</u> (EUS)), as high cystic <u>amylase</u> differentiates pseudocyst from <u>pancreatic cystic tumors</u>.
- <u>ERCP</u> avoided unless transpapillary drainage considered, or diagnosis unclear, as may introduce infection.

Management

- Pancreatic rest (e.g., with nasojejunal feeding) may hasten resolution of <u>acute pancreatitis</u> and associated pseudocyst.
- Asymptomatic pseudocysts < 6 cm can be managed conservatively, because most will resolve spontaneously (but may take months).
- Drainage considered (without clear scientific basis) for symptomatic, > 6 cm pseudocysts, present for > 6 weeks. Approaches include:

- **Linear EUS**. Favored approach by specialist units, as linear EUS allows cyst drainage into stomach/duodenum, delineation and avoidance of pericystic varices (common in view of PVT). Less than 1 cm between gastric and pseudocyst wall necessary.
- **Transpapillary** drainage via <u>pancreatic stent</u> insertion at ERCP depends on cyst–duct communication.
- **Percutaneous**. Effective, but may develop cutaneo-pancreatic fistula if pancreatic duct leak continues, so percutaneous, transgastric puncture ideal (allowing drainage into stomach after drain removal, or endoscopic internalization of drain).
- **Surgery** with internal cyst drainage may provide resolution, but 24% complication rate. Persistent or recurrent pseudocysts may ultimately require pancreatic resection if duct rupture does not resolve (<u>Whipple's procedure</u> for cysts in head, distal pancreatectomy if in tail).
- Pseudoaneurysm treated with angiographic embolization, rarely surgery.
- ERCP and plastic stent insertion for biliary obstruction.

Pancreatic stents

- Vary in shape and size. Temporary (e.g., polyethylene) or permanent (e.g., wall stents). Used to treat pancreatic duct strictures in setting of refractory abdominal pain associated with chronic pancreatitis, pancreatic duct disruptions, <u>pancreatic pseudocysts</u> or fistulae,prevention of post-ERCP pancreatitis.
- In patients with <u>pancreatic pseudocyst</u> or fistulae, pancreatic stent insertion, particularly across the point of duct disruption, may accelerate resolution. Should only be undertaken by endoscopists with specialist experience of pancreatic endotherapy.
- Insertion of small 3–5F polyethylene stents into main pancreatic duct at ERCP increasingly used to prevent post-ERCP pancreatitis, particularly in high risk patients (e.g., suspected <u>sphincter of Oddi dysfunction</u>, previous post-ERCP pancreatitis—also see <u>endoscopic complications</u>). In series from specialist centers, pancreatic stent insertion does seem to reduce risk, but unsuccessful attempts at insertion may worsen outcome further, with risk of pancreatic trauma. 80% of stents fall out within three weeks, but checking X-ray at this time is essential, with endoscopic stent removal if stent still *in situ*.
- Long-term pancreatic duct stenting for relapsing or <u>chronic pancreatitis</u> not of proven benefit, and may cause further duct stricturing.

Pancreatitis

See: <u>acute pancreatitis</u>, <u>autoimmune pancreatitis</u>, <u>chronic pancreatitis</u>, and <u>hereditary pancreatitis</u>.

Steatorrhea

Steatorrhoea is the passage of bulky, pale, foul-smelling stools that float and are difficult to flush away (in fact, most stools float due to gas, not fat content). A greasy film or even droplets of oil may be seen in the toilet pan. More than 90% of daily dietary fat is absorbed into the general circulation, but any defects in the processing or absorption of fat can reduce this uptake and lead to fatty diarrhea.

Causes

- Pancreatic insufficiency, e.g., chronic pancreatitis - reduced lipase and co-lipase production impairs fat hydrolysis.
- Bile salt deficiency e.g., intrahepatic cholestasis, cirrhosis or biliary obstruction – less bile salts reduces micelle formation
- Small-intestinal disease e.g., celiac disease - impaired global absorption of lipids, carbohydrates, proteins and minerals occurs with severe disease
- Other causes include postsurgical, drug-induced, diarrhea-induced and hyperthyroidism

Clinical clues

- A history of pale, bulky, terribly smelly stools that are difficult to flush suggests steatorrhea.
- Abdominal discomfort, bloating, and flatulence can occur.
- Ask about symptoms related to fat-soluble <u>vitamin</u> (A, D, E, K) deficiency:
  - Bleeding, easy bruising, night blindness, metabolic bone disease), low calcium, magnesium, phosphate (e.g., tetany, muscle weakness), iron (microcytic anemia), vitamin B12 (macrocytic anemia, glossitis, angular stomatitis).
- Is there a history of weight loss, failure to thrive (in children), or primary/secondary amenorrhea?
- Does patient have a clinical problem known to predispose to malabsorption (e.g., <u>chronic pancreatitis</u>, <u>celiac disease</u>, small bowel <u>Crohn's disease</u>)?

Confirming Steatorrhea

- **Sudan III stain.** This qualitative test of fecal fat is positive in > 80% of patients with true steatorrhea, provided they are ingesting 75–100 g of fat/day).
- **Three-day fecal fat** is the "gold standard" to confirm steatorrhea, with >7 g stool fat/24 hours abnormal.
- **Fecal fat concentration.** Gut mucosal disease usually leads to malabsorption of water and electrolytes, and so fat is relatively diluted within stool. This is in contrast to maldigestion (e.g., in <u>pancreatic insufficiency</u>), when fecal fat concentration > 9.5 g/100 g stool is characteristically seen.

Identifying etiology

Clues to the etiology in history and initial results will lead to tests being tailored to each case. The aim should be to confirm fecal fat elevation on an adequate fat diet, then tailor tests to likely source, e.g., pancreatic, bile salt or small bowel (see also <u>Diarrhea</u> in "Top 10" section).

The following investigations for common causes of steatorrhea should be performed:
- Stool for ova, cysts and parasites, fecal pancreatic elastase-1
- Direct bilirubin, alkaline phosphatase, gamma-GT for biliary obstruction
- Immunoglobulin (Ig) A-tissue transglutaminase (tTG) titer for celiac disease
- Abdominal CT scan with oral and IV contrast to look for small bowel lymphoma, Crohn's disease, pancreatic abnormalities
- Magnetic resonance cholangiopancreatography (MRCP) or ERCP to look for biliary disease
- Hydrogen breath test for bacterial overgrowth.

Management
- Where the etiology of malabsorption is difficult to establish, therapeutic trials may direct clinician to the etiology, e.g.,:
  - PANCREATIC ENZYME SUPPLEMENTS in suspected pancreatic insufficiency may lead to rapid improvement in steatorrhea.
  - Antibiotics may improve <u>bacterial overgrowth</u>.
  - Bile acid sequesters (e.g., CHOLESTYRAMINE) may improve diarrhea/steatorrhea related to <u>bile acid malabsorption</u>.
- Vitamins, micronutrients, and hematinics need replacing if deficient.
- Consider effects of bone loss (see <u>osteoporosis</u>), so arrange <u>bone densitometry</u>, and provide fracture prophylaxis as necessary.

Biliary tree

Biliary atresia

Congenital anomaly affecting 1:14,000 live births, with fibrosis and destruction of biliary tree at different sites.
● Type I – common bile duct.
● Type II – common hepatic duct.
● Type III – liver hilum (85% of cases).
Presents with progressive jaundice and hepatomegaly by second week postpartum, with other defects (e.g., dextrocardia) in 25%. Diagnosis suggested by abdominal U/S or hepatobiliary scintiscan in neonate with persistent jaundice, and made by cholangiography, either via ERCP, transhepatic puncture, or more usually intraoperatively. Liver biopsy may be characteristic (portal tract expansion, bile plugging of ducts).

Treatment is surgical, usually through Roux-en-Y anastomosis, with loop of small bowel anastomosed to hepatic ducts at hilum (Kasai porto-enterostomy). This is effective in > 50%, but only 35% 10-year survival due to complications, including secondary biliary cirrhosis. Liver transplantation may be required.

Biliary bypass procedures

Resection of extrahepatic bile duct, or biliary diversion, may be indicated for a range of biliary problems, including:
● Iatrogenic/traumatic bile duct injury (e.g., postcholecystectomy), which is not amenable to endoscopic stent insertion.
● Biliary stone disease (e.g., Mirrizzi's syndrome).
● Persistent biliary stricture (e.g., secondary to pancreatic cancer or chronic pancreatitis).
● Choledochal cyst.

Operative approaches include:
● Whipple's procedure (distal common bile duct (CBD), duodenum, and pancreatic head resection).
● Hepatico-jejunostomy: Roux-en-Y anastomosis, with jejunal loop on to common hepatic duct.
● Choledochoduodenostomy: usually side-to-side anastomosis of lower CBD on to duodenal bulb. Used for very distal strictures.
● Cholecyst–enterostomy: anastomosis of gallbladder on to small bowel—rarely performed.

Practical point. In patient with hepaticojejunostomy, subsequent ERCP to access biliary tree is often impossible, due to Roux-en-Y anastomosis and long jejunal loop.

Biliary reflux

- Refers to the reflux into the stomach and esophagus of biliary fluid from the duodenum. Alkaline bile is an irritant to esophageal squamous mucosa. Factors associated with biliary reflux include duodenal pathology (e.g., distal duodenal stricture), hiatus hernia, and surgery (e.g., Billroth II partial <u>gastrectomy</u>, with reflux of bile from afferent loop into stomach). Symptoms are similar to those of gastro-esophageal reflux, but pH esophageal monitoring (also see <u>esophageal manometry</u>) demonstrates increased pH in association with reflux symptoms, and acid suppression provides no benefit.
- Treatment includes prokinetic agents (metaclopramide, domperidone (see <u>DOPAMINE RECEPTOR ANTAGONISTS</u>)) and mucosal protection (<u>sucralfate</u> 2 g bd PO). Surgery is sometimes necessary—a <u>Roux-en-Y anastomosis</u> allows diversion of bile flow further down jejunum.

Biliary strictures

May develop at any point within biliary tree, but site may give some clue to etiology (see Table 5.2.1): e.g., low common bile duct (CBD) stricture more likely due to <u>pancreatic cancer</u>, chronic <u>pancreatitis</u>; mid-CBD due to <u>Mirrizzi's syndrome</u>, <u>gallbladder cancer</u>; and hilar structuring may be due to <u>primary sclerosing cholangitis</u>, <u>cholangiocarcinoma</u>.

Clinical features

Jaundice (see <u>Recent onset jaundice</u>), right upper quadrant pain, <u>cholangitis</u> (fever, rigors), abnormal <u>liver function tests</u>, or rarely the complications of secondary biliary cirrhosis.

Investigations

- Bloods may show ↑Bn, cholestatic LFTs (↑ALP, GGT).
- U/S accurately demonstrate biliary dilatation, presence of gallbladder stones, and possible mass lesions.
- <u>CT scan</u> and <u>MRI/MRCP</u> are noninvasive tests of choice to define exact site of stricture, etiology, and surrounding structures.
- <u>ERCP</u> allows delineation of stricture/biliary tree, cytological brushings, endobiliary biopsies, and therapy (e.g., stone extraction, biliary stenting).
- <u>Endoscopic ultrasound</u>, including intraductal miniprobe ultrasound, may be available in specialist units, and may delineate nature of stricture further (e.g., <u>cholangiocarcinoma</u>).

Management
Depends on defining the cause of the stricture (see relevant sections). Simplistically, treatment involves endoscopic resolution of stricture (e.g., sphincterotomy for ampullary stenosis, balloon dilatation of benign stricture), endoscopic stenting, or surgery (which may include cholecystectomy for Mirizzi's syndrome, or biliary bypass procedure).

Table 5.2.1 Causes of biliary strictures

Primary sclerosing cholangitis	HIV cholangiopathy (see HIV and the liver)
Cholangiocarcinoma	Autoimmune pancreatitis
Gallbladder cancer	Pancreatic cancer
Extrinsic compression by hilar nodes	Ampullary cancer/stenosis
Mirizzi's syndrome	Bile duct stone-related stricture
Cholecystectomy-related bile duct injury	Clonorchis infection
Ischemic stricture	Bile duct (peri-dochal) varices/cavernoma
Acute/chronic pancreatitis	

Biliary tree variations

- Most variations in the anatomy of the biliary tree appear to result from alterations in the budding from the foregut of the embryonic liver and biliary tract. Minor anomalies usually cause no clinical problems, but may be of great relevance to the biliary surgeon.
- An accessory bile duct from right hepatic duct to cystic duct/gall bladder ("duct of Lushka") may result in biliary leak post-cholecystectomy. In 5% the right hepatic duct inserts low down in common hepatic duct, and may be mistaken for cystic duct. In 20% the cystic duct does not pass straight into the common hepatic duct, but runs parallel to it, down toward the papilla ("low inserting cystic duct"), with a risk of incorrect ductal ligation at surgery, and incorrect stent placement at ERCP.
- Gall bladders may be congenitally bilobed, double, intrahepatic, or absent. Other congenital abnormalities may cause symptoms through predisposing to bile stasis, stone formation, or malignancy (see Caroli's disease; choledochal cysts).

Cholangiocarcinoma

Definition and pathogenesis
- Primary malignancy arising from intrahepatic or extrahepatic biliary tree, which causes 1.5% of all cancers; the rate is increasing. An important cause of biliary strictures.

- Associations include <u>primary sclerosing cholangitis</u> (PSC) (> 20% of cases of longstanding PSC develop cholangiocarcinoma, but PSC associated with only 5% of cases), <u>gallstones</u>, <u>choledochal cysts</u>, <u>Caroli's disease</u>, and biliary infestation with oriental liver fluke <u>Clonorchis</u> *sinensis*.
- Approximately 20–25% of tumors intrahepatic, 50–60% perihilar ("Klatskin" tumors involve confluence of left and right hepatic ducts in 20%), and 20–25% distal bile duct.

Clinical features

Abdominal discomfort, weight loss, and obstructive jaundice are the commonest presenting symptoms, similar to those of <u>pancreatic cancer</u>.

Investigations

- See <u>Recent onset jaundice</u>
- Site, size, and vascular involvement of tumor may be demonstrated with <u>CT</u> and <u>MRCP</u>. Biliary anatomy well shown with MRCP, but <u>ERCP</u> allows intraductal U/S and endoscopic stenting to be performed. <u>PET scanning</u> may find a role.
- Tissue diagnosis may be made by endoscopic biopsies or brushings, or percutaneous biopsy. Diagnosis particularly difficult to confirm in patient with PSC and intra/extrahepatic duct strictures.
- Tumor marker CA19-9 ↑ in 85% of cases, but diagnostic role limited because it may be elevated in biliary obstruction *per se*. Staging by TNM (see <u>tumor staging</u>).

Management

- Surgical resection possible in only 10–15% of cases. five-year survival postsurgery 9–18% for proximal tumors, 20–30% for distal bile duct lesions. <u>Liver transplantation</u> is rarely performed (because of very high rates of recurrence, but very highly selected patient groups may show up to 53% five-year survival, with emerging data on aggressive neoadjuvant therapy prior to transplantation showing some promise.
- Effective palliative endoscopic or percutaneous transhepatic stenting (plastic or self-expanding metal stents) is vital to preserve liver function and prevent cholangitis.
- Conventional chemotherapy (e.g., gemcytabine regimens) may provide partial response in 20–30% of cases. Palliative <u>photodynamic therapy</u> shows promise and may help to maintain duct patency.

Cholangitis

Infection of the biliary tree, usually arising from combination of biliary obstruction (e.g., <u>biliary stricture</u>) and presence of bacteria (usually Gram-negative gut flora).

Etiology + pathogenesis

Causes of obstruction include stones (see <u>choledocholithiasis</u>), biliary strictures (e.g., <u>primary sclerosing cholangitis</u>, <u>pancreatic cancer</u>, <u>cholangiocarcinoma</u>), infestation (e.g., <u>Clonorchis</u>), and following instrumentation (particularly if incomplete drainage achieved at <u>ERCP</u>).

Clinical features

Classic Charcot triad includes fever (>90% of cases), jaundice (65%), and right upper quadrant pain (>40%). The presence of all three strongly favors the diagnosis, but this combination occurs in <20% of cases at presentation. Septic shock and confusion may occur.

- Secondary complications include acute renal failure, disseminated intravascular coagulation (DIC), and <u>liver abscess</u> formation.

Investigation

- CBC shows ↑WCC (↑ neutrophils).
- BUN & Creatinine - Renal failure associated with septic shock.
- LFTs: ↑Bn, and predominantly cholestatic pattern (↑↑ALP/GGT), but ↑ALT, AST often present.
- Blood cultures positive in up to 50% of cases.
- Urgent <u>U/S</u> or <u>CT scan</u> showing biliary dilatation in correct clinical setting strongly supports diagnosis. Loss of aerobilia (air in biliary tree) in patient with biliary stent *in situ* suggests blocked stent.
- After demonstration of dilated bile ducts, <u>ERCP</u> allows confirmation of biliary obstruction and therapy.

Management

- Fluid resuscitation and management in high dependency area if hypotensive with signs of septic shock.
- Broad spectrum IV antibiotics (e.g., IV <u>CEPHALOSPORIN</u> + <u>METRONIDAZOLE</u>, or <u>PIPERACILLIN/TAZOBACTAM</u>), but note that antibiotics alone rarely resolve cholangitis in the presence of ongoing biliary obstruction.
- ERCP with biliary decompression (e.g., biliary sphincterotomy and stone removal/stent insertion) essential. Percutaneous transhepatic drainage (PTC) only used if ERCP fails/technically impossible, as complications higher (and puncture often increases bacteremia acutely).
- Mortality rate 7–40%, with poor outcome closely correlated with delays in definitive management.

Cholecystectomy

- 700,000 cholecystectomies a year performed in the United States, mainly for <u>gallstones</u>.
- Laparoscopic cholecystectomy (LC) in > 80% of cases, but conversion to open cholecystectomy (OC) needed in 5–10%. In patients with bile duct stones (<u>choledocholithiasis</u>), duct clearance and sphincterotomy usually done by <u>ERCP</u> prior to surgery, but laparoscopic bile duct clearance increasingly performed at time of LC.
- Major complications include wound infection, bleeding, abscess formation, or bile leak (arising from cystic duct stump, damaged common bile duct, or aberrant bilary ducts (e.g., duct of Lushka)). See <u>biliary tree variants.</u> Bile duct injury occurs in 0.1–0.2% of OC, 0.5–1% of LC. Complications due to <u>biliary strictures</u> may develop immediately or up to 20 years later. Mortality for cholecystectomy 0.2% overall (0.03% in those < 65 years old).

Cholecystitis

Defined as inflammation of the gallbladder, which results from obstruction of the cystic duct by gallstones in 90% of cases, and occurs in 30% of patients with gallstones. Acalculous cholecystitis is related to biliary stasis (e.g., major surgery/trauma, sepsis, parenteral nutrition, sickle cell disease, diabetes mellitus). Bacterial infection is thought to be secondary to obstruction.

Clinical features

Most patients have a prior history of biliary colic (see gallstones), but pain of acute cholecystitis is more constant and severe and lasts for > six hours. It settles in most cases after 1–4 days.

- Fever, nausea, and vomiting often present.
- Examination may reveal fever and tachycardia, with tenderness in the right upper quadrant (Murphy's sign), with guarding and rebound. Palpable gallbladder in 30% of cases.
- Jaundice suggests choledocholithiasis or Mirizzi's syndrome.
- Gallbladder perforation occurs in 10–15% of cases, and gallbladder empyema may occur.

Investigation

- ↑ WCC (neutrophilia) is common.
- ↑ ALP in 25% of cases, but deranged liver function tests usually suggest associated biliary obstruction (CBD stones in 10% of patients with calculous cholecystitis).
- Transabdominal ultrasound is >90–95% sensitive, 80% specific for cholecystitis. Diagnosis suggested by pericholecystic fluid, gallbladder wall thickening >4 mm, and presence of gallstones. Wall thickness unreliable in patients with ascites and hypoalbuminemia.
- CT scan 95% sensitive and specific for cholecystitis. Although less effective than U/S in detecting gallstones, it is more accurate in identifying complications (e.g., gallbladder perforation, empyema).
- Hepatobiliary scintigraphy (HIDA scan) may show impaired gallbladder emptying in an acalculous cholecystitis.

Management

Cholecystectomy.

Choledochal cyst

Cystic dilatation of the intra/extrahepatic bile ducts. Particularly reported in the Far East. Classified into several types (see Box 5.2.1).

Clinical features

Majority of patients present at <30 years, with pain and jaundice. Complications include rupture, cholangitis, cirrhosis, acute pancreatitis, portal hypertension, and cholangiocarcinoma (up to 50% of untreated patients by age 50).

Investigation
Diagnosis usually made by CT scanning, MRCP, or ERCP.

Management
Complete cyst excision is essential (in part to reduce risk of cholangiocarcinoma), with Roux-en-Y hepaticojejunostomy (see biliary bypass procedures). Recurrent symptoms are common, and secondary biliary cirrhosis may require liver transplantation.

Box 5.2.1 Classification of choledochal cysts

Type 1: Diffuse or fusiform dilatation of extrahepatic bile ducts (93% of cases)

Type 2: Diverticulum arising from bile duct

Type 3: Cystic dilatation of distal bile duct, within the duodenum

Type 4: Type I and an intrahepatic cyst

(Type 5: Caroli's disease)

Double duct sign

Term used to describe appearance on ERCP, MRCP, or CT, of stricture (and upstream dilatation) of common bile duct and pancreatic duct, usually in patients with biliary obstruction. Often associated with pancreatic cancer (in head of pancreas, as shown on ERCP in Fig. 2.11 opposite), but rarer causes include focal pancreatitis or ampullary cancer/stenosis.

Gallbladder cancer

Epidemiology
Rare malignancy, usually affecting elderly patients. Associated with gallstones in 70–90% of cases, calcified ("porcelain") gallbladder (gallbladder cancer in 25%), and gallbladder polyps > 1 cm in diameter (malignant in 23–88% of patients). Prophylactic cholecystectomy should particularly be considered for the last two risk factors. Tumor found in fundus in 60%, body in 30%, neck in 10%.

Clinical features
Right upper quadrant discomfort, weight loss, and jaundice. A hard, tender mass is sometimes felt in region of the gallbladder. Occasionally condition is asymptomatic, with diagnosis made following 1–3% of cholecystectomies performed for gallstones.

Investigations

CT and U/S may show thickened gallbladder wall and mass within gallbladder lumen. Local spread well shown with CT. ERCP may show obstructed cystic duct, and mid-common bile duct stricture. Percutaneous biopsy may make histological diagnosis.

Management

Surgical resection rarely curative unless diagnosis made incidentally at time of <u>cholecystectomy</u>, as cancer spreads early to surrounding structures, including liver. Radical surgery (including right hepatectomy) rarely of benefit, and no clear role for systemic chemotherapy or radiotherapy. Palliative approaches include biliary stenting to relieve jaundice, and <u>photodynamic therapy</u> may find a role in maintaining bile duct patency. Overall mean survival rate is six months, and the five-year survival rate < 5%.

Gallbladder empyema

Refers to the presence of pus within the gallbladder. It usually develops following acute <u>cholecystitis</u>, but cystic duct obstruction due to tumor (e.g., <u>cholangiocarcinoma</u>) may also occur. Infection may arise from <u>cholangitis</u>. Usually presents with right upper quadrant pain and signs of sepsis. Gallbladder perforation with subsequent peritonitis is an important complication if left untreated. CT or U/S may show a distended, fluid-filled gallbladder, with pericholecystic fluid. Treatment is with IV antibiotics (e.g., third-generation <u>CEPHALOSPORIN</u> and <u>METRONIDAZOLE</u>) and percutaneous gallbladder drain insertion (cholecystectomy is usually delayed because of high rate of post-operative septic complications).

Gallbladder polyps

- Refers to any mucosal projection into lumen of gallbladder. Prevalence 1–4%. More than 90% not neoplasms at all (e.g., cholesterol "polyp" arising from wall of gallbladder), and < 5% are true adenomas. Difficult to accurately define different types on imaging (usually ultrasound), but malignant change very rare in any gallbladder polyp < 10 mm.
- Usually asymptomatic, or found in association with symptomatic <u>gallstones</u>.
- Prudent management is to perform <u>cholecystectomy</u> if polyp > 10 mm (and certainly if > 18 mm, as these polyps carry significant risk of invasive adenocarcinoma). In those with polyps < 10 mm, ultrasound every six to twelve months may be considered to exclude an increase in size.

Gallstones

Epidemiology + pathogenesis

Present in 10–20% of the world's adult population. Increased prevalence in women, first-degree relatives of sufferers, obesity, and pregnancy. Terminal ileal disease, including <u>Crohn's disease</u>, and surgical resection associated with increased risk (possibly due to reduced bile acid absorption, increased cholesterol:bile acid secretion, and supersaturated bile). High-carbohydrate, low-fiber diet may be linked. Pigment stones linked with hemolysis (e.g., sickle cell anemia) and chronic biliary infection (e.g., <u>Clonorchis</u> infection). Cholesterol-predominant stones account for 75% of cases; pigment stones (calcium bilirubinate, mucin glyocoprotein, bacterial products) account for 25%.

Clinical feature

Range of clinical scenarios in patients with gallstones, and pattern determines specific investigation and management. Symptoms develop in 1–3% of patients per year with gallstones.

Asymptomatic gallstones. Up to 80% of gallstone carriers remain asymptomatic, with incidental diagnosis made on imaging.

Symptomatic gallstones

- Biliary colic refers to 1–5 hours of constant severe, dull, or boring pain, most commonly in the epigastrium or right upper quadrant. Pain may radiate to right scapular region. Severe biliary colic occurs in 1–8%/year, and other complications (e.g., <u>acute pancreatitis</u>, <u>cholecystitis</u>) in 1–3%/year.
- Acute <u>cholecystitis</u> presents with biliary colic-type pain, except that it lasts hours–days, and is commonly associated with nausea, vomiting, and fever.
- Jaundice ± right upper quadrant suggests <u>choledocholithiasis</u>, or more rarely <u>Mirizzi's syndrome</u>, and evidence of sepsis points to <u>cholangitis</u>.
- <u>Acute pancreatitis</u>.

Investigations

Imaging

- Transabdominal <u>ultrasound</u> is > 92% sensitive, and 99% specific for gallbladder stones > 2 mm, and is usually the only modality required. It is much less sensitive (approximately 50%) at detecting common bile duct (CBD) stones.
- AXR rarely of use as only 10% of gallstones are radiolucent.
- <u>CT scanning</u> may miss 20% of gallbladder stones, but is better at detecting complications of cholecystitis (e.g., perforation, empyema).
- <u>Endoscopic ultrasound</u> is highly accurate in detection of gallbladder stones or sludge, but is invasive and rarely necessary in uncomplicated cases.

Blood tests

- In patients with asymptomatic gallstones or biliary colic all blood tests should be normal.
- See also <u>cholecystitis</u>, <u>choledocholithiasis</u>, <u>cholangitis</u>.

Management
Cholecystectomy rarely indicated for asymptomatic gallstones (but needless and ineffective surgery often erroneously performed upon finding them), but indicated for symptomatic disease (see cholecystitis, choledocholithiasis).

Hemobilia

- Bleeding into the biliary tree is an unusual cause of acute upper GI tract bleeding. Causes include blunt or penetrating trauma, instrumentation (e.g., liver biopsy, ERCP, TIPSS), gallstones, hepatic artery aneurysms, bile duct ('peridochal') varices, liver abscesses, and tumors (e.g., hepatocellular carcinoma).
- May be associated with right upper quadrant discomfort and jaundice (due to intraluminal blood clot or underlying disease, such as tumor).
- Making diagnosis often requires consideration of possibility (e.g., in patients with ↓ BP and Hb post-liver biopsy). At endoscopy, finding of blood in second part of duodenum without clear bleeding point should be followed by close inspection of ampulla with duodenoscope ± ERCP, if any risk factors for hemobilia. Source of bleeding may be suggested on CT, and bleeding point may be defined by angiography.
- Management involves correcting any coagulopathy and biliary decompression with endoscopic stent if obstructed. Hemobilia usually settles spontaneously, but may require angiographic embolization and rarely surgery.

Sphincter of Oddi dysfunction (SOD)

Definition + clinical features
Hypertension of biliary/pancreatic sphincter may cause episodic pancreatico-biliary-type pain, and biliary SOD is categorized into 3 clinical groups:
- **Type I:** biliary pain, plus liver function tests (LFTs) > ×2 ULN on > 1 occasion, and dilated common bile duct.
- **Type II:** biliary pain, and one of the above.
- **Type III:** biliary pain only.

Investigation
- Dilated CBD may be seen on U/S, CT, or MRCP (CBD normally < 7 mm in diameter, but may be slightly wider (up to approximately 9 mm) postcholecystectomy and in extreme elderly, in the absence of other pathology.
- LFTs may be elevated during attacks of pain.
- Sphincter of Oddi manometry (SOM) at ERCP is the "gold-standard" investigation. Baseline sphincter pressure > 40 mmHg, or sustained peaks > 100 mmHg are consistent with the diagnosis, but the technique is technically difficult.
- Hepatobiliary scintigraphy (e.g., HIDA scan) may show delayed biliary emptying.

Management
- Definitive treatment for proven SOD is biliary (& pancreatic) sphincterotomy, but risks of <u>ERCP</u>-related complications are particularly high in this patient group (up to 20% <u>acute pancreatitis</u>). Safety of procedure, probability of abnormal SOM, and response to sphincterotomy are lowest for type III SOD. <u>Pancreatic stent</u> insertion may lower risks of procedure.
- Before ERCP/SOM, many physicians would try empirical medical therapy for SOD II/III (e.g., antispasmodics/tricyclic antidepressants), and consider <u>cholecystectomy</u> if any evidence of <u>gallstones</u>/sludge on transabdominal or <u>endoscopic ultrasound</u> (passage of microcalculi may mimic SOD).

Table 5.2.2 Biliary SOD categorized into three types

SOD type	Frequency of abnormal manometry (%)	Benefit of sphincterotomy based on manometry findings (%)	
		Abnormal	Normal
I	75–95	90–95	90–95
II	55–65	85	35
III	25–60	55–65	<10

Colon

Adenoma-to-carcinoma hypothesis

There is good epidemiological, clinical, pathological, and molecular evidence that most colon cancers arise within previously benign adenomas. Cancer cells in a malignant polyp share the same molecular alterations as in surrounding adenoma cells, but have additional mutations that are critical for malignant behavior.

There are two general stages in colon carcinogenesis. **Tumor initiation** involves the formation of an adenoma. All adenomas are thought to arise from an initial loss of APC gene function. Sporadic adenomas arise through acquired somatic mutations of both alleles; this takes years to occur so these polyps occur late in life and are relatively uncommon. In familial adenomatous polyposis, one APC allele is inherited in a mutated form, the second mutation takes much less time to acquire, so polyps occur at a younger age—FAP is a disorder of tumor initiation. The progression to cancer is a consequence of number of polyps rather than increased malignant potential of individual adenomas.

The second step involves progression from adenomas to carcinoma and is termed **tumor promotion**. It involves mutations or deletions in tumor suppressor genes located on chromosomes 17 (p53) and 18 (Deleted in colon cancer or DCC gene). Hereditary nonpolyposis cancer (HNPCC) is marked by an accelerated tumor promotion stage: adenomas progress more rapidly to cancer, which is why surveillance intervals in HNPCC need to be shortened.

Antibiotic-associated diarrhea (AAD)

Common—occurs after 5 to 25% antibiotic courses. Two main forms:
- Idiopathic, with no known pathogen (90% cases). Characteristic features are onset during antibiotic exposure, dose-related frequency, resolution when the antibiotic is discontinued, absence of inflammation on colonic biopsy or stool examination for leucocytes, and a benign course.
- Diarrhea associated with *Clostridium difficile* (about 10% of all cases of AAD), which may present with pseudomembranous colitis. See clostridial infections of GI tract.

Mechanisms
- Direct effects of antibiotics on intestinal mucosa.
  - E.g., neomycin and clofazimine.
  - Erythromycin is prokinetic because of motilin receptor stimulation.
- Possible effects on gut ecology.
  - Altered bile acid metabolism.
  - Altered carbohydrate fermentation.
  - Overgrowth of pathogens.

Management
- Meta-analyses show a benefit of probiotic administration with lactobacillus or Saccharomyces in AAD.
- AAD due to direct antibiotic effect may respond rapidly to cessation of antibiotic.
- Also see clostridial infections of GI tract and Acute diarrhea.

Appendix and appendicitis

Acute appendicitis remains the most common surgical emergency and may involve gangrene or perforation into the abdominal cavity. Although its function remains unknown, the high concentration of lymphoid tissue has always suggested an immune regulatory function. Recent epidemiological data shows that appendectomy has a protective effect in <u>ulcerative colitis</u> and <u>Crohn's disease</u>, and the course of ulcerative colitis seems milder following a history of appendectomy.[1] At present it is not clear if it is the appendectomy itself or the prior appendicitis that is protective.

Carcinoembryonic antigen (CEA)

A glycoprotein discovered in 1965 in association with <u>colorectal cancer</u> and embryonic and fetal gut tissues. Elevated in various malignant diseases (breast, lung, <u>gastric</u>, and <u>pancreatic cancers</u>) and also in nonmalignant conditions (heavy cigarette smoking, chronic bronchitis, and pancreatitis). Measuring CEA is not useful as a screening test, even when applied to patients with gastrointestinal signs or symptoms. CEA level is a poor measure of tumor bulk because the level is highest when the liver is involved, even to only a minor degree, and may be barely elevated in patients with a bulky intra-abdominal recurrence. With these caveats, there are some defined roles for CEA (see Box 6.1.1)

Box 6.1.1 Rules for measuring CEA

1. Preoperative CEA level is related to the stage of <u>colon cancer</u> and may serve as a predictor of surgical incurability: values greater than 5.0 ng/ml have been associated with a poor prognosis, independent of surgical stage

2. Postoperative CEA level may serve as a measure of the completeness of tumor resection. If a preoperatively elevated CEA value does not fall to normal levels within four weeks (a period that is twice the plasma half-life of CEA) after surgery, the resection was probably incomplete or occult metastases are present

3. The CEA level may serve as a useful monitor of tumor recurrence

4. The CEA assay may serve as a monitor of response to treatment of metastatic disease. Serial CEA values parallel either tumor regression or tumor progression. A rising CEA level is incompatible with tumor regression, whereas CEA values decrease in most patients who have responded to treatment.

1 Sacher, DB (2002). *Gut* 51: 764.

Collagenous colitis

See: <u>microscopic colitis</u>.

Colonic cancer

Epidemiology and pathogenesis

As with other malignancies, colonic cancer is an acquired genetic disease produced by exposure to environmental carcinogens; the damage caused by these accrues over many years. No single gene is so crucial that a mutation results in cancer.

In the United States there are approximately 135,000 new cases of colon cancer and 60,000 deaths from colon cancer per year (for the UK, figures are 30,000 and 16,000). Attack rates are lower in Japan and most developing countries. <u>Rectal cancer</u> is different in epidemiology, pathogenesis, and treatment.

Risk factors include:

- Cancer family syndromes: <u>familial adenomatous polyposis (FAP)</u> or <u>Gardner's syndrome</u>, <u>HNPCC</u>.
- Prior polyps (main determinants of risk are polyp size >1 cm and tubulovillous or severely dysplastic histology) and cancers (metachronous cancers in 5%).
- <u>Inflammatory bowel disease</u>: main determinants are duration of disease and extensive disease (approximately 10% after 30 years in patients with pancolitis).
- Diet: risk is modest at most. High fat and low fiber are the most common associations. Current advice is to reduce caloric intake, reduce dietary fat to less than 25% of total calorie intake, enrich diet with five portions of fruit and vegetables per day, and include 25 g fiber in the diet per day.

Clinical features

Change of bowel habit in people >40 years is the classic symptom. Tumors often grow slowly and produce four main symptom patterns:

- Obstruction. Distension, pain, nausea, and vomiting. Obstruction is more common in the (narrower) sigmoid, descending and transverse colon than the cecum or ascending colon.
- Bleeding: usually occult but if visible, blood tends to be mixed in with the stool.
- Local invasion: often produces pain but can lead to e.g., ureteric obstruction, bladder invasion, or malignant fistulation.
- Wasting syndrome. Loss of appetite, weight, and strength. Can occur with any GI tract (and many other) malignancy: particularly involves loss of subcutaneous fat.

Investigations

- <u>Colonoscopy</u> is the most accurate and sensitive diagnostic modality: even if distal colonic tumors are found, full colonoscopic evaluation is required to detect synchronous lesions (5%).

- Barium enemas are still frequently used, but biopsy is not possible, patients find them unpleasant, and the diagnostic sensitivity is less (approximately 85%).
- CT pneumocolon (CT with air distension of the bowel) is increasingly used and some centers are combining CT scanning with positron emission tomography (PET): labeling of intestinal contents with oral contrast media and removal of these from CT scans by digital image manipulation should allow accurate radiological imaging of the bowel without the need for bowel cleansing in the near future.

Management

Central aim is to detect tumors early in their natural history and to intervene with appropriate surgery.

Preoperative workup includes:
- CT scan of chest, abdomen, and pelvis to exclude metastases.
- Full colonoscopy to exclude a synchronous colonic tumor.
- Other tests include routine hematology (?iron deficient anemia) and biochemistry and (arguably), testing for CEA.

Management depends on staging (see Dukes staging and tumor staging), and evidence of local or metastatic disease.

Local disease

Surgery. Curative treatment is surgical: local resection of tumor and regional nodes with clearance margins of 5 cm is the aim. Tumors proximal to the splenic flexure are removed by right hemicolectomy: tumor of the left colon are removed by left hemicolectomy. Sigmoid cancers are treated with low anterior resections but very low tumors may require a colostomy. The overall operative mortality for colorectal cancer is about 5%. Treatment of rectal cancer is covered elsewhere.

Adjuvant chemotherapy after "curative" surgery. There is benefit in treating patients with Dukes stage C disease with 5FU and levamisole. No evidence of survival benefit is found in stage B disease. Newer regimens including oxaloplatin and irenotecan are being evaluated and may alter recommendations. Adjuvant radiotherapy for colon cancer outside rectum has no benefit.

Follow-up. 30% of patients undergoing "curative" surgery develop metastases. Colonoscopy should be carried out 3–6 months postoperatively and again at 12 months. A rise in CEA may indicate metastatic disease. Intensive follow-up with either ultrasound or CT scanning has a minor impact, at considerable expense, on patient outcome.

Metastatic disease

Surgery. A single or small number of hepatic metastases should be considered for surgical resection because some patients will go on to experience a prolonged disease-free interval. A solitary lung metastasis less than 3 cm can also be considered for surgery but the impact on survival and cure rates is less clear.

Chemotherapy or nonsurgical ablation techniques. Intra-arterial infusion of chemotherapeutic agents is reported to ablate or shrink a small number of tumors with less systemic drug toxicity. Radiofrequency ablation using transcutaneously positioned needles may also be effective.

Immunostimulant therapy is an attractive but unproven treatment option.

Prognosis

The pathological stage (see Dukes staging) is the best predictor of outcome. Crude 5-year-survival rates (i.e., not adjusted for age-related mortality) are 85, 65, 40, and <5% for stages A, B, C, and D, respectively.

Metastatic disease occurs in 25% and carries an adverse prognosis; the mean survival period for patients with hepatic metastases (the commonest site) at diagnosis is 4.5 months. Other metastatic sites include regional lymph nodes, lung, peritoneum, and adrenals. There is a suggestion that with improving chemotherapy the natural history is changing so that metastatic disease to the lungs and brain, previously rarely seen, is becoming more common. CT is the most sensitive test for detecting occult metastases, but addition of PET scanning may further enhance early detection.

Prevention of colonic cancer

Diet. There is no clear association with high fat or low fiber intake that can be separated from overall calorie intake.

Micronutrients. There are theoretical benefits to calcium and selenium supplementation, not supported by clinical trials. Anti-oxidants including vitamins A, E, and beta-carotene have not been proven beneficial or to reduce the rate of polyp recurrence.

Aspirin and NSAIDs. Aspirin takers get fewer colon cancers and NSAIDs inhibit tumor development *in vitro*. The nonsteroidal drug SULINDAC reduces polyp formation in familial adenomatous polyposis, but has shown conflicting results for sporadic colonic polyps.

There is early data suggesting that statins have a protective effect on cancer development: more data are awaited.

Colonic inertia

Defined as a delayed transit of radio-opaque markers through the proximal colon (see Box 6.1.2). Classically found in about 70% of patients (most often young to middle-aged women) consulting for infrequent defecation who are nonresponsive to therapy. Unlike patients with normal colonic transit, they show no sign of psychological distress and may have a physiological basis to their symptoms. Although resting motility appears normal, there seems to be a failure to increase motility after meals. This suggests an abnormality of the enteric plexus. Patients with severe colonic inertia may have reduced esophageal motility, delayed transit through the small intestine, and a high incidence of bladder dysfunction.

Colonic polyps

There are four common types (only adenomas are neoplastic).
● Adenomas.
● Benign hyperplastic polyps.
● Hamartomatous polyps.
● Inflammatory polyps.

Adenomas

Can be peduncular or sessile but are very common (up to 50% in autopsy studies, frequency increasing with age). Importance lies in the risk of malignant transformation, which relates to size (adenoma >2 cm has significant risk of containing cancer) and histology (can be tubular, villous [often sessile, more likely to contain focus of cancer], or tubulo-villous).

Etiology. There is disordered and persistent cell replication coupled with retarded cell maturation.

Genetic factors include aneuploidy, tetraploidy, DNA hypomethylation. Altered expression of oncogenes *fos*, *myc*, *ras* occurs. Mutations in APC, DCC, p53 have been reported. See adenoma–carcinoma sequence.

Environmental factors may include diet (some but not conclusive evidence for the role of fat, fiber, bile acids, fecal bacteria). Nonsteroidal anti-inflammatory drugs may retard polyps in familial syndromes (familial adenomatous polyposis (FAP), hereditary non-polyposis colon cancer (HNPCC), but seem ineffectual in sporadic adenomas.

Clinical features. Usually asymptomatic. Symptoms of rectal bleeding, prolapse, abdominal pain, or change in bowel habit usually occur with large polyps. There is no correlation with histology or location. Only polyps over 1.5 cm are associated with positive fecal occult blood tests. Large villous adenomas can produce watery diarrhea and hypokalemia.

Diagnosis. Barium radiology, endoscopy (sigmoidoscopy/colonoscopy), and more recently CT colonography can produce a diagnosis: endoscopy is currently the most sensitive and only endoscopy allows biopsy and therapeutic excision.

Box 6.1.2 Colonic transit studies

Technique used to study patients with severe constipation and otherwise normal GI investigations. Patient takes a high fiber diet and avoids laxatives, enemas, or any medications that may affect bowel function. Results can only be interpreted if procedure is strictly adhered to:
● **Day 1:** Patient takes 1 capsule (containing 20 radio-opaque markers) in water at 0900 h
● **Day 5:** 0900 h. Supine abdominal X-ray. If no markers seen, discontinue study (as no evidence of slow transit)
● **Day 7:** 0900 h. Supine abdominal X-ray. Slow transit constipation diagnosed if >80% of markers retained

Box 6.1.3 When is a colonic polyp not a polyp?

Polyp means any tissue protrusion above the mucosal surface into the lumen.

Neoplastic polyps
(Adenomas and cancers): see text

Nonneoplastic polyps
Hyperplastic, inflammatory, hamartomatous

Other lesions
- Lipomas, fibromas, leiomyomas, and Kaposi's sarcoma are usually submucosal and less often diagnosed by biopsy
- Pneumatosis can also appear polypoid
- Angiomas can sometimes be sampled by hot biopsy but there is a risk of bleeding
- Benign lymphoid nodules can be mistaken for neoplasms or polyps, especially in the terminal ileum
- Occasionally metastatic tumors may be seen on colonoscopy
- Carcinoids

Natural history. Adenoma–carcinoma progression probably takes 5–10 years, possibly less in the case of HNPCC/microsatellite instability. Although polyps grow slowly and only perhaps 5% is destined for malignancy, the necessity of excision for histology underlies current advice that all colonic polyps should be removed if possible.

Therapy. See polypectomy.

Benign hyperplastic polyps
Usually <5 mm, often multiple, commonest in recto-sigmoid. About 50% of all polyps <5 mm are hyperplastic. Arise because of an increased number of epithelial cells per unit length, which causes buckling and a serrated surface. Traditionally thought not to be premalignant, but some genetic changes occur that overlap with adenoma–cancer sequence.

Hamartomatous polyps
An abnormal mixture of benign cells. See juvenile polyps, Peutz–Jeghers, and Cowden's disease.

Inflammatory polyps
Also called pseudopolyps. Common in ulcerative or Crohn's colitis but also seen after infective or ischemic colitis. They represent islands of residual mucosa in a sea of previously sloughed healed mucosa.

Polypectomy follow-up
About 30% of people undergoing colonoscopic polypectomy will develop recurrent adenomas (although any lesions missed at index examination will be considered a recurrence).

Predicting recurrence

Risk factors for recurrence are the presence of multiple adenomas at index examination, polyp size over 10 mm, villous histology, or cancer in the polyp.

Frequency of surveillance colonoscopy

This is fertile ground for issuing of guidelines (ACG, AGA[1]). It is sensible to base frequency of surveillance on risk of recurrent polyps.

- Low-risk patients – follow up colonoscopy in five years.
- High-risk patients should have a short interval follow-up based on clinical judgment.
- Colonoscopy should be performed within three to four months after colonoscopic removal of a large (>2 cm) sessile polyp if there is concern that the adenoma has not been completely removed.

Risk for developing further adenoma or cancer after colonoscopic polypectomy

Low risk

- 1–2 adenomas less than 10 mm diameter

High risk

- Multiple (3 or more) adenomas
- Large adenoma over 10 mm
- Adenomas with villous component
- Adenoma with high grade dysplasia
- First-degree relative with colon cancer

Colorectal cancer screening and surveillance

- **Screening.** Testing of apparently healthy people who may be at average or increased risk of disease.
- **Surveillance.** Periodic testing of people at high risk for the disease who have previously tested negative.

Colorectal cancer (CRC) screening (see algorithm Fig. 6.1.1)

Average risk

(i.e., background population risk in people with no risk factors)

- Two screening modalities reduce mortality from colon cancer.
  - <u>Fecal occult blood test</u> (FOBT) provides up to 30% reduction in mortality if done annually with rigorous follow-up of positives with endoscopy.
  - Endoscopic examination of the colon. Endoscopy reduces mortality from colon cancer; although this would seem to be confined to area of bowel visualized at endoscopy, controversy exists about the incidence of proximal tumors out of reach of the flexible

1 Winawer S, Fletcher R, Rex D, et al. (2003). AGA colorectal cancer screening and surveillance: clinical guidelines and rationale—update based on new evidence. *Gastroenterology* 124:544.

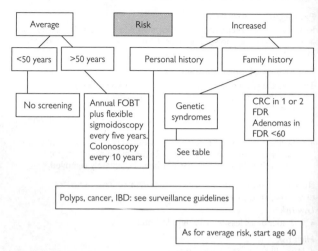

Figure 6.1.1 Algorithm for colorectal cancer screening based on American Gastroenterology Association guidelines. CRC, colorectal cancer; FOBT, fecal occult blood testing; FDR, first-degree relatives; IBD, inflammatory bowel disease.

sigmoidoscope. One study reports less than 2% of people with a normal sigmoidoscopy have proximal tumors.[1]
- Other methods such as CT pneumocolon ("virtual colonoscopy") are still being evaluated.
- The best screening method for colon cancer has not been determined.
- Criteria include sensitivity, specificity, patient acceptability, and affordability.
- Recommendations published by the American Gastroenterology Association (AGA) are shown in the algorithm.

Increased risk

Family history (excluding cancer family syndromes)
Familial clustering of colorectal cancer is common. Risk is increased depending on the number of affected relatives, their age of diagnosis, and the presence of adenomatous polyps in a first-degree relative under the age of 60 (see Table 6.1.1).

How this affects screening is controversial and depends on the cutoff of acceptable risk. A family history of colon cancer should lead to screening with regular FOBT and sigmoidoscopy every five years. Patients with multiple affected family members or an affected first-degree relative <55 years should have colonoscopy five years earlier than the earliest age of occurrence of cancer in the family.

1 Imperiale, TF et al. (2000) *N. Engl. J. Med.* 343: 169.

Cancer family syndromes

Genetic screening is valuable for syndromes relating to <u>familial adenoma-tous polyposis</u> (FAP); referral to a geneticist should be considered for confusing histories.

Table 6.1.1 Familial colon cancer: relative risk

Relatives affected	Risk
None-1	in 35
One first-degree	1 in 17
One first-degree and one second-degree	1 in 12
One first-degree under 45	1 in 10
Both parents	1 in 8.5
Two first-degree	1 in 6
Three first-degree	1 in 2

Table 6.1.2 Colorectal cancer surveillance

Condition	Recommendation
<u>Familial adenomatous polyposis</u>	Genetic testing for APC mutations age 12. Yearly flexible sigmoidoscopy starting at age 12 in people with a family history of FAP. If polyps found, full colonoscopy with a view to prophylactic colectomy and surveillance of remaining rectum. In addition, upper endoscopic surveillance of stomach, duodenum, and periampullary region. Consider AFP for hepatoblastoma
<u>Hereditary nonpolyposis colorectal cancer</u>	Individuals identified by family history (see Amsterdam criteria in <u>hereditary nonpolyposis colorectal cancer</u>). Start colonoscopic surveillance (**not** flexible sigmoidoscopy because many tumors are right-sided) at 20–25 years at intervals of 1–2 years. Offer genetic testing to first-degree relatives of patients with known inherited mismatch repair defect
<u>Peutz–Jegher's syndrome</u>	Every two years upper and lower GI endoscopy, barium follow-through (?video <u>capsule endoscopy</u>). Polypectomy for large polyps to avoid intussusception. Surveillance for gonadal, breast, cervical cancer
<u>Juvenile polyposis</u>	Rare. No firm guidelines

Colorectal cancer surveillance (see Table 6.1.2)

High risk
- **Highly penetrant autosomal dominant syndromes.**
  - Familial adenomatous polyposis.
  - Hereditary nonpolyposis colorectal cancer.
- Hamartomatous polyposis syndromes (Peutz–Jeghers syndrome, juvenile polyposis, Cowden's disease).
- Longstanding history of inflammatory bowel disease of the colon.
- Patients with acromegaly. Current recommendations are for colonoscopy every three years from age 40.

Moderate risk

Prior history of adenomatous colonic polyps
- Solitary adenomas <1 cm diameter do not predict recurrent neoplasia and these lesions, especially in the elderly, do not need follow-up.
- Surveillance colonoscopy is indicated for:
  - Adenomas >1 cm.
  - Villous or tubulo-villous histology.
  - Multiple adenomas.
  - Advanced dysplasia.
- Three-year interval is adequate for follow-up colonoscopy if the colon has been cleared of polyps, with subsequent intervals of five years.

Prior history of colon cancer
- The anastomosis site should be examined at three to six months and perhaps again at one year (little evidence for this recommendation).
- After this, examination is recommended every three to five years as for patients with advanced adenomas.

Inflammatory bowel disease. See Box 6.1.4.

Cowden's disease

Autosomal dominant condition relating to juvenile polyposis. Associated with a mutation of the PTEN gene on chromosome 10, resulting in multiple hamartomas of skin and mucous membranes. The hallmark is multiple trichilemmomas around the eyes, nose, and mouth. About one-third of affected people have hamartomas scattered through upper and lower GI tract. They can be 1 mm to several cm diameter and include lipomas, juvenile polyps, inflammatory polyps, ganglioneuromas, and lymphoid hyperplasia. Glycogenic acanthosis can be seen in esophageal lesions.

There is no increased risk of GI cancer but a 10% risk of thyroid cancer and a 50% risk of breast cancer.

Crohn's disease

After Burrill B. Crohn, a New York physician who published in 1932 on "regional ileitis" with Ginsberg and Oppenheimer. Many believe Dalziel described the disease in 1912.

Box 6.1.4 Colorectal cancer surveillance in patients with IBD

This is a controversial area. Extensive <u>ulcerative colitis</u> or <u>Crohn's</u> colitis of long duration (>10 years for patients with disease proximal to splenic flexure, >15 years in patients with left-sided disease above the sigmoid: no increased risk in patients with proctitis alone) have an increased risk of colon cancer.

The magnitude of increased risk varies in different studies, partly due to referral bias reflecting hospital rather than community prevalence studies. Commonly quoted figures are an incidence of colon cancer of 7–15% at 20 years after diagnosis of UC with an increasing incidence of about 1% per year after this. Long-term treatment with 5-ASA may decrease the risk of colon cancer associated with IBD.

Risk is further increased in patients with
• <u>Primary sclerosing cholangitis</u>
• A family history of <u>colon cancer</u>
• (Possibly) young onset of disease
• Colonic stricturing

There is no evidence that endoscopic surveillance improves mortality from colon cancer in IBD. Areas of dysplasia are difficult to see macroscopically, so standard guidelines recommend surveillance with colonoscopic biopsies taken from four quadrants every 10 cm.

<u>Dysplasia</u> is a recognized predictor of malignancy, but there is interobserver variabwility in interpretation. Alternative markers of precancer include detection of aneuploidy, abnormal mucins, genetic markers, and optical reflectance characteristics ("optical biopsy").

Definition. A chronic inflammatory condition that can affect any part of the gut from mouth to anus but most frequently the distal small intestine and proximal colon.

Epidemiology

• Accurate figures are difficult because of lack of gold standard for diagnostic criteria and global variations in case ascertainment.
• Found worldwide but incidence varies. In high incidence areas (United States, UK, northern Europe) the incidence is about 4–8/100,000. In Australasia and in white South Africans it is about 2/100,000. Low incidence areas include Asia, Japan, and South America, with estimates of 0.05 to 0.8/100,000 per year. In careful studies of stable populations in high incidence areas (United States and Denmark) the incidence increased sixfold from 1950s to 1980s and appears to have stabilized since.
• Slightly more common in women, with peak incidence age 20–40 and a second smaller peak in older adults.

Etiology and pathogenesis

- Almost 100 years after initial description, whether Crohn's disease represents an appropriate response to an unrecognized pathogen or an inappropriate response to an innocuous stimulus is not resolved.
- Resemblance of Crohn's disease to some animal diseases with known bacterial causes (John's disease in goats) and the proven role of gut pathogens in inducing inflammation in genetically susceptible animal models of inflammatory bowel disease strongly suggest a central role for bacterial antigens as triggering factors.
- A huge amount of experimental work has helped to define cellular and humoral immune events underlying mucosal inflammation. Evidence points to over-responsiveness of T cells to enteric flora in IBD, with T cells producing a Th1 cytokine response profile in Crohn's disease.
- Genetic diseases involving defects in bacterial killing and degradation (e.g., chronic granulomatous disease) produce a phenotype very like inflammatory bowel disease and this supports experimental evidence that the interaction between T cells and macrophages also appears central to the pathogenesis of Crohn's disease.
- The recent rise in incidence supports the importance of environmental factors.
- Diet and smoking are particularly important; some evidence suggests Crohn's patients have a problem handling saturated fatty acids, while smoking worsens disease, possibly due to its effect on microvasculature.

Genetics versus environment

- Strong genetic component in predisposing to Crohn's disease, with a high concordance rate among identical twins and higher incidence among Ashkenazi Jews. Techniques of genome-wide screening for linkage and association studies of candidate genes have revealed association with a locus on chromosome 16 as being due to gene CARD-15 (NOD-2), which codes for receptor for muramyl dipeptide (MDP) a component of bacterial cell walls.
- The recent rise in incidence supports the importance of environmental factors.
- Diet and smoking are particularly important; some evidence suggests Crohn's patients have a problem handling saturated fatty acids, while smoking worsens disease possible due to its effect on microvasculature.

Pathology

The hallmark is focal intestinal inflammation: disease is classically discontinuous giving rise to "skip lesions" unlike ulcerative colitis (UC), which is continuous. Early lesions include aphthous ulcers overlying lymphoic aggregates and support a role of luminal antigens initiating immune activation. Noncaseating granulomas, although characteristic of Crohn's disease are neither unique to the disease nor universally found (occur in up to 70% of surgical resection specimens).

TNF is involved in granuloma formation: this is how anti-TNF strategies were developed for Crohn's.

Inflammation is transmural, and accounts for late development of large ulcers, sinus tracks, anal fissures, and anorectal fistulae. Concomitant attempts at healing lead to extensive fibrosis as major component of Crohn's disease. TGF beta is a key cytokine involved in this process.

Clinical features

Disease distribution. 40% have disease confined to terminal ileum and proximal colon, 30% have disease confined to the small bowel, and 20% have disease confined to the colon. The remaining 10% have disease elsewhere in the GI tract, particularly perianal disease although the mouth, esophagus, and stomach can also be affected.

Symptoms. Classical symptoms are **abdominal pain and diarrhea**. Weight loss, anorexia, and fever may be seen, and growth retardation is common and important in children. Gross rectal bleeding and acute hemorrhage are uncommon.

- **Anemia** occurs in 30%, mainly as a result of iron deficiency but sometimes as a result of <u>vitamin B12 deficiency</u> in ileal disease or <u>folate</u> deficiency in proximal small bowel disease.
- Patients can present with small-bowel **obstruction** or symptoms relating to small-bowel **stricturing**. Colonic Crohn's disease may present with bloody diarrhea but tenesmus is less common than in <u>ulcerative colitis</u> because the rectum is less commonly affected (although about 30% of patients with ileal disease have some degree of proctitis).
- Gastroduodenal Crohn's disease can present as *Helicobacter*-negative peptic ulcer disease.

Extraintestinal manifestations

Pauciarticular **arthropathy** affects 6% of patients with Crohn's, usually accompanying active intestinal disease and may include sacroilitis. There is an association with ankylosing spondylitis: nearly all patients with ankylosing spondylitis and Crohn's are HLA B27 positive. Polyarticular arthropathy affects about 4% of Crohn's patients.

- **Metabolic bone disease** is common, with osteopenia (T score on DEXA scanning of −1 to −2.49) found in up to 50% of patients; steroid usage is the main risk factor, but loss of bone density is an independent feature of disease.
- There is an association with venous and arterial **thrombo-embolic disease**. Hospitalization, immobility, and malnutrition contribute, but in addition platelets can be high and many clotting factors are increased. There is no independent association with factor V Leiden. Treatment with prophylactic anticoagulants is safe and effective.
- Mucocutaneous manifestations include aphthous ulceration, <u>pyoderma gangrenosum</u>, and <u>erythema nodosum</u>.
- Ocular manifestations (scleritis, episcleritis, and uveitis) occur in about 5% of Crohn's patients.
- <u>Gallstones</u> are twice as common in Crohn's as a control population, There is an association with <u>fatty liver</u> and <u>autoimmune hepatitis</u> as well as with <u>primary sclerosing cholangitis</u>.
- Terminal ileal disease is associated with renal <u>oxalate stones</u>.

Behavior of disease

Disease can be stricturing, penetrating, or neither. This has been incorporated into recent classifications of Crohn's such as the Vienna classification (see Table 6.1.3).

Fistulae reflect the transmural character of Crohn's. Perianal fistulaes may occur in 15–30%, and enteroenteric, entero-vaginal, and entero-cutaneous fistulas can occur.

Establishing the diagnosis and evaluating the disease

History and examination. Focus on recent travel, antibiotic use, diet, family history, sexual activity, and ask about smoking. Examine carefully for signs of obstruction, tenderness, or a mass. Always examine the perianal region.

Laboratory tests. **Stool culture** is important, including examination for parasites and *Clostridium difficile* toxin. Check **full blood count** (look for anemia, raised platelets as a surrogate sign of inflammation, leucocytosis) **hematinics** including iron and TIBC, B12 and folate levels, **LFT** (best test of liver function are albumin and INR; liver often switches out of synthesizing albumin and switches into making inflammatory mediators like CRP). Also remember to look for **vitamin and micronutrient** deficiency; calcium and magnesium levels can be low: zinc may be low in extensive small-bowel disease and is a critical factor in tissue healing.

Special investigations
- Ultrasound, endoscopy, radiological (CT and barium) studies, and histopathology are all used to make the diagnosis.
- Endoscopy is probably the gold standard for diagnosing colonic and terminal ileal disease; it is the only diagnostic modality that readily permits mucosal biopsy and also allows for balloon dilatation of any strictures.
- Barium follow through is still a standard method for evaluating the small bowel, although capsule endoscopy may have an important role if stricturing can be excluded.
- CT does not show mucosal detail but is very helpful in discerning extraluminal features. There is interest in using CT or MRI to assess regional blood flow in attempting to distinguish fibrostenotic Crohn's from inflammatory disease causing stricturing as the treatment implications are very different. MRI is the modality of choice for imaging perianal or pelvic fistulating disease (Color plate 3).
- Ultrasound is very useful in expert hands and is reported as having high sensitivity and specificity for detecting thickened bowel, abscesses, and fistulae.

Differentiating Crohn's from ulcerative colitis

This can be an issue when IBD is confined to the colon. Discriminating features include small-bowel disease, mainly right-sided colonic disease, rectal sparing, fistulization, perianal disease, and granulomas, all of which favor Crohn's disease. Immunological markers may be of some help; pANCA is found in 70% of UC but only 15% of Crohn's and antibodies to

Table 6.1.3 Vienna classification of Crohn's disease

Age at diagnosis	1 = <40 years 1 > 40 years	Time of histological, surgical, radiological, or endoscopical diagnosis; no retrospective time of diagnosis
Location		
	1 = Terminal ileum 2 = Colon 3 = Ileocolon 4 = Upper GI-tract	Maximum extent of the lesions at any time before resectionAphthous lesions or ulcerations of any size (mucosal erythema is not enough)
Behaviour	1 = Nonstricturing, nonpenetrating 2 = Stricturing 3 = Penetrating	Inflammatory masses, abscesses, fistulae, perianal ulcers are defined as penetrating Strictures can be diagnosed radiologically, endoscopically, or surgicallyPostoperative complications are excluded

Reprinted with permission from Gasche, C. et al. A simple classification of Crohn's disease: Report of the Working Party for the World Congresses of Gastroenterology, Vienna 1998. *Inflamm. Bowel Dis.* 2000; 6: 8–15.

Saccharomyces cervisiae are found in up to 50% of Crohn's but less often in UC. When done together, specificity is further improved.

Assessing disease activity

It is usually sufficient to follow the patient's response to treatment, as well as simple markers of inflammatory activity such as the CRP. There are a number of scoring systems that are important research tools: see <u>Crohn's disease activity indices</u>.

Aims and principles of management

Because a cure is not available, goals of therapy are to induce and maintain remission. Medical therapies include <u>AMINOSALICYLATES,</u> <u>ANTIBIOTICS, CORTICOSTEROIDS</u>, and immunosuppressants including <u>AZATHIOPRINE/6-MERCAPTOPURINE</u>, and <u>METHOTREXATE.</u>
- <u>AMINOSALICYLATES</u> are superior to placebo in treating colonic disease and pentasa is effective for ileal disease in a dose of 4 g/day. The data about the efficacy of <u>5-ASA</u> in maintaining remission are contradictory: one meta-analysis has suggested some benefit in patients after ileal resection, but a prospective randomized trial has not confirmed this result and the benefits seem marginal at best for this group of patients.
- <u>ANTIBIOTICS</u> have a role in treating infectious complications of Crohn's disease.

- <u>METRONIDAZOLE</u> is of proven efficacy in reducing postsurgical endoscopic recurrence after ileal resection and probably also has an effect in healing perianal fistulae. The effect may not be totally due to its antibacterial properties, because *in vitro* it inhibits neutrophil margination across endothelium. <u>CIPROFLOXACIN</u> is also used in treating complications of Crohn's with good effect.
- Claims have been made for multiple antibacterial therapy targeted against mycobacteria but the data to date are not compelling.
- Novel <u>CORTICOSTEROIDS</u> such as budesonide have been shown to be almost as effective as prednisolone with fewer side effects, but budesonide is not effective as maintenance therapy.
- <u>CORTICOSTEROIDS</u> still play a central role in many physician's management of Crohn's disease, although they do not heal the disease and the adverse side effects are well known. They are not effective as long-term therapy, although many patients find difficulty in tapering the dose without recurrent symptoms.
- Convincing evidence of efficacy exists for azathioprine/6-mercaptopurine and <u>METHOTREXATE</u>. These drugs are widely and increasingly used in patients with active Crohn's who fail to respond to first-line therapies or who fail to taper steroids.
- Data on cyclosporin and mycophenolate do not indicate a major role for these drugs in the management of Crohn's.
- <u>ANTI-TNF</u> therapy includes monoclonal antibodies against TNF (Infliximab, Adalimumab, and Certolizumab). They are indicated for moderate to severe disease where conventional agents have failed. There is some indirect evidence they may alter the natural history of Crohn's disease
- <u>ANTI-INTEGRIN</u> antibodies (Natalizumab) are also effective, and approved for patients who have failed anti-TNF therapy. Patients need to be advised about the small risk of Progressive Multifocal Leukoencephalopathy (PML) which developed in one patient with Crohn's disease in clinical trials.

Nutritional therapy

targets both repletion of specific nutrient deficits and also primary therapy of the disease. Elemental diets are as effective as corticosteroids in inducing remission, particularly in children.

Surgery

- Up to 75% of Crohn's patients will have surgery within 20 years of diagnosis. Indications for surgery include complications such as intra-abdominal masses, medically intractable fistulae, fibrotic strictures with obstruction, toxic megacolon, hemorrhage, and cancer.
- Details of surgical procedures vary with site of disease and to some extent with country, but can be classified as:
  - Resections with or without anastomoses.
  - External or internal bypass surgery.
  - Surgical procedures to repair or resect fistulae.

- Recurrent disease is common after surgery and has been assessed endoscopically as approaching 80%. About 50% of patients undergoing surgery will need another operation within 10 years.

Crohn's disease in pregnancy

Active disease is probably associated with reduced fertility, which may relate to chronic inflammation, undernutrition, or reduced libido. Women with quiescent disease at conception have the same rate of recurrence as nonpregnant women. Among women with active disease at conception, one-third get better, one-third get worse, and one-third do not change during pregnancy. Most pregnancies carried by women with Crohn's are normal, and perianal complications develop infrequently in women who deliver vaginally with an episiotomy.

Course and prognosis

The rate of relapse in the first 1–2 years correlates with the risk of relapse in the ensuing five years. About 25% of patients will maintain long periods of remission, 25% experience chronically active symptoms, and 50% have a course that fluctuates between active and inactive disease.

Risk of cancer

When Crohn's affects the colon, the risk of <u>colon cancer</u> appears to be similar to that for cancer in <u>ulcerative colitis</u>. Surveillance colonoscopy is recommended from 10 years after diagnosis. Data from radiological studies in the 1970s suggests that stricturing disease of the colon has a higher risk of malignancy, of approximately 7%. There is an increased risk of small bowel adenocarcinoma in small bowel Crohn's disease, and probably a small increased risk of Hodgkins and non-Hodgkins lymphoma.

Crohn's disease activity indices

Symptoms and clinical signs of Crohn's disease do not always correlate with inflammatory severity; the cardinal features of abdominal pain and diarrhea may be due to superimposed irritable bowel, previous surgical resection, or complications such as strictures or fistulae.

The most widely used activity index is the **Crohn's disease activity index (CDAI)** developed by Best (see Box 6.1.5). The main criticisms are the excessive weight put on the number of bowel actions per day, which can be influenced by many factors apart from disease activity, and the inclusion of hematocrit as a marker of activity. Many research studies use a fall in the CDAI as a primary endpoint of efficacy: traditionally a fall of 70 points has been required, but recently this has been revised so that a fall of 100 points is currently required for evidence of efficacy.

The **Harvey–Bradshaw index**, proposed in 1980, is a simplified form of the CDAI and also in widespread use in research studies of disease intervention.

Endoscopic activity scores such as the **Crohn's disease endoscopic inflammation score** (CDEIS) are also widely used, as for instance in the work of Rutgeerts showing early endoscopic recurrence after resectional surgery for Crohn's disease that predates symptomatic recurrence.

Box 6.1.5 Calculating the Crohn's disease activity index

$$\text{CDAI} = 2 \times 1 + 5 \times 2 + 7 \times 3 + 20 \times 4 + 30 \times 5 + 10 \times 6 + 6 \times 7 +$$
$$\text{(weight factor)}_8$$

where

1 = Number of liquid or very soft stools in one week

2 = Sum of seven daily abdominal pain ratings:
   (0 = none, 1 = mild, 2 = moderate, 3 = severe)

3 = Sum of seven daily ratings of general well-being:
   (0 = well, 1 = slightly below par, 2 = poor, 3 = very poor, 4=terrible)

4 = Symptoms or findings presumed related to Crohn's disease
   (score 1 for each)
   • arthritis or arthralgia
   • iritis or uveitis
   • erythema nodosum, pyoderma gangrenosum, aphthous stomatitis
   • anal fissure, fistula, or perirectal abscess
   • other bowel-related fistula
   • febrile (fever) episode over 100 degrees during past week

5 = Taking lomotil or opiates for diarrhea

6 = Abnormal mass
   0 = none; 0.4 = questionable; 1 = present

7 = Hematocrit [(Typical − Current) × 6]
   Normal average: for male = 47, for female = 42

8 = 100 × [(standard weight − actual body weight)/standard weight]

An on-line calculator for this index can be found at: www.ibdjohn.com/cdai

This box was published in Best, WR et al. Development of a Crohn's disease activity index. National Cooperative Crohn's Disease Study. Gastroenterology 1976; 70(3): 439–44. Copyright Elsevier 1976.

Diversion colitis

Development of inflammation in the distal bypassed colon after colostomy or ileostomy performed for cancer, diverticulitis, inflammatory bowel disease, or trauma. First reported by Morson in 1972.

Inflammation is seen endoscopically in 90% of patients: most (95%) are mild or moderate, with only 5% severe. However, symptoms present in a minority—less than 10%. Symptoms are more common in patients operated on for IBD and develop within one to nine months after fecal diversion.

Pathogenesis. Because inflammation resolves after restoration of the fecal stream, luminal nutrient deficiency is the favored mechanism. Roediger showed that luminal short-chain fatty acids (SCFA) are the main fuels for the distal colonocyte (butyrate provides 70% oxidative energy for epithelial cells: acetate, ketone bodies, and glutamine are alternatives). SCFA enemas can be therapeutic but do not always work. Other luminal factors (growth factors, dietary constituents, or bacterial products) may be involved in the pathogenesis. See short chain fatty acids.

Diagnosis and pathological findings. Where there was no preoperative inflammation, diagnosis is straightforward: flexible sigmoidoscopy with biopsy and culture of stools for ova cysts, parasites, and pathogens (including C. difficile toxin) will establish the severity of inflammation. Radiology does not help unless a fistula or abscess is suspected, in which case CT is indicated; remember to consider radiation or ischemic colitis in the appropriate clinical context.

Differentiating recurrent Crohn's disease from diversion colitis. This can be difficult; endoscopic features favoring Crohn's disease are longitudinal ulcers and strictures. Ulcers are usually small in diversion colitis. Absent preoperative rectal involvement can be helpful. Pathological features are compared in Table 6.1.4.

Treatment. SCFA enemas may work (60 mM lactate, 30 mM proprionate, 40 mM butyrate) but the putrid smell of these agents lead to high degrees of patient noncompliance. Steroid enemas do not work but 5-ASA enemas have been used successfully. Therapy using probiotics is also currently under investigation.

Diverticular disease (diverticulosis, diverticulitis, and diverticular bleeding)

A diverticulum (pleural: diverticula) is a saclike protrusion of the intestinal wall. Most diverticula of clinical interest occur in the colon, but also see duodenal diverticulum, Meckel's diverticulum, jejunal diverticulum, and Zenker's diverticulum (see pharyngeal pouch).

Colonic diverticula do not contain all bowel-wall layers because the mucosa and submucosa herniate through the muscle layers of the colon at the points where the vasa recta penetrate the circular muscle layer. Colonic diverticula may thus be considered to be psuedodiverticula.

Diverticulosis. Prevalence increases with age (5% at age 40: 65% by age 85) and also seems to have increased markedly in the last century. In Western countries it is common and usually left-sided: in the Far East it is rarer, more commonly right-sided, and affects younger people. Pathogenesis is commonly held to relate to low dietary fiber.

Table 6.1.4 Differentiating recurrent Crohn's disease from diversion colitis

Diversion colitis	Crohn's disease
Granulomas can occur but are usually mucinous. Transmural changes usually absent	Transmural inflammation, crypt architectural changes (suggests lonstanding inflammation) and epithelioid granulomas
Lymphoid hyperplasia with frequent germinal centers is very prominent	Lymphoid hyperplasia can occur
Very few macrophages and plasma cells	

Diverticulitis. Inflammation of the wall and surrounding tissues leads to a variable clinical picture ranging from subclinical inflammation to life-threatening peritonitis.

Simple diverticulitis is characterized by constant left lower-quadrant pain, nausea, or vomiting in 20–60%, and change of bowel habit. Physical signs include lower abdominal tenderness and an abdominal mass (in about 20%). Low grade fever and leucocytosis are common but about 50% have a normal white cell count. Urinalysis may reveal sterile pyuria secondary to adjacent inflammation. **Complicated diverticulitis** may be accompanied by signs of peritonitis, abscess formation, or fistulation. Fecal discharge from the vagina is diagnostic of a colo-vaginal fistula.

Diagnosis. Plain abdominal films can help in excluding other causes of abdominal pain and in showing free intraperitoneal air. For further diagnostic information, contrast-enhanced <u>CT scan</u> is preferred. CT can identify complications: peritonitis, fistula formation, obstruction, and abscess formation. It can also function as an aid to therapeutic abscess drainage. In about 10%, CT is unable to distinguish acute diverticulitis from <u>colon cancer</u> as both produce focal bowel-wall thickening.

Treatment
- Depends on the individual and severity of inflammation. Most patients with simple diverticulitis can be treated conservatively with broad spectrum <u>ANTIBIOTICS</u> with cover directed toward Gram-negative rods and anaerobes (e.g., <u>CEFUROXIME</u> or <u>CIPROFLOXACIN</u> plus <u>METRONIDAZOLE</u>).
- Patients with complicated diverticulitis (free intraperitoneal perforation, obstruction, abscess, or fistula formation) will often need surgery. In the emergency situation, a two-stage procedure is commonly employed, with resection of the diseased colon, oversewing of the rectum, and an end colostomy (a Hartmann procedure). The colostomy can be closed three months later.

Diverticular bleeding. Local trauma to the vasa recti within diverticula can lead to arterial bleeding. Diverticular bleeding is the commonest cause of acute massive colonic blood loss. Although bleeding may stop spontaneously, rebleeding is common and often comes from the right colon, even though most diverticula are left-sided.

Management of diverticular bleeding. After resuscitation, the principles are to diagnose and locate the source of bleeding, and to treat the cause (see also <u>acute lower GI bleeding</u>). <u>Colonoscopy</u> is reasonable in most patients because blood is cathartic and visualization of a bleeding source may allow <u>endoscopic hemostasis</u> to be achieved. Some clinicians employ rapid <u>bowel preparation</u>: recommendations include the use of balanced electrolyte solutions, e.g., kleenprep given via NG tube. In patients for whom colonoscopy is unsuccessful, the bleeding is massive, or the patient remains hemodynamically unstable, options include angiography or surgery. Diagnostic angiography can be combined with a trial of octreotide infusion to stop the bleeding and allow bowel prep for future operative intervention, or selective embolization of a bleeding vessel or area of angiodysplasia. It is, however, important to exclude upper GI sources of bleeding. Surgical options usually involve segmental colectomy.

Diet and Diverticular Disease: Individuals with diverticular disease had frequently been counseled that they should avoid all nuts and certain seeds. Recent published data has shown that the ingestion of nuts and/or seeds does not increase the risk of developing diverticulitis in individuals with known diverticular disease.

Dukes staging system

Cuthbert Esquire Dukes, 1932. A classification of <u>colon cancer</u> invasion still in routine use because the relation of advancing stage to cancer mortality has been repeatedly demonstrated.

- **Stage A** tumors are mucosal (may invade into the submucosa but do not reach the muscularis propria). Five-year survival 95–100%.
- **Stage B1** tumors invade the muscularis propria, and B2 lesions completely penetrate the smooth muscle layer to the serosa but without lymph node involvement. Five-year survival 80–85%.
- **Stage C** lesions are defined by regional lymph node involvement. They are further divided into primary tumors limited to the bowel wall (C1) and those that penetrate the bowel wall. Five-year survival 50–70%.
- **Stage D** lesions include all those with metastases. Five-year survival 5–15%.

The American Joint Commission on Cancer devised the TNM classification (see <u>tumor staging</u>), which has largely replaced the Dukes staging system, for randomizing patients into clinical trials. Comparison of Dukes with TNM yields the following: Dukes A = T1/2, N0, M0. Dukes B = T3/4, N0, M0. Dukes C = T1–4, N1 or N2, M0. Dukes D = M1.

Familial adenomatous polyposis (FAP)

Etiology + pathogenesis. FAP is the most common adenomatous polyposis syndrome (others include <u>juvenile polyposis</u>, <u>Peutz–Jeghers</u>, <u>Gardner's</u>, and <u>Turcot's syndromes</u>). Autosomal dominant inheritance, with prevalence 1:7500, and 80–100% disease penetrance. APC (adenomatous polyposis coli) gene located on chromosome 5 encodes for a protein that functions as a tumor suppressor protein, probably through interaction with β-catenin. If APC protein mutated, β-catenin no longer downregulated, allowing it to upregulate target genes that then promote adenoma formation.

Clinical features. Patients may present with rectal bleeding and diarrhea, but many identified for screening/surveillance on basis of a careful family history from an affected index case (nevertheless, 20% of patients with FAP have no family history, suggesting germline mutations).

Colonic disease. Hundreds to thousands of adenomatous <u>colon polyps</u> develop after puberty, and diagnosis is usually made at age 20–30 years. <u>Colonic cancer</u> is an inevitable part of the disease course, approximately 10 to 15 years after the onset of the polyposis. 90% of cases of FAP are diagnosed < 50 years.

Gastroduodenal disease. Duodenal adenomas occur in 60–90%, and duodenal/periampullary cancers develop in 5–12%. Following the widespread use of prophylactic colectomy, duodenal cancer is now the major cause of cancer death in FAP. Spigelman classification assesses duodenal FAP according to number, distribution, and histology of polyps. Endoscopic assessment (with duodenoscope, not gastroscope, in view of peri-ampullary involvement) is advised every 1–3 years following colectomy or > 20 years of age. Very poor prognosis following radical surgery in FAP patients with duodenal carcinoma, and >30% risk of developing cancer in those with "Spigelman IV" disease has led most specialist units to advise prophylactic <u>Whipple's resection</u> for extensive premalignant duodenal FAP. <u>Gastric polyps</u> are common, but <u>gastric cancer</u> occurs rarely.

Cancer in other sites. Although less common than luminal GI cancers, other associations with FAP include pancreatic cancer, hepatoblastoma, diffuse mesenteric fibromatosis (desmoid tumors), and cancers of the thyroid and brain.

Box 6.1.6 Limitation of fecal occult blood tests and recommendations for correct use

False positive tests
- Endogenous peroxidase (e.g., vegetable peroxidase in broccoli, turnips, cauliflower, radishes, melon)
- Nonhuman hemoglobin: red meat
- Any source of GI bleeding (epistaxis, gingival bleeding, hemorrhoids)
- Aspirin and NSAIDs, which increase upper GI bleeds
  - **Recommendation:** patients should avoid red meat, peroxidase containing vegetables and vitamin C and NSAIDs for three days before and during testing. Avoiding iron preparations is also recommended, although the evidence for this is weak.

False negative tests
- Hemoglobin degradation by storage or fecal bacteria
- **Recommendation:** develop slides within 4–6 days. Do not rehydrate slides for average risk screening
- Ascorbic acid (vitamin C) interferes with indicator dye
- Lesion not bleeding at time of sampling
  - Recommendation: Two samples of each of three consecutive stools should be tested.

Investigation. In an affected individual with no family history, diagnosis is suggested by finding hundreds of adenomatous polyps on colonoscopy/sigmoidoscopy. Most polyps are < 1 cm, and individually are identical to adenomatous polyps found in general population.

Management

- Where diagnosis is established, there is no specific merit in waiting before advising colonic resection in the postpubertal patient, in view of near certainty of developing malignancy.
- Colectomy with ileorectal anastomosis maintains continence, but cancer recurrence occurs in rectal stump in 15%, even with regular surveillance, and carries a dismal prognosis. Colectomy with ileoanal anastomosis, or total colectomy with ileostomy are usual advised.
- Polyp regression has been shown with sulindac (which may act through COX-2 inhibition), but reliable prevention of progression to malignancy has not been shown, and medical management cannot be used in place of surgery. It has been used to reduce development of new polyps in rectal stump. Its role in inducing regression of gastroduodenal polyps is under assessment.

Screening. A genetic diagnosis of APC mutation can be made in > 98% of patients using exhaustive genetic techniques. The commercially available "truncated protein test" for APC mutations will be positive in 80% of FAP families. When it is in a family member, gene carriage in other family members can be demonstrated with near 100% accuracy. A negative test in a family member removes need for regular surveillance, but in those tested positive, sigmoidoscopy should be performed yearly from age 10–12 years. If affected family member is negative for genetic test, screening relies on clinical assessment (i.e., sigmoidoscopy). Genetic counseling is a vital component of screening.

Gardner's syndrome

A familial disease consisting of gastrointestinal polyposis and osteomas associated with several benign soft tissue tumors such as desmoids, epidermoid cysts, fibromas, lipomas, dental impactions, and congenital hypertrophy of the retinal pigment epithelium. It is a variable manifestation of a mutation in the APC gene.

Hereditary nonpolyposis colon cancer (HNPCC)

- An autosomal dominant condition, causing about 5% of colon cancers. Cancer arises in discrete adenomas but polyposis does not occur. About 80% are caused by germline mutations in genes involved in repair of DNA damaged during replication (this tends to occur at repetitive DNA sequences called microsatellites). These genes are called mismatch repair genes and include hMSH2 on chromosome 2 (40–50%) and hMLH1 on chromosome 3 (20–30%).

- The best known criteria for defining HNPCC are the "Amsterdam" criteria (see Box 6.1.7). However these criteria do not account for the frequent occurrence of noncolonic cancers in these families. There may be early onset of endometrial, ovarian, upper urinary tract, small-intestinal, and stomach cancer.
- **Clinical features** of HNPCC compared with sporadic cancers are shown in the table. There is a high incidence of synchronous and metachronous tumors (mean annual rate of about 3%).
- **Diagnosis** of HNPCC is still made on clinical grounds, but identification of the responsible genes suggests that genetic testing will become available.
- **Screening.** Lifetime risk for colorectal cancer is about 1 in 2: start colonoscopy screening at 25 years old or five years before earliest age occurrence of colon cancer in family; repeat every two years (upper GI screening also required).

Box 6.1.7 Amsterdam II criteria for hereditary non-polyposis colorectal cancer

At least three relatives with HNPCC-associated cancer (colorectal cancer, cancer of the endometrium, small bowel, ureter, or renal pelvis) plus all of the following:
1 One affected patient is a first-degree relative of the other two
2 Two or more successive generations affected
3 One or more cases of colon cancer diagnosed before age 50
4 FAP excluded
5 Tumors verified by pathological examination

Table 6.1.5 Clinical features of HNPCC compared with sporadic colon cancer

	HNPCC	**Sporadic cancer**
Mean age at diagnosis (years)	45	65
Multiple cancers	35%	4–11%
Proximal location	72%	35%
Excess malignancy at other sites	Yes	No
Mucinous tumors	Common	Rare
Prognosis	Favorable	Variable

This table was published in Feldman M, et al. Sleisenger and Fordtran's gastrointestinal and liver disease, 7th ed. Copyright Elsevier 1998.

Hereditary polyposis

Inherited polyposis may be broadly considered in terms of adenomatous and hamartomatous syndromes.

Adenomatous polyposis syndromes

Range of inherited adenomatous polyposis syndromes characterized by the development of large numbers of adenomatous polyps in the colon, and high risk of <u>colon cancer</u>.

- <u>Familial adenomatous polyposis</u> (FAP).
- <u>Gardner's syndrome</u>. Similar intestinal polyp pattern to that of FAP, with additional thyroid/adrenal tumors, fibromas, desmoid tumors, and bone tumors. Associated with APC gene.
- <u>Turcot's syndrome</u>. Colonic adenomas (usually fewer than in FAP), with medulloblastoma.

Hamartomatous polyposis syndromes

Hamartomas are of mesenchymal origin, and carry lower risk of malignant change than adenomas. However, increased cancer risk (GI and non-GI seen in these conditions).

- <u>Peutz Jeghers syndrome</u>.
- <u>Juvenile polyposis syndrome</u>.
- <u>Cowden's disease</u>.

See also <u>hereditary nonpolyposis colon cancer</u> (HNPCC).

<u>Cronkite–Canada</u> syndrome is a rare, noninherited cause of polyposis.

Irritable bowel syndrome (IBS)

A common, chronic recurrent illness (rather than a specific medical disease: there being no recognized pathology and no specific cause) characterized by abdominal pain or discomfort and a disturbed bowel habit (see Boxes 6.1.8 and 6.1.9 for diagnostic criteria).

Epidemiology

Found all over the world but different cultures have varying perceptions of disease and illness seeking behavior. In the West, more common in women and more common in those under 50 years. Most commonly diagnosed gastrointestinal condition; comprises 25 – 50% of referrals to gastroenterologists

Pathophysiology

Remains uncertain. Hereditary and environmental factors likely to have a role. Many studies report abnormal gastrointestinal motility, visceral hypersensitivity, psychological abnormalities, and emotional stress in patients with IBS.

Motility

Intestinal contractile and electrical activity is increased in patients with IBS, but this is probably an exaggerated response to stimuli rather than physical pathology. There is increased sensitivity to visceral stimulation, although there are wide variations in subgroups of IBS patients with diarrhea or constipation.

Triggers for sensitization

There is currently much interest in the role of inflammatory cells or mediators in at least some types of IBS. Proliferation of intestinal mast cells, or sympathetic afferent excitation via increased neuropeptide release have been proposed as mechanisms by which food or stress may trigger symptoms.

There is an association between emotion and gut motility and this has been proposed as a further factor in IBS.

Postinfective sensitization

Culture positive gastroenteritis is a very strong risk factor for IBS, which does not seem linked to continuing infection. A change in microbial flora seems to be associated with changes in colonic transit and rectal sensitivity but the mechanisms are largely undefined.

Small-bowel bacterial overgrowth

More recent studies suggest that a significant number of patients with IBS have small bowel bacterial overgrowth and that they may respond to antibiotics (particularly rifaximin)

Food intolerance

Studies of dietary restriction followed by reintroduction suggest food intolerance in 30–60% of IBS patients. Immunological or biochemical correlation has been lacking: despite a reported association with atopy, skin testing with food-derived allergens is of dubious relevance. A recent study reports positive results of food elimination based on serum IgG antibodies in IBS patients.[1]

Symptoms

Patients present with a wide array of symptoms that include both gastrointestinal and extraintestinal complaints (e.g., psychiatric, impaired sexual function). Chronic abdominal pain and altered bowel habits (diarrhea, constipation) are characteristic.

Diagnosis

- IBS is not a diagnosis of exclusion. Diagnosis is based on criteria agreed at a conference in Rome (Boxes 6.1.8 and 6.1.9).
- Consensus statement by the AGA recommends that the diagnosis of IBS should be based upon symptoms consistent with the condition (as summarized by the Rome criteria) and excluding in a cost-effective manner other conditions with similar clinical presentations.
- The decision to investigate is based on the age of the patient, family history, and the presence of "alarm" symptoms (see Boxes 6.1.8–6.1.11).
- Routine labs including inflammatory markers and TTG seems reasonable in the absence of alarm symptoms. A position statement

---

1 Atkinson, W et al. (2004). *Gut* 53: 1459.

issued by the ACG suggests that in patients without alarm features, the routine use of flexible sigmoidoscopy, barium enema, colonoscopy, fecal occult blood tests, stool for ova and parasites, stool for culture, or thyroid function tests cannot be recommended.

- Patients with alarm features should undergo the appropriate endoscopic, stool, and radiologic testing: serum B12, folic acid, iron studies, thyroid function, and stool microsopy should be done and colonoscopy should be considered to exclude <u>microscopic colitis</u>.
- Fecal urgency or incontinence suggests a need for <u>anorectal manometry</u>

Treatment

Successful management combines individualizing treatment of predominant symptoms and conferring insight on how symptoms may related to emotional stresses. Time spent in exploring association between symptoms and life events often pays dividends. Establishment of a therapeutic physician-patient relationship is extremely important. Realistic expectations with consistent limits should be established. The patient should be involved in treatment decisions.

Box 6.1.8 Rome II criteria for irritable bowel syndrome

At least twelve weeks in the preceding twelve months of abdominal discomfort or pain with two or more of the following features:
- Relief by defecation
- Onset associated with a change in stool frequency
- Onset associated with a change in stool appearance

Symptoms supporting a diagnosis of IBS:
- Abnormal stool frequency
- Abnormal stool form
- Difficulties in evacuation
- Passage of mucus
- Bloating or feelings of distension

Box 6.1.9 Rome III criteria for irritable bowel syndrome

Recurrent abdominal pain or discomfort at least three days per month in the last three months associated with two or more of the following:
- Improvement with defecation
- Onset associated with a change in stool frequency
- Onset associated with a change in stool appearance (form)

Criteria fulfilled for the last three months with symptom onset at least six months prior to diagnosis. Discomfort means an uncomfortable sensation not described as pain.

Box 6.1.10 Clinical features supporting the diagnosis of irritable bowel syndrome

- Rome III criteria
- Long history with relapsing and remitting course
- Exacerbations triggered by life events
- Coexistence of anxiety and depression
- Associated with symptoms in other organ systems
- Symptoms aggravated by eating

Box 6.1.11 Clinical features suggesting organic disease other than IBS

- Onset in old age
- Progressive deterioration
- Fever
- Weight loss greater than 10 pounds
- Anemia
- Family history of colon cancer
- Rectal bleeding (not caused by fissures or hemorrhoids)
- Chronic severe diarrhea
- Steatorrhea
- Dehydration

Medications are an adjunct to the treatment of IBS and should be aimed at the predominant symptom. There is little evidence that drugs are particularly effective. Evidence for efficacy of therapies is complicated by a high placebo effect with all modes of treatment. This may relate to the benefit observed with complementary remedies (see Box 6.1.13).

Drugs useful in managing IBS are shown opposite. Sometimes drugs useful for one symptom can make another worse. In particular, dietary fiber or stimulant laxatives can make bloating and abdominal pain worse. We recommend the use of nonstimulant osmotic laxatives such as miralax for constipation. Antidepressants used in low doses have a visceral analgesic effect that should be explained to the patient as this often facilitates acceptability. Tricyclics can have a supplemental effect in relieving insomnia.

Newer drugs (e.g., alosetron, tegaserod) are aimed at modifying visceral sensitivity and reactivity by using ligands for intestinal serotonin receptors. The long-term benefit of this approach remains to be determined.

Alosetron (5-hydroxytryptamine-3 receptor antagonist) was shown to be effective in female diarrhea predominant-IBS patients. However, the drug was associated with ischemic colitis and was removed from the market by the FDA. It has since been brought back to the market under tight control.

Tegaserod (5-hydroxytryptamine-4 receptor agonist) was approved for IBS and constipation but removed from the market in March 2007 because of cardiovascular side effects.

Lubiprostone is a locally acting chloride channel activator that enhances chloride-rich intestinal fluid secretion. It was initially FDA approved for treatment of chronic idiopathic constipation but later also received approval for treatment of IBS with constipation in women 18 years and older.

There is also some evidence that patients with IBS may respond to treatment with antibiotics (particularly rifaxamin)

Diet and IBS

Patients often believe that <u>food intolerance</u> contributes to their symptoms and some sufferers benefit from eliminating certain foods from the diet. Detection of food intolerance is often difficult, even with the help of food diaries and dieticians. Consider trial of lactose free diet to exclude <u>lactose intolerance</u>. Exclusion of foods that increase gas should be excluded in patients who complain of bloating/flatulence. Whether elimination of other foods is beneficial is unclear. Exclusion diets are labor-intensive and time-consuming. They depend on the principle of stabilizing the patient on a very bland diet for a few days and then gradually introducing favorite foods one or two per day.

Prognosis in IBS

There is a high probability of remaining free of severe symptoms in IBS patients but symptoms usually persist for a long time (5% free of symptoms at five years). Medical intervention relieves or improves symptoms and quality of life in about two-thirds of patients with IBS. Outcome is best in males with a short history, predominant constipation, and a good initial response to treatment. Long-term response is best where psychosocial issues have been explored and patient education emphasized.

Box 6.1.12 IBS: all in the mind?

- IBS is more common in those attending psychiatric clinics, and there is an association with psychological factors including anxiety and depression. The only prospective data comes from IBS triggered by an episode of gastroenteritis: psychological factors at onset of infection appear to predict development of chronic bowel symptoms.
- IBS patients appear to show particular illness behavior; they consult doctors more frequently about minor ailments and there is an overlap with illnesses such as chronic fatigue syndrome and fibromyalgia.
- IBS patients report more stressful life events, ranging from loss to familial disruption, domestic or career dissatisfaction, or abuse (physical or sexual). Loss of self-esteem and autonomy is frequently manifest in somatic symptoms including those of IBS.

Box 6.1.13 **Complementary and alternative therapies in IBS**

Evidence is accumulating that a variety of therapies can modulate stress hormones and other physiologic functions. Different therapies are directed at different aspects of healing.
- **Physical therapies** (massage, acupuncture, reflexology, shiatsu) may work on the release of tension.
- **Meditation and hypnotherapy** produce focused relaxation that may facilitate cognitive behavioral change.
- **Biofeedback** may help patients gain control over their symptoms.

Box 6.1.14 **Drugs useful in managing IBS**

- **Antispasmodics** for abdominal pain: dicyclomine
- **Antidiarrheal agents:** <u>LOPERAMIDE</u>, <u>CHOLESTYRAMINE</u>
- **Anticonstipating agents:** miralax
- **Antidepressants:** tricyclics, SSRIs
- **Serotonin-4 receptor agonists** for diarrhea: tegaserod
- **Serotonin-3 receptor antagonist** for constipation: alosetron
- **Chloride channel activator** for diarrhea: lupiprostone
- **Antibiotics:** Rifaxamin

Juvenile polyps and polyposis

Juvenile polyps are mucosal tumors consisting of excess lamina propria and dilated cystic glands rather than epithelial cells. They are hamartomas and appear to be acquired, being most common from ages 1–7. They usually regress spontaneously but can occur in adults. They are usually single, range in size from 3 mm to 2 cm, and are commonest in the rectum. They may prolapse during defecation.

They have no malignant potential when single but removal is suggested because of their blood supply and tendency to bleed. Association with proximal adenomas is rare.

Juvenile polyposis syndrome is defined by 10 or more juvenile polyps; juvenile polyps occurring throughout the GI tract; or any number of juvenile polyps with a family history of juvenile polyposis. 1/3 cases have history of first degree relative with juvenile polyposis. Autosomal dominant. Associated with germline mutations in PTEN and DPC4, which are tumor suppressor genes (DPC4 has a role in signaling through TGF). Association with <u>HHT</u>. Symptoms usually begin between ages 4–14. Rectal bleeding and anemia most common presentation. When juvenile polyps are multiple, there is an increased risk of cancer because of the adenomatous tissue present in some polyps rather than the juvenile polyps *per se*. The lifetime risk of cancer is approximately 20%.

No consensus for optimal screening or surveillance. Screening is recommended in early teens with surveillance colonoscopy every two years.

Upper GI endoscopy, SBFT, possibly capsule endoscopy should be done every 1-2 years. Colonoscopy with polypectomy likely adequate if small numbers of polyps. Asymptomatic first degree relatives of patients with FJP are at risk for juvenile polyposis and colorectal cancer and should be screened for the disease. Consider colonoscopy every one to two years from age 14–35 and then less frequently.

Laxative abuse

Also see <u>LAXATIVES</u>.

Patients abusing laxatives fall into one of four categories (see Table 6.1.6). Detection depends on a high level of suspicion. Hypokalemia may complicate purgative abuse. Melanosis coli suggests ingestion of anthracene laxatives. A large fecal osmotic gap may suggest magnesium ingestion. Fecal osmolality less than 290 mOsm/kg suggests dilution of the stool with water. Mixing stool with hypertonic urine gives a very high fecal osmolality, with a negative fecal osmotic gap because of the high urinary concentrations of Na^+ and K^+.

Table 6.1.6 Groups of patients abusing laxatives

Group	Characteristics
Patients with <u>bulimia</u>	Usually adolescent/young adult women concerned about weight
Secondary gain	May have disability claim pending, or abuse laxatives to induce concern in others
Munchausen's syndrome	Feigned illness to confound physicians
Munchausen's syndrome by proxy	Poisoning by caregivers

This table was published in Feldman M, et al. Sleisenger and Fordtran's gastrointestinal and liver disease, 7th ed. Copyright Elsevier 1998.

Megacolon

Defined as a radiological diameter of the rectosigmoid or descending colon of >6.5 cm, ascending colon of >8 cm, or cecal diameter >12 cm. Can be **congenital** (<u>Hirschsprung's</u>, and may be subtle congenital abnormalities resulting in autonomic denervation) or **acquired** (can be associated with any cause of <u>constipation</u>, and rarely with infection by <u>trypanosomiasis</u> in Chagas's disease). See also <u>toxic megacolon</u>.

- Acquired megacolon is assumed if there is no congenital lesion or when symptoms did not appear in infancy. Look for an underlying cause (see Box 6.1.15).

- Idiopathic megarectum and megacolon relate to dilatation of the rectum and/or colon in the absence of demonstrable organic disease. Patients with megarectum tend to present with fecal soiling and impaction and are young.

Diagnosis. Water soluble contrast media are useful in defining colonic anatomy. <u>Anorectal manometry</u> is useful in differentiating congenital from acquired causes: an intact recto-inhibitory reflex depends on intact ganglia and if present the patient does not have Hirschsprung's disease. <u>Colonic transit</u> is usually delayed in those with megacolon but may be normal in those with isolated megarectum. The gold standard for diagnosis of <u>Hirschsprung's</u> is a rectal biopsy, which can be obtained using a mucosal suction technique. Need to rule out obstruction.

Management. Optimal treatment is to empty the bowel completely (phosphate enemas) and then titrate an osmotic laxative. Disimpaction may be required: stimulant laxatives should be avoided. Usually lifelong laxatives are needed and follow up is important. Behavioral treatment and surgery may be helpful. Mainstay of treatment of <u>Hischsprung's</u> is surgery.

Acute or <u>toxic megacolon</u> is covered separately.

Box 6.1.15 Causes of acquired megacolon

Neurologic: Chagas's disease, Parkinson's disease, myotonic dystrophy, diabetic neuropathy

Smooth muscle: scleroderma, <u>amyloidosis</u>

Metabolic: hypothyroidism, hypokalemia, <u>porphyria</u>, pheochromocytoma

Drugs

Mechanical obstruction

Melanosis coli

Brown discoloration of colonic epithelium, caused by accumulation of lipofuscin pigment in lamina propria macrophages resulting from laxative-induced apoptosis. Found in 70% of people who use anthroquinone laxatives (cascara, aloe, senna, rhubarb). It does disappear within 12 months of stopping laxatives. Colonic tumors lack pigment-containing macrophages and are thus very easily seen.

Microscopic colitis

Comprises two distinct diseases, **<u>collagenous colitis</u>** and **lymphocytic colitis**, united by their clinical presentation of watery diarrhea with macroscopically normal colonic mucosa on endoscopy but evidence of histological inflammation.

Epidemiology

Initially thought commoner in women (collagenous colitis) age 50–70, but recognized in both sexes. Prevalence as high as 10–15 per 100,000. Historically probably underreported because of failure to biopsy normal appearing mucosa in patients with watery diarrhea. Association with <u>celiac</u> and autoimmune diseases.

Pathology

Increased CD8 T cells, plasma cells, macrophages. In collagenous colitis, there is a thickened subepithelial collegan layer, greater than 10 μm thick (Color plate 11). It tends to be collagen type I and III rather than the normal type IV, and is commoner on the right side of the colon than the left.

Etiology and pathogenesis

Thought broadly to involve epithelial immune responses to antigens derived from luminal contents. Fecal diversion produces improvement but the condition relapses once intestinal continuity is re-established. Dietary factors, intestinal pathogens, drugs (particularly NSAIDs), and toxins have all been proposed as important causative factors. The collagen band may be partly a result of reduced collagenases rather than increased deposition, and its thickness does not relate to clinical severity; it may be a secondary phenomenon rather than causative for the diarrhea.

Clinical features

Usually chronic watery diarrhea sometimes associated with crampy abdominal pain and weight loss. Examination normal, routine blood tests normal, stool microscopy negative for blood but 50% positive for leucocytes. Colonoscopy is normal or only mildly and variably abnormal endoscopically. Usually intermittent course.

Treatment

Stop NSAIDs and other drugs associated with microscopic colitis. The range of therapies tried (<u>METRONIDAZOLE</u>, <u>BISMUTH</u>, <u>5-ASA</u>, bile acid resins, <u>CORTICOSTEROIDS</u> or other immunosuppressants, as well as simple anti-diarrheal agents such as loperamide) reveals that the diseases are poorly understood. First line agents include anti-diarrheals and <u>bismuth</u>. If those fail, one can consider trial of 5-ASA and then metronidazole. There is good data for the use of <u>BUDESONIDE</u>. If diarrhea continues, make sure to rule out associated <u>celiac disease</u>.

Ogilvie's syndrome (acute pseudo-obstruction)

Acute pseudo-obstruction localized to the colon, precipitated by trauma, orthopaedic surgery, infection, obstetric procedures, pelvic surgery, or electrolyte disturbances such as hypokalaemia. The precise cause is not known, but the condition results from a dilatation of the colon in response to non-mechanical factors. All patients present with abdominal distention.

Patients may also have nausea, vomiting, abdominal pain, constipation, and, paradoxically, diarrhea.

Diagnosis is by abdominal X-ray, which shows gaseous distension of the colon, with no bowel sounds on examination. Need to rule out mechanical obstruction and toxic megacolon.

Treatment
- NPO, <u>nasogastric tube</u>, IV fluids. Water soluble contrast exam to exclude mechanical obstruction: hyperosmolarity often helps to evacuate colon. Eliminate possible precipitants (e.g., electrolyte repletion).
- Try and decompress the colon with a rectal decompresson tube. Neostigmine (2.5 mg IV over 1–3 minutes) can be very helpful in management of acute colonic pseudo-obstruction. Patients should be on an ECG monitor: have IV atropine available in case of bradycardia. Response is usually within 20 minutes: treatment can be repeated up to three times until successful.
- **Surgery** is rarely required. Advisable for patients with cecal diameter over 11 cm and refractory to medical or endoscopic management. Tube cecostomy can be helpful: for patients with fever, leucocytosis, or peritoneal signs, right hemicolectomy may be required.

Perianal Crohn's disease

Incidence. Reported rates vary from 4% to 60%. More common with colonic disease, particularly rectal <u>Crohn's disease</u>. Usually, perianal disease presents concurrently or after intestinal disease but in 25% of patients perianal disease can precede intestinal manifestation by several years.

Spectrum of disease
- **Skin lesions** include skin tags and abscesses that are usually linked to a fistula.
- **Anal canal lesions** include fissures, ulcers, and stenosis. Fissures tend to be eccentric rather than midline. Stricture can relate to smooth muscle spasm or to extramucosal fibrosis.
- **Perianal fistulae.** Often accompany perianal abscesses. Classified by Parks in 1976: see <u>anorectal fistulae</u>. Rectovaginal fistulation occurs in about 5–10% with perianal disease.

Assessment of severity
- Conventional scoring systems like the <u>Crohn's disease activity index</u> correlate poorly with severity. A perianal disease activity index (PDAI) has been developed and validated by a Canadian group.[1]
- If examination is painful, examination under anaesthetic is appropriate.

---

1 Irvine, E J. et al. (1995). *J. Clin. Gastroenterol.* 20: 27.

- Imaging includes endoanal ultrasound (see <u>endoscopic ultrasound</u>) and <u>MRI</u>. Ultrasound is very useful at characterizing sphincter defects while MRI is useful for assessing sphincter integrity as well as defining fistula tract anatomy.

Treatment

Medical

- **Immunomodulators.** Azathioprine/6MP will heal about 30% of fistulae, and methotrexate probably has similar efficacy.
- **Anti-TNF treatment** has been evaluated in perianal Crohn's. <u>INFLIXIMAB</u> has been shown to be highly effective in treating fistulae. Adalimumab also appears effective in treating perianal fistulae.
- **Antibiotics** are useful. Usually recurrence of symptoms once antibiotics are stopped. Long-term metronidazole has been associated with a risk of neuropathy (particularly doses > 1 g). Ciprofloxacin has little effect against anaerobes but is of proven use in perianal Crohn's.
- Fissures are increasingly treated with pharmacological therapy including topical nitrates (GTN), botulinum toxin, and topical niphedipine.
- **Topical aminosalicylates** may be effective in rectal disease.
- **Steroids** can prevent fistula healing and may lead to abscess formation.

Surgical

Surgical options range from drainage of abscesses, fistulectomies, to major interventions such as proctocolectomy with stoma formation.

- Emergency treatment of sepsis may involve incision of an abscess, with antibiotics. Fistulae after drainage often treated by placing a <u>seton suture</u>, aimed at preventing further abscess formation.
- Operations for fistulae are complex and out of our scope here. Simple perianal fistulae are often amenable to fistulectomy. For extensive disease, an obvious concern and principle of surgery is the maintenance of fecal continence.

Pneumatosis intestinalis

Presence of gas in the wall of the small intestine or colon. Clinical sign, not a disease itself. May be incidental or indicate presence of life-threatening intra-abdominal catastrophe. Most cases involve the small intestine and only 5% of cases affect the colon. Pathogenesis poorly understood; likely multifactorial. Clinical features: commonest in the 60s, no sex difference, usually asymptomatic but can be associated with diarrhea, mucous discharge, rectal bleeding, constipation, abdominal pain. **Need to rule out intra-abdominal catastrophe** (e.g., bowel infarction) requiring emergency exploratory laparotomy versus conservative therapy for non-life-threatening disease. Those symptomatic patients without intra-abdominal catastrophe can be treated by breathing high flow oxygen for several days or <u>METRONIDAZOLE</u> can also be effective. Complications are rare, but include obstruction, volvulus, intussusception, hemorrhage.

Polyposis syndromes

See: colonic polyps and hereditary polyposis.

Pseudomembranous colitis

See: clostridial infections of GI tract.

Pseudo-obstruction

Symptoms and signs of intestinal obstruction in the absence of an occluding lesion. Caused by disorders of smooth muscle, myenteric plexus or extra-intestinal nervous system. (See Box 6.1.16.) Ogilvie's syndrome is acute pseudo-obstruction localized to the colon, precipitated by trauma, orthopedic surgery, obstetric procedures, pelvic surgery, or electrolyte disturbances (e.g., $\downarrow K^+$).

Clinical features

Varying degrees of abdominal pain, distension, and vomiting depending partly on which part of bowel is involved. Small-bowel involvement with stasis and bacterial overgrowth may lead to steatorrhea. This can lead to weight loss and malabsorption. There may be gastroparesis or esophageal involvement. There may be a succussion splash and obstructive sounding bowel sounds.

Investigations

As well as blood tests directed to various diagnoses listed in the Box 6.1.16, barium or cross-sectional imaging of the whole GI tract is indicated. The aim is to make a diagnosis where possible but mainly to exclude mechanical obstruction. One should also assess nutritional status, confirm dysmotility with a transit test (scintigraphy), and consider manometry.

There may even be a need for brain MRI; electromyography, or nerve conduction studies; and autonomic function tests. There is an association with urinary tract involvement such as megacystis or megaureters.

Box 6.1.16 Causes of chronic intestinal pseudo-obstruction

- Disorders of smooth muscle (either primary due to rare visceral myopathies, or secondary to amyloid, radiation, SLE, muscular dystrophy, or systemic sclerosis)
- Disorders of the myenteric plexus
- Neurological problems: Parkinson's, autonomic dysfunction
- Small-bowel diverticulosis
- Endocrine: hypothyroidism, porphyria
- Drugs (OPIATES, phenothiazines, ANTICHOLINERGICS, tricyclics, calcium channel blockers)

Treatment

Chronic

- **Nutritional support**
- **Electrolyte balance**, especially potassium, calcium, and magnesium is important.
- Drug treatment with <u>PROKINETICS</u> is attractive but <u>METOCLOPRAMIDE</u> and <u>DOMPERIDONE</u> rarely work: cisapride is more effective but is now unavailable. Erythromycin is a motilin agonist and is sometimes tried. <u>OCTREOTIDE</u> in small doses can induce migrating motor complexes in the small intestine.
- Broad spectrum antibiotics are useful in treating patients with <u>bacterial overgrowth</u> due to stagnant loop syndrome.
- Surgery is rarely required and does not always remove symptoms. A small number of patients need home <u>parenteral nutrition</u>.

Acute

- **Colonoscopic decompression** can be tried although is not universally effective.
- Treatment with neostigmine, 2.5 mg IV over two to three minutes (patient should be on a monitor with atropine ready in case of bradycardia) has been shown effective in a prospective controlled study[1] and is probably underutilized.

TNM classification

See: <u>tumor staging</u>.

Toxic megacolon

- Defined as a transverse colonic diameter of > 6 cm with loss of haustration in a patient with colitis. It occurs in about 5% of cases of severe attacks and can be triggered by opiates or hypokalemia.
- Feared complication of fulminant inflammatory bowel disease that can also complicate infectious colitis (e.g., *Campylobacter, Shigella*) and acute distal obstruction (e.g., volvulus). Can occur in patients without obvious colonic disease or mechanical obstruction (see <u>Ogilvie's syndrome</u>).

Treatment

If dilatation occurs during treatment of an acute attack of colitis, surgery is indicated. If the dilatation is present when the patient is first seen, medical treatment with IV fluids and steroids can be tried. Many clinicians try to decompress the colon with a colonic tube: air accumulates in the transverse colon because it is the most anterior portion of the colon, and rolling of the patient into a prone position for 15 min every 2 h is also advocated. 50% respond with therapy; urgent colectomy is required for those who do not improve after 24–72 h of medical therapy.

1 Ponec, RJ et al. (1999). N. Engl. J. Med 341: 137.

Tumor staging

TNM classification widely applied to staging of solid tumors (e.g., colo-rectal [but also see <u>Dukes classification</u>], <u>esophageal</u>, <u>gastric</u>, <u>pancreatic</u> <u>cancer</u>), because it is of prognostic value and guides management.

T—Primary tumor

T0	No evidence of primary
Tis	Carcinoma *in situ*
T1	Invasion of lamina propria or submucosa
T2	Invasion of muscularis propria
T3	Invasion of adventitia
T4	Invasion of adjacent structures

N—Regional lymph nodes

0	No regional nodal metastases
N1	Regional nodal metastases

M—Distant metastases

MX	Cannot be assessed
M0	No distant metastases
M1	Distant metastases

Table 6.1.7 Tumor staging (TNM classification)

Stage	T	N	M
0	Tis	N0	M0
IA	T1	N0	M0
IIA	T2,T3	N0	M0
IIB	T1, T2	N1	M0
III	T3	N1	M0
	T4	Any N	M0
IV	Any T	Any N	M1

Turcot's syndrome

A syndrome of familial colonic polyposis with primary tumors of the CNS. The commonest group has a germline mutation, and the CNS tumors tend to be medulloblastomas. The second group has germline mutatons in mismatch repair genes typical of HNPCC and is associated with glioblastoma multiforme.

Typhlitis

Background

- From Greek *typhlon,* meaning "cecum," but also known as ileocecal syndrome and neutropenic enterocolitis.
- Occurs almost exclusively in immunocompromised patients (e.g., HIV, post-bone-marrow transplant).
- Rarely diagnosed by gastroenterologists, but accounts for 10% of deaths in children with leukemia during chemotherapy.
- Etiology unknown, but important factors may include mucosal injury due to cytotoxics, *cytomegalovirus* or bacterial infection, and mucosal ischemia. *Pseudomonas* has been implicated.

Clinical features

- Nausea, vomiting, fever.
- Generalized or right-sided abdominal pain + tenderness.
- Diarrhea with blood.
- Shock, due to secondary sepsis or cecal perforation.

Investigations

- Important to exclude other causes (e.g., *Clostridium difficile* toxin for pseudomembranous colitis).
- Neutrophil count almost always < 0.1 x 10^9/l.
- Abdominal X-ray may show free air (perforation) or "thumb-printing."
- CT scan may show cecal distension, and cecal, right-colon, or terminal-ileum wall thickening.

Management

- NPO, NG tube, and gastric decompression.
- IV fluid replacement and consideration for TPN.
- Broad spectrum antibiotics (e.g., third-generation <u>CEPHALOSPORIN</u> + <u>METRONIDAZOLE</u>).
- Surgery necessary for perforation (and some advocate it at diagnosis in view of 40–50% mortality associated with cecal perforation, bowel necrosis, and sepsis).

Ulcerative colitis

First recognized as different from infectious colitis in 1859 by Samuel Wilks.

Definition. An inflammatory condition that affects the rectum and extends proximally to affect a variable amount of the colon.

Epidemiology

Found worldwide but incidence varies about tenfold between high incidence areas (UK, United States, Northern Europe, Australia; approximate incidence 10 per 100,000 per year, approximate prevalence 100 per 100,000 population) and low incidence areas (Asia, Japan, South America).

In contrast to the rising incidence of <u>Crohn's</u>, the incidence has remained steady over the last 50 years. Affects men and women equally, with peak incidence age 20–40 and a second smaller peak in older adults. Said to affect (Ashkenazi) Jews more frequently, but the lower incidence among Jews in Israel compared to the United States suggests that environmental factors play a role.

Genetics

There is a genetic component (concordance rates for identical twins are 13% and 2% for monozygotic and dizygotic twins; more than allowable by chance but less than occurs in <u>Crohn's</u>) but inheritance is not simply Mendelian. Several genes may be involved in disease susceptibility. Several linkage studies suggest a susceptibility locus on chromosome 12 and other loci on 2, 3, 6, and 7 have been implicated. Other genes may influence disease behavior independently of susceptibility.

Etiology

Unknown; hypotheses include infection, sensitivity to food components (no evidence to support this), immune response to bacterial or self-antigens, and the role of the central nervous system ("stress") and a possible abnormality in colonic epithelial cells. Few attempt to explain the mainly left-sided nature of the disease.

- **Infection.** No specific pathogen has been identified. There may be differences in adhesions of *E. coli* from patients compared to controls, and attempts at altering the luminal environment with probiotic bacteria suggest that the luminal microflora are relevant to disease pathogenesis.
- **Immunopathogenesis.** There are increased IgG1- and IgG3-secreting plasma cells. There are autoantibodies to components of epithelial cells and also to p-ANCA in 60–80% patients. Changes in T cells and intraepithelial lymphocytes are confusing and have an uncertain relevance to pathogenesis. There is strong epithelial expression of MHC class II antigens in active colitis, which may relate to antigen expression to local T cells. Many of the changes in immune cell function may be secondary to increased levels of pro-inflammatory cytokines (IL-1, IL-6, interferon gamma).

Clinical features

Symptoms. Bloody diarrhea and mucus per rectum. Urgency of defecation is common and may give abdominal discomfort but pain is not usually a prominent symptom (although abdominal cramps may accompany severe disease). Symptoms do not always correlate with endoscopic severity of disease. Onset is classically slow and insidious but acute onset can happen and UC can be precipitated by an acute infectious colitis.

Blood and pus are usually mixed with the stool but pure blood alone may be seen in disease localized to the rectum (proctitis). Diarrhea is common, but patients with proctitis may complain of constipation or hard stools.

Systemic symptoms are common in severe attacks; there may be anorexia, vomiting, fever, and symptoms of anemia.

Signs. Affected bowel may be tender. Bowel sounds are usually normal.

Signs of dehydration, fever, evidence of weight loss, tachycardia are evidence of a severe attack.

There may be extraintestinal manifestations of colitis (see later section).

Assessing disease severity. Although there are endoscopic and histological scoring systems, the clinical criteria of Truelove and Witts[1] are still used as a guide to decide on admission and intravenous therapy.

- **Mild:** less than 4 stools/day, no systemic disturbance.
- **Moderate:** 4–6 stools/day, minimal disturbance.
- **Severe:** over 6 stools/day, with blood and systemic disturbance (fever, tachycardia, anemia, or ESR over 30). Note that it is unclear how many systemic features are required.

   Laboratory markers of severity include ↑CRP, ↑platelet count, ↓albumin.

Diagnosis and differential diagnosis

The diagnosis rests on the clinical picture, especially the history, the endoscopic appearance, (Color plate 18) histologic appearance of colonic biopsy specimens, and microbiological exclusion of infectious colitis. The endoscopic appearances vary with severity of disease from mild (edema, loss of vascularity, and patchy subepithelial hemorrhage) to severe (loss of vascular pattern, hemorrhage, mucopus, ulceration, and loss of epithelium, sometimes with small islands of residual mucosa that can be mistaken for polyps and are, therefore, called "pseudopolyps")

Always consider Crohn's colitis in the differential diagnosis; ileoscopy or radiological small-bowel evaluation is often necessary (especially if inflammation appears confined to the rectum but there are raised inflammatory markers, low albumin, or anemia). Exclude other forms of segmental colitis, such as ischemia, radiation colitis, microscopic colitis, and drug-induced colitis.

Investigations

Laboratory tests. Check for anemia or iron deficiency. Thrombocytosis, eosinophilia, leucocytosis may all reflect active disease. Hypokalemia, hypoalbuminemia, and abnormal liver blood tests may be associated with severe disease. Liver blood tests may be abnormal reflecting primary sclerosing cholangitis in about 5% of cases.

Colonoscopy is not usually necessary for diagnosis (sigmoidoscopy, either rigid or flexible, is often sufficient for this) but can be helpful for determining the extent of disease. Although colonoscopy is safe in expert hands, in severe disease it cannot be recommended for general use. In the assessment of chronic colitis and in surveillance for dysplasia as a complication of long-standing colitis, colonoscopy is still essential.

1 Truelove, SC and Witts, LJ (1995). *Br. Med. J.* 2: 1041.

Radiology. A plain abdominal X-ray is useful in excluding a perforation, assessing the amount of fecal loading, excluding toxic dilatation, and giving some evidence of extent of disease. Contrast barium radiology has very little role in assessing ulcerative colitis. In the case of an acutely tender abdomen, CT with contrast gives much more information and can show colonic wall thickening and hyperemia.

Biopsies. Always take a biopsy since there is often disparity between endoscopic appearance and histology.

Pathology
50% have disease confined to the sigmoid or rectum, 30% have disease beyond the sigmoid but not affecting the whole colon, and 20% have a pancolitis. Rectal sparing can be seen as a result of topical treatment with steroids or 5-ASA. Although shortening and narrowing of the colon can occur as a result of chronic colitis, fibrosis and stricturing is uncommon. Microscopic features: inflammation is confined to the mucosa, with neutrophils, lymphocytes, macrophages, and eosinophils. There is inflammation of the crypts and depletion of goblet cells.

Extraintestinal manifestations
See Box 6.1.18. There is an important association between UC and thrombo-embolism (DVT and PE). Hospitalization, immobility, and malnutrition contribute, but, in addition, platelets can be high and many clotting factors are increased. There is no independent association with factor V Leiden. Treatment with prophylactic anticoagulants is safe and effective.

Management
Medical <u>CORTICOSTEROIDS</u> (see Box 6.1.19) have reduced mortality of acute attacks from over 35% to less than 1% and are effective in about 70% of acute attacks. 5-ASA (see 5-<u>AMINOSALICYLATES</u>) has significantly reduced relapse rate and improved quality of life. Immunosuppressant drugs (azathioprine/6-mercaptopurine, methotrexate) have been introduced for the management of chronic active disease, because they have a steroid-sparing effect, and to maintain remission. <u>CYCLOSPORINE</u> is being increasingly used in severe ulcerative colitis. Suggested treatment

---

Box 6.1.17 **Histological differentiation of ulcerative colitis from infectious colitis**

This is difficult, but the following features suggest chronicity and help to make the diagnosis of ulcerative colitis with a probability of more than 80%:
- Distorted crypt architecture
- Crypt atrophy
- Irregular mucosal surface
- Basal lymphoid aggregates
- Chronic inflammatory infiltrate

Box 6.1.18 Extraintestinal manifestations of ulcerative colitis

Related to activity of colitis
- Peripheral arthropathy
- Erythema nodosum
- Episcleritis
- Aphthous mouth ulcers

Usually related to activity of colitis
- Pyoderma gangrenosum
- Anterior uveitis

Unrelated to colitis
- Sacroiliitis
- Ankylosing spondylitis
- Primary sclerosing cholangitis

Rare
- Pericarditis
- Amyloidosis

regimens for proctitis, mild disease, severe disease, chronic active disease, and maintenance therapy are shown in Box 6.1.19. Recent data suggest INFLIXIMAB may be useful in moderate to severe colitis.

Surgical
Indications for surgery in ulcerative colitis include:
- Severe attacks not responding to medical therapy.
- Complications of a severe attack (perforation, acute colonic dilatation).
- Chronic continuous disease with impaired quality of life.
- Dysplasia or carcinoma.

Choice of operation
- Total colectomy with permanent ileostomy.
- Total colectomy with ileo-anal pouch formation.

Colectomy with pouch formation is the operation of choice except for the elderly, those with impaired sphincter pressures, and those who do not wish to have a restorative proctocolectomy.

Complications, course, and prognosis

Most (80%) patients have intermittent attacks with varying lengths of remission. A few have chronic continuous disease, and the remainder have a severe first attack with toxic megacolon or disease refractory to medical treatment that requires colectomy. The extent of the disease can change with time: about 20 patients with proctitis will extend their disease after 10 years. Disease extending past the rectosigmoid is associated with a risk of malignant transformation; this risk relates principally to the duration and extent of disease of disease.

Colitis in pregnancy
Fertility is normal. Pregnancy is not a risk factor for relapse. Disease has no adverse effect on developing fetus. Steroids, 5-<u>ASA</u>, and even <u>AZATHIOPRINE</u> appear safe in pregnancy. <u>METHOTREXATE</u> is teratogenic and is contraindicated.

Box 6.1.19 Treatment regimens for ulcerative colitis

Proctitis
Most respond to topical 5-ASA or steroid enemas or a combination of both (e.g., colifoam enema in the morning and 5-ASA enema at night. Suppositories are effective for pure proctitis. If symptoms continue, add in oral 5-ASA. **Remember to check for proximal constipation above the inflammation**: this is common and stops patients improving. Most clinicians treat proximal constipation with fiber but there is emerging evidence that this is poorly tolerated: an osmotic laxative such as polyethylene glycol (Miralax) should be used instead.

Mildly active disease
Use oral mesalazine, oral steroids in moderate doses (prednisone 20 mg/day) and consider topical therapy if the disease is confined to the left colon.

Severe disease
Admit to hospital, replace fluid and electrolyte losses. Give IV steroids (hydrocortisone 100 mg qid). Continuing oral nutrition appears not to influence outcome of a severe attack.

  Treatment with IV steroids should be continued for five to seven days if the patient is improving. If the patient does not improve, then decision often lies between starting cyclosporine or sending the patient for surgery (total colectomy with a view to ileo-anal pouch formation).

Chronic active disease
Two flares within 12 months or disease that relapses rapidly on tapering steroids is an indication for starting second-line treatment with an immunosuppressive agent. Persistent chronic disease in patients receiving steroids and immunosuppressive drugs is an indication for surgery.

Maintenance treatment
Use mesalazine indefinitely in a dose of 1,200–1,600 mg/day. Monitor renal function yearly because of the low risk of interstitial nephritis.

Box 6.1.20 When to start cyclosporine? When to refer for surgery?

Difficult and controversial. Data from the 1980s suggested that if mucosal islands, colonic dilatation, or small-intestinal loops were visible on abdominal X-ray, there was an over 70% chance of the patient needing colectomy.

The best recent data on prognosis in severe colitis comes from Travis, SP *et al.* (1996) *Gut* 38: 905; the following factors if present on third day give an 85% prediction of needing surgery:

• Stool frequency >8 x per day
• CRP > 45 in those passing three to eight stools per day

These factors are used by many to allow a decision on third day after admission on starting cyclosporine. Trials are underway to assess whether cyclosporine on admission confers added benefit.

Volvulus

A twisting of the gut around one axis causing lumen occlusion and sometimes strangulation. Can affect the stomach or colon.

Gastric volvulus

Most common in fifth decade, affects men and women equally. In 60% the stomach twists about its long axis. This is usually associated with a diaphragmatic hernia and is commonly an acute event; classically, there is upper abdominal or retrosternal pain and unproductive retching. Gastric infarction can occur. In 40% the stomach twists about its short axis. This is more likely to be incomplete, intermittent, and to present with chronic symptoms.

Acute gastric volvulus is an emergency and has a high mortality if untreated. Nasogastric intubation is indicated, and if there is no infarction, upper GI endoscopy is indicated to attempt detorsion. Surgery, if necessary, can be open or laparoscopic; repair of associated hiatus hernia is necessary.

Colonic volvulus

Can occur where there is a loop of bowel that is movable in the peritoneal cavity with close approximation of the fixation points. Commonest in the sigmoid colon (75%) and cecum (20%). Rarely may affect the transverse colon and splenic flexure. A history of chronic constipation and laxative abuse is common; patients with sigmoid volvulus are often elderly and abdominal tenderness is present only in a minority.

Management of colonic volvulus. Sigmoidoscopic decompression of the colon with placement of a rectal tube into the obstructed segment works in about 60% patients with sigmoid volvulus. The risk of recurrence is 40–50%, which suggests elective resection of the volvulus following successful decompression. Strangulated sigmoid volvulus requires emergency laparotomy with end colostomy.

Colonoscopic decompression of cecal volvulus can be successful but the risk of perforating the thinned, often ischemic, cecum is higher. The best surgical option is controversial but right hemicolectomy is often performed.

Overall mortality approaches 10%, the major predictive factor being the presence of gangrenous bowel, which occurs in about 20%.

Rectum

Anal cancer

Rare (incidence 1 per 100,000 per year comprises 1–2% of <u>colonic cancers</u>). Risk factors include genital warts and history of receptive anal sex; human papilloma virus type 16 for squamous tumors.

- Mean age at presentation 60 years, with bleeding, pain, and pruritus, but 25% of patients are asymptomatic. Adenocarcinomas of the anal canal behave like adenocarcinomas of the rectum and are treated in a similar way with abdomino-perineal resection and pre- or postoperative chemoradiation for large or invasive tumors.
- 80% of cancers are squamous cell cancers and for this group treatment with chemoradiotherapy has replaced aggressive surgery and results in improved five-year survival rate of 70%.
- Nonepidermal tumors are very rare, and include melanomas, intraepithelial neoplasia (also known as Bowen's disease), and Paget's disease, which is an intraepithelial mucinous adenocarcinoma arising from dermal apocrine sweat glands.

Anal fissure

Epidemiology + pathology

Painful linear ulcers in the anal canal. Young and middle-aged adults most commonly affected (M = F). 90% of primary fissures are in the posterior midline. Fissures can also be secondary to <u>Crohn's disease</u>, <u>anal cancer</u>, and infection (e.g. syphilis, TB)—in which case they are usually more lateral.

The elliptical arrangement of the fibers of the anal sphincter is supposed to offer less muscular support to the mucosa posteriorly, predisposing to traumatic tears after passage of a large hard stool. Repeated trauma can lead to chronic fissures—in these patients, resting anal tone is high (though whether this is cause or effect is unclear) and this may produce a degree of ischemia that can lead to fibrosis.

Clinical features

The hallmark is severe sharp pain during and after defecation with scanty bright red bleeding. Digital examination or proctoscopy is usually too painful without topical anesthesia. Simple inspection may reveal the diagnosis. A sentinel pile (fibrotic nubbin of skin at the anal verge) is common.

Treatment

Stools must be made soft and easy to pass (ensure high fluids: use non-stimulant osmotic <u>LAXATIVE</u>). Topical anesthetics and frequent baths can reduce sphincter spasm. Medical treatment with topical nitrates or diltiazem is effective at increasing fissure healing. Surgical therapy includes sphincterotomy, which lowers sphincter tone; lateral sphincterotomy has better results than midline sphincterotomy with fissurectomy. The procedure of manual dilatation under anesthetic produces very uncontrolled results, frequent complications, and is now discredited.

Anorectal abscesses

Usually result from infection of the anal glands along the dentate line. Acute infection may cause an abscess and lead to a chronic anorectal fistula. Abscesses are classified according to where they extend to and may be perianal, ischiorectal, intersphincteric, or supralevator (see Fig. 6.2.1). Commonest type is perianal (40–50%) and least common type is supralevator (5–10%).

Diagnosis can be difficult because there may be no external signs and rectal examination may be painful. Examination under anesthetic, MRI scanning or intra-anal ultrasound can all be very helpful in establishing a diagnosis.

Treatment requires incision and drainage. Culture of pus is not usually necessary. Antibiotics alone are inadequate, although <u>METRONIDAZOLE</u> and <u>CIPROFLOXACIN</u> have an important adjunctive role; in particular, intravenous antibiotics may be needed if the patient is immunocompromised diabetic or shows sign of systemic sepsis.

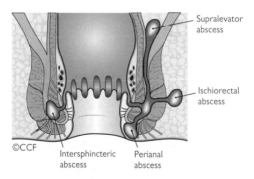

©CCF

Supralevator abscess

Ischiorectal abscess

Intersphincteric abscess

Perianal abscess

Figure 6.2.1 Classification of anorectal abscesses. Reproduced from Feldman M, Friedman LS, and Sleisenger MH (2003). *Sleisenger and Fordtran's Gastrointestinal and Liver Diease*, p. 2286, with permission from Elsevier

Anorectal fistulae

A complication of a perianal abscess, resulting in a connection between the anorectum and the skin at the anal verge or elsewhere in the perineum. Any discharging area or area of granulation around the anus should be assumed to connect with the anorectum unless proved otherwise. Operative exploration or <u>MRI</u> are very useful in defining complex cases. The external and internal openings must be defined and the presence of any extensions established. An underlying disease process such as <u>Crohn's disease</u>, ongoing infection of the presence of a foreign body must not be missed. Biopsy is often needed.

Classification[1] is by their relation to the internal and external sphincters. There are four major categories: intersphincteric, trans-sphincteric, extrasphincteric, and suprasphincteric.

Preoperative assessment of sphincter function by anorectal manometry and an anorectal ultrasound is wise when any degree of sphincter damage is anicipated. Only those tracks passing through distal parts of the sphincter can be laid open without fear of incontinence. For fistulae not amenable to fistulotomy, rather than cutting and repairing the sphincter, which often does not heal well, the insertion of a *seton suture* is a safer option. Complex or high fistulae require complex surgery.

Fecal incontinence

- A common problem, but often difficult for patients to discuss with doctors or close relatives.
- Direct questioning of the patient is often necessary, as is an understanding of continence mechanisms (see Box 6.2.1).
- Continence depends on the sphincter muscles, stool consistency, and cognitive factors.

Clinical Evaluation

History—Ask about passive incontinence and urge incontinence. Ask, also, about duration and severity (solid, liquid, or gas? a slight stain on underpants or the whole stool?). Ask about coincident urinary incontinence.

Ask about potential causes: obstetric history (maximum birth weight, instrumentation, tears/episiotomies, presentation of baby, e.g., occipito-posterior); previous anal surgery; other sytemic/neurological diseases.

Examination—Routine examination including perianal examination, rectal exam (look for fecal impaction), and sigmoidoscopy (rectal inflammation, mucus-secreting polyp such as villous adenoma) is essential. It's important to assess anal tone and squeeze pressure but digital examination correlates poorly with operative and histological findings.

---

1 Parkes, AG et al. (1976) *Br. J. Surg.* 63: 1–12.

Box 6.2.1 Continence mechanisms

- Spongy vascular tissues within the anal canal play a minor role in continence by assisting with anal closure. Minor degrees of seepage may be seen after partial excision of this tissue at hemorrhoidectomy.
- The major mechanisms of continence depend on the anal sphincters. The internal sphincter is the continuation of the circular muscle layer and is under autonomic control. It contributes 70% of resting anal tone. The external sphincter is striated, supplied by sacral nerves S2–4. Tonic neural activation contributes 30% of resting tone, but voluntary squeeze of the external sphincter at times of distension can double normal resting tone.
- The puborectalis muscle wraps around the anorectal junction, forming a sharp angle between the rectum and anal canal. Relaxation of puborectalis allows straightening of the recto-anal angle for defecation.
- The anal canal is very sensitive to touch, pain, and temperature, and this allows for discrimination of solid, liquid, and gas contents, which can allow selective passage of these materials.
- Rectal sensation and compliance is important in maintaining continence. Neuropathies can impair sensation and compliance may be reduced by radiation, colitis, or ischemia.

Investigations—include <u>anorectal physiology</u> and <u>endoanal ultrasound.</u>
  See Table 6.2.1 for causes of incontinence.

Treatment
Conservative
Conservative treatments include ANTIDIARRHEAL AGENTS, e.g., lopera-mide tablets or syrup titrated to achieve beneficial effect, mechanical barriers, or behavioral treatments including <u>biofeedback</u>, which is effective even in patients with structural sphincter damage.

Surgical
As a minimally invasive surgical approach, sacral nerve stimulators may help and have the benefit that a temporary wire can initially be tried to assess for efficacy. Surgery should be reserved for patients with major fecal incontinence in whom conservative methods have failed. The external sphincter can sometimes be repaired after obstetric disruption with an overlap repair. The internal sphincter is not amenable to surgical repair. Repair of a prolapse may be possible by rectopexy. Other surgical treatments undergoing evaluation include dynamic graciloplasty and the artificial bowel sphincter. Colostomy remains an alternative that can return the patient to a near normal lifestyle.

Table 6.2.1 Causes of fecal incontinence

Internal anal sphincter degeneration	Most common cause—elderly
Obstetric trauma	One-third of primiparous women have some damage to the anal sphincter after their first delivery. Forceps delivery, a large baby, and occipito-posterior position are further risk factors.
Surgical damage	Surgically induced sphincter damage can occur after lateral sphincterotomy or major colonic resection
Anal dilatation	Incontinence may complicate manual dilatation of the anus (which used to be performed for <u>anal fissures</u>) or anal fistulae passing through the sphincter muscles. Receptive anal intercourse is also a risk factor.
<u>Rectal prolapse</u>	Incontinence in 30–80%. EUS can help in the diagnosis.
Congenital	Half of all patients with spina bifida soil regularly. One-third of children operated on for <u>Hirschsprung's</u> are incontinent at age 4. Soiling may complicate surgery for sacral tumors.
Spinal injury	Soiling occurs in 30% patients with multiple sclerosis
Radiation injury	Radiation to the anorectum combined with proctitis and reduction in compliance can produce incontinence
Systemic disease	Diabetics can have somatic and autonomic neuropathy. In scleroderma, internal sphincter muscle atrophy, acquired megacolon, and bacterial overgrowth can all occur.

Hemorrhoids

- Dilated vascular channels located in left lateral, right posterior, and right anterior positions within anal canal. A normal part of human anatomy, when diseased, can lead to prolapse, bleeding, and itching (very common: 10–25% adult population). External hemorrhoids are covered with squamous epithelium, while internal hemorrhoids are classified into four groups (see Box 6.2.2).
- Exact pathogenesis is not clear, but may be due to failure of supporting structures; upright posture and prolonged time straining at stool do not help.

Treatment is based on grade (see Box 6.2.2).

Grade 1 and 2 usually respond to diet: increase fiber and fluid intake to ensure soft, easy-to-pass stool. Over-the-counter preparations often contain lubricants, astringents, vasoconstrictors, and antiseptics. Important constituents in prescribed preparations are steroids and local anesthetics to reduce inflammation and provide relief from painful defecation. Don't use topical steroids for longer than a few days and beware of the possibility of perianal candidasis, which should be treated with oral and topical nystatin.

If these fail and patient does not have grade 3 or 4 hemorrhoids (which usually need surgical hemorrhoidectomy) aggressive nonsurgical treatments include sclerosing agents, band ligation, cryotherapy, electro-coagulation, and use of heater probe. Only first two in common use.

- Sclerosing agents. Aim is to inject irritant (e.g., arachis oil containing 5% phenol) into submucosa above hemorrhoid to create fibrosis and prevent prolapse. Pelvic sepsis is rare, but usually occurs three to five days postprocedure, and can be life threatening.
- Band ligation. Widely used for second and third degree hemorrhoids. Stop aspirin and NSAIDs for five days before and after treatment. Immediate pain signifies too close placement to the dentate line: band needs to be removed. Complications include bleeding (usually controlled by balloon tamponade with a Foley catheter balloon, but sometimes needing adrenaline injection or even a small suture) and sepsis.
- External hemorrhoids are visible and palpable on wiping, but cause few symptoms apart from slight interference with personal hygiene. However they may thrombose, causing rapid appearance of a lump and pain. This usually subsides after a few days.

Box 6.2.2 Classification of internal hemorrhoids

Grade 1 Bleeding with defecation

Grade 2 Prolapse with defecation but return naturally to their normal position

Grade 3 Prolapse at any time, especially with defecation, and can be replaced manually

Grade 4 Permanently prolapsed

Hirschsprung's disease

Harald Hirschsprung (1830–1916)—the first pediatrician to be appointed in Denmark.

An important cause of congenital <u>megacolon</u>. Hirschsprung's occurs in 1:5,000 live births. Autosomal dominant or recessive inheritance, with low penetration (30%). Absence of ganglion cells from myenteric and submucosal plexuses, extending proximally from internal anal sphincter, is characteristic.

Clinical features. Usually presents after birth with failure to pass meconium, and later in childhood with recurrent fecal impaction, constipation, and malnutrition. May be complicated by enterocolitis in infancy. Overflow rarely occurs. Associated with multiple endocrine neoplasia (MEN)-2 and <u>Down syndrome</u>.

Investigation

- Barium enema may show a narrowed distal rectum free of feces, with proximal colonic dilatation.
- Procto-sigmoidoscopy normal, with deep rectal biopsy showing absence of ganglion cells in submucosa.
- Anorectal manometry may show that resting internal anal sphincter pressure is normal/elevated, and that, in response to rectal distension, internal anal sphincter contracts (rather than relaxes, with compensatory external sphincter contraction, as in normal 'rectal inhibitory reflex').

Management

Primary treatment is surgery, aimed at excising the aganglionic segment. Colostomy prior to definitive surgery may be required. Persistent problems with soiling may occur in approximately 10%.

Pouchitis

Inflammation occurring in an ileal pouch after proctocolectomy with <u>ileal pouch–anal anastomosis</u> or Kock's continent ileostomy. Risk of pouchitis is highest in first 12 months after ileostomy, ranging from 20–35%. Patients with IBD (especially those with extra-intestinal manifestations) are more commonly affected than patients with <u>familial adenomatous polyposis</u>. After 10 years of a pouch, at least 50% of patients will have had at least one episode. Acute episodes of pouchitis do not affect long-term pouch function. Chronic pouchitis (affecting 10% of patients) can be as symptomatic as the previous UC. About 1% of patients may require removal of pouch secondary to chronic pouchitis.

Etiology is unknown, but probably relates to anaerobic colonization of the pouch mucosa and subsequent colonic metaplasia. Exclusion of other superimposed infections is a concern, as is the possibility that the patient has had <u>Crohn's disease</u> all along.

Clinical features include diarrhea, urgency, abdominal pain, and bleeding. Accurate diagnosis requires a combination of endoscopic, clinical, and histological assessment: reliance on clinical assessment alone results in overdiagnosis and unnecessary treatment. Scoring systems have been developed to standardize evaluation and response to treatment: the best is the pouchitis disease activity index (PDAI, see Table 6.2.2). Pouchitis is defined as a score over 7; remission is a score less than 7 in a patient with a history of pouchitis.

Treatment

Simple antidiarrheal agents may help diarrhea but for true pouchitis, antibiotics (metronidazole or ciprofloxacin) are the first line of treatment. Topical treatment with 5-ASA enemas or steroid enemas can help. Treatment with bismuth subsalicylate (pepto bismol) is not supported on current evidence. Oral probiotic therapy has been shown with at least one preparation (VSL-3) to maintain remission in patients with chronic pouchitis after treatment with antibiotics. One study also suggested that VSL-3 given after IPAA may prevent the development of pouchitis.

For a review see Mahadevan, U and Sandborn, WJ (2003) Gastroenterology 124: 1636.

Table 6.2.2 Pouchitis disease activity index

Criteria	Score
Clinical	
Stool frequency (usual: 1–2 more than usual; 3 or more than usual)	0–2
Rectal bleeding (none/rare: present daily)	0–1
Fecal urgency/cramps (none: occasional: usual)	0–2
Fever	1 if present
Endoscopic	
Oedema, granularity, friability, loss of vascular pattern, mucous exudates, ulceration	1 for each if present
Histologic	
Polymorph infiltration: mild, moderate, severe	1–3
Average ulceration per low power field: < 25%, 25–50%, > 50%	1–3

Reprinted with permission from Sandborn WJ, et al. Pouchitis after ileal pouch-anal anastomosis: a Pouchitis Disease Activity Index. Mayo Clin Proc 1994; 69(5):409–415

Pruritus ani

Perianal area is commonest site for intractable itching of the skin, due to:
- Benign anorectal condition such as <u>hemorrhoids</u> or anal fissure.
- Neoplasia such as Bowen's disease, Paget's disease, or <u>anal cancer</u>.
- Dermatological disease (dermatitis, lichen sclerosis).
- Infection: *Candida*, threadworm (more common with underlying systemic disease such as diabetes).
- Possible dietary components: coffee has been implicated as a common irritant.
- Before labeling the condition as idiopathic, consider fecal leakage
- Treatment involves identifying the cause. An advice sheet may help (see Box 6.2.3); most important single piece of advice is to avoid vigorous wiping or polishing.

Box 6.2.3 Advice sheet for pruritus ani

1. Avoid creams and ointments if possible. Short-term steroids (1% hydrocortisone ointment) can help; long-term use thins the skin
2. Wash the skin with water after each stool; pat dry, do not rub
3. Wear cotton underclothing. Try stockings rather than tights (note: this mainly applies to women)
4. Avoid hot and spicy foods that cause wind and loose stools
5. Wear a cotton pad or folded sheet of toilet paper to absorb any mucus or moisture seeping from the anus
6. Avoid scratching at all costs

Rectal cancer

Accounts for one-third of colorectal cancer. Epidemiology, etiology, pathogenesis, and screening recommendations are common to <u>colon cancer</u>. Aspects meriting specific discussion include:

Imaging. Preoperative staging includes digital rectal examination, <u>CT</u> or <u>MRI</u> scanning of abdomen and pelvis, endoscopic evaluation with biopsy, and endoscopic ultrasound (EUS). EUS is accurate at evaluating tumor stage and perirectal node involvement.

Staging. Treatment decisions should be made with reference to the TNM classification (see <u>tumor staging</u>) rather than Dukes staging. The American joint committee on cancer has designated staging as stage I (T1 or T2, N0, M0), stage II (T3 or T4, N0, M0), stage III (any T, nodal involvement, M0), and stage IV (distant metastases).

Surgery. Resection is indicated for removal of primary tumor and regional lymph nodes for localized disease. Transanal excision can be used for early cancers confined to the rectal submucosa. The technique of excision can affect the rate of local recurrence: total mesorectal excision with colo-anal anastomosis is associated with low incidence of local recurrence (4%) but there is a risk of anastomotic dehiscence of up to 15%. Abdomino-perineal resection with end-sigmoid colostomy is indicated in patients with lower-third rectal cancers who cannot undergo a sphincter-saving procedure because there is less than 2 cm disease-free distal margin.

Adjuvant therapy. Because of the increased risk of local recurrence (up to 50% for stage II or III disease), peri-operative radiation has a greater effect in rectal cancer than, colon cancer. Pre- and post-operative radiation therapy decrease risk of tumor recurrence in stage II or III but increased patient survival has not been shown. Because pre-operative radiotherapy delays surgery and makes pathological staging difficult, post-operative radiotherapy may be preferable. Combined therapy with 5FU and radiation is widely used for stage II and III disease but further studies are needed to determine long-term results.

Palliative and experimental treatments. Endoscopic therapy using Nd:YAG laser can recanalize the rectum in patients with obstructing cancers who are unfit for surgery. Mesh metal stenting and photodynamic therapy have been used in small numbers of patients.

Prognosis. Overall five-year survival rates are 72% for stage I, 54% for stage II, 40% for stage III, and 7% for stage IV.

Rectal prolapse

Intussusception of the rectum through the anal canal can vary from rectal mucosa only, to full thickness of rectum and sigmoid colon. Causal factors include any neurological or muscular disease leading to weakness of the pelvic floor, impaired function of the anal sphincters, chronic constipation with resultant straining, and colorectal tumors.

Clinical features and diagnosis. Presenting symptoms may include pain, incontinence, or a sensation of "something coming down." Demonstration can be helped by having the patient strain in a sitting position or by defecography; proctoscopy is important in excluding internal hemorrhoids and anal tumors. Colonoscopy to exclude a tumor is indicated, as is a complete pelvic floor examination because of the risk of associated bladder or uterine prolapse. Anorectal manometry, with testing of pudendal nerve function, may be necessary because the nerve can be injured by chronic traction by a prolapse.

Treatment. Surgery is central to management. There are many different procedures depending on age and etiology. Both abdominal (anterior repair and rectopexy) and perineal approaches (usually resection of the prolapse, possibly with pelvic floor repair) are possible: there is interest in laparoscopic repair of prolapse but long-term outcome data are needed.

Rectocele

In women, the anterior rectal wall above the perineal body is unsupported and the rectovaginal septum may bulge anteriorly to form a rectocele. This can give symptoms of incomplete evacuation of stool, a lump appearing at the introitus with straining, and sometimes having to support the posterior vaginal wall with finger or thumb, or digitally evacuate stool, to enable defecation. The rectocele is most easily demonstrated on a <u>defecography</u> study. Surgical repair can be done via endorectal, transvaginal, or transperineal approaches and is beneficial in about 75% of selected patients.

Solitary rectal ulcer syndrome

Rare (incidence 1:100,000, equal in men and women, can be seen in all age groups) but also frequently misdiagnosed. The cardinal feature is isolated erythema or ulceration of part of the rectum, usually the anterior wall.

Clinical features
- Passage of blood and mucus PR with straining and a feeling of incomplete evacuation.
- Evidence of rectal prolapse.
- **Sigmoidoscopic appearances** are classically a single ulcer on the anterior rectal wall at 5–10 cm from the anal verge but a polypoid lesion may be seen in 25% or an isolated patch of hyperemia in 20%.
- Histology shows distortion of glands with edema and fibrosis of the lamina propria. The muscularis mucosa is thickened and muscle fibers extend up between the crypts.

Pathogenesis
Prolapse of rectal mucosa (possibly occurring internally and, therefore, not visible or palpable) and paradoxical contraction of the pelvic floor are thought to be important, possibly leading to ischemia of the mucosa. Direct trauma due to rectal digitations has been implicated but many of the lesions are above the reach of a finger.

Investigations
Symptoms, sigmoidoscopic appearances, and histology are the most important. Endo-anal ultrasound may show thickening of the internal sphincter, and <u>defecography studies</u> may show abnormal patterns of defecation. Barium studies and anorectal physiology are not helpful.

Treatment
Topical treatments do not help. Dietary supplementation with fiber is disappointing, especially if there is associated rectal prolapse. <u>Biofeedback</u> may help those with paradoxical puborectalis contraction. Surgical options include rectopexy and resection of the prolapsing muscosa. Rectopexy helps about 50% but increases symptoms in some. Surgery has a minor role and should be reserved for those with intractable symptoms and good evidence of prolapse.

Intestinal infections

Actinomycosis

Subacute or chronic inflammatory disease caused by a variety of fermentative actinomycetes causing multiple abscesses and draining tracts. Requirements for active tissue invasion in humans include a prior break in epithelium (e.g., postsurgery), tissue ischemia, or prior infection by other organisms. Most cases involve the face or neck. Abdominal involvement is rare and is usually associated with perforating/fistulating GI conditions (appendicitis, diverticulitis, surgery, foreign bodies—such as fish bones). May present as slowly growing tumors. Classically, sinus tracts contain sulphur granules. Diagnosis made by culture and microscopy. Antibiotic treatment includes augmentin + metronidazole possibly with an aminoglycoside (e.g., gentamicin).

Adenovirus

- Serotypes 40 and 41 of subgroup F of this large family of DNA viruses are known as enteric adenoviruses because of an association with acute watery diarrhea in infants and children (incidence 4–10% in developed countries, second in importance to rotavirus as viral cause of infectious diarrhea). Nonenteric adenovirus types have been found in AIDS patients with diarrhea.
- Symptoms include watery diarrhea and vomiting, with respiratory symptoms and low grade fever. Diagnosis requires immune electron microscopy. Incubation period 7 days; virus shed in stool for 10–14 days.

No specific treatment: goals of therapy are to prevent dehydration and maintain nutritional intake. Complications can include lactose intolerance and malabsorption. See also Acute diarrhea.

Amoebiasis

Epidemiology + pathology. *Entamoeba histolytica* is pathogenic in man and causes amoebic colitis and liver abscess. Cysts can live outside the hosts or be carried asymptomatically in the stool, while trophozoites, passed by people with invasive disease, cannot survive outside the host. The presence in stool of trophozoites with intracytoplasmic red blood cells is pathognomonic for infection by *E. histolytica*.

Clinical features. Varies from asymptomatic to a life-threatening fulminant colitis. Misdiagnosis as ulcerative colitis and treatment with CORTICOSTEROIDS may predispose to perforation and systemic sepsis.

- Colonoscopic appearance of shallow ulcers, commonest on right side of colon. Ulcers may erode into blood vessels or cause intestinal perforation and peritonitis.
- Systemic dissemination may involve brain, lungs, pericardium, liver.
- Liver abscess in approximately 4% of patients, with male predominance (despite equal sex distribution for colitis). Clinical features of abdominal pain, fever, and constitutional symptoms, but jaundice in < 15%.

- Colonic narrowing may be due to amoeboma (this should be managed medically because surgical resection has high complication rate).

Investigation. Diagnosis involves careful stool microscopy to look for cysts or trophozoites. Usually few leucocytes in the stool. Sigmoidoscopy can help but rectal involvement is less frequent than cecal involvement; colonoscopy is, therefore, investigation of choice. Liver abscess identified on <u>ultrasound</u> or <u>CT scan</u>, and enzyme immunoassay (EIA) serological test has sensitivity of 99% and specificity > 90% in patients with amoebic liver abscess, and is more reliable than stool microscopy.

Management is with <u>METRONIDAZOLE</u>: cure in 90%; treatment usually given for 10 days for intestinal disease. Diloxanide is recommended to eradicate cysts. Therapeutic needle aspiration/catheter drainage of liver abscess only considered if:

- Abscess > 5 cm, therefore, at risk of rupture.
- Left lobe liver abscess, which carries increased risk of intraperitoneal/pericardial rupture.
- Failure to gain a clinical response to therapy within one week.

Bilharzia

See: Schistosomiasis.

Blastocystis

Previously considered a yeast; recently reclassified as a protozoan. Associated with GI symptoms, but may simply be an indicator of exposure to fecal infection with "true pathogens," such as *E. histolytica*. 60% of patients with *Blastocystis hominis* but no other stool pathogens have underlying disease associated with some immunosuppression, and most have symptoms lasting 3–10 days. Reasonable to treat symptomatic patients where no other stool pathogens have been identified and who have moderate to heavy infection (more than 5 *B. hominis* per high-power field on microscopy). Treatment is usually with <u>METRONIDAZOLE</u>; furazolidone and co-trimoxazole are inhibitory *in vitro*.

Botulism

Rare food-borne illness usually due to neurotoxins produced by *Clostridium botulinum*, although there are recent cases due to contaminated drugs injected subcutaneously (also see <u>Clostridial infections in GI tract</u>). Toxin produces gastrointestinal symptoms within 18 to 36 h, followed by constipation with dry mouth, diplopia, blurred vision, dysarthria, dysphagia, and muscle weakness, with a classical symmetrical descending paralysis.

Therapy includes supportive ventilation and antitoxin if disease is diagnosed early.

Campylobacter

Motile Gram-negative rods that have emerged since the 1970s as a major cause of acute dysentery, accounting for up to 20% of positive stool cultures in patients with acute infective bloody diarrhea. Two main species are responsible, *C. jejuni* and *C. coli*: both affect the colon, producing an acute febrile syndrome in children and adults resembling <u>*Shigella*</u> infection.

Epidemiology. Similar to *Salmonella*. Person-to-person transmission is common: poultry and eggs the commonest source of infection.

Pathogenesis may involve epithelial invasion or toxin production.

Clinical features. Children and young adults are most susceptible. Incubation period 1–6 days. There is a prodrome of fatigue and myalgia for 24 hours; then nausea, abdominal cramps, tenderness, and bloody diarrhea are typical. Disease spectrum ranges from asymptomatic carriage to life-threatening colitis with toxic megacolon. Reiter's syndrome and hemolytic–uremic syndrome can all occur. About 30% of patients with Guillain–Barré syndrome have evidence of Campylobacter infection (either stool culture or antibodies to C. jejuni). Antibodies to C. Jejuni share epitopes with brain gangliosides suggesting that cross-reacting antibodies may contribute to the development of nerve damage following campylobacter enteritis.

Diagnosis. Made on stool cultures, which seldom remain positive for more than two weeks. 90% have negative stool cultures after five weeks.

Therapy. Mainstay is replacement of fluids and electrolytes. Recurrent or severe disease, or arguably disease that is diagnosed early, can be treated with antibiotics: erythromycin 250 mg Po qds for five days and ciprofloxacin 500 mg Po bd are effective: ciprofloxacin has the advantage of being effective against entero-toxigenic E.coli, Shigella, and *Salmonella*. Quinolone resistance reaches 50% in some areas but most are sensitive to azithromycin. Also see <u>acute diarrhea</u>.

Candida

Epidemiology. A frequent commensal of healthy people (found in 40–65% normal fecal flora), it is also the commonest fungal human pathogen. The clinical syndrome depends largely on the host immune status, although there are also fungal virulence factors.

Clinical features. Two main patterns:
- Mucocutaneous candidiasis rarely causes death, although in patients with refractory HIV infection it can become resistant to antifungal therapy and lead to severe oropharyngeal/esophageal involvement.
- Disseminated candidiaisis has a high mortality but is comparatively rare.

In the GI tract the commonest lesions associated with *Candida* are single or multiple ulcerations: white plaque and thickened mucosal folds can be seen at endoscopy. Apart from oropharynx, the esophagus is the most commonly affected site within the GI tract, but gastric and small-intestinal infection can also occur. The commonest symptom associated with intestinal candidiasis is diarrhea; since the organism is so often present, a small-bowel biopsy with histologic evidence of invasion is necessary for diagnosis.

Differential diagnosis includes other diseases affecting the GI tract in immunocompromised hosts: other mycoses, TB, ischemic bowel, typhlitis, *Mycobacterium avium*.

Treatment. Fluconazole and nystatin commonly used for mucocutaneous disease including oropharyngeal candidiasis. For disseminated disease, amphotericin B is recommended with fluconazole as second-line therapy. See ANTIFUNGALS.

> **Box 7.1 Risk factors for *Candida***
>
> - HIV (see HIV and the gut)
> - Immunosuppression
> - Parenteral feeding
> - Urinary catheters
> - Broad spectrum antibiotics
> - CORTICOSTEROIDS
> - Burns, trauma
> - Recent surgery
> - Hemodialysis

Cestodes

See: tapeworms.

Cholera

Kills 100,000 per year in Asia, Africa, and Latin America. Children aged two to nine and women of child-bearing age are most at risk; mortality in children is 3–5% but in adults effective fluid replacement has reduced mortality to less than 1%.

Pathogenesis. There are about 10 species of *Vibrio* pathogenic to humans: *V. cholerae* and *V. parahaemolyticus* are the most important. Serotyping of *V. Cholerae* is according to O antigen of cell surface lipopolysaccharide: cholera is caused by group O1. Contaminated water is the main route of transmission: person-to-person transmission is rare.

Diagnosis is usually made presumptively or by laboratory identification of toxigenic vibrios.

Clinical features. Ingested cholera produces a toxin that switches on adenyl cyclase: the resulting increase in cAMP stimulates chloride secretion and reduces sodium reabsorption, producing large volume watery diarrhea. The risks are those of metabolic acidosis, hyponatremia, hypokalemia, hypoglycemia, and fits. Fever and abdominal pain are rare.

Outcome. Hypoglycemia and altered conscious level are risk factors for death. Full recovery without antibiotics can be expected in one to six days with adequate fluid replacement.

Therapy. Oral rehydration (WHO) solution is effective in 95% cases.

Vaccination. There is an oral vaccine available for travelers to endemic or epidemic areas. The injectable vaccine uses a killed whole-cell vaccine, gives only 50% protection for three to six months, and does not prevent the transmission of disease. CDC does not recommend cholera vaccines for most travelers, nor is the vaccine available in the United States.

Clonorchis infection

Chinese liver fluke (*Clonorchis sinensis*) infects 30 million people worldwide, mainly in SE Asia. Life cycle involves passage of eggs in human feces, ingestion by snail, subsequent ingestion of cercariae by fish, and consumption of fish and encysted larvae by man. 10–25 mm adult worms induce inflammatory response in biliary tree where they may persist for 30 years, leading to biliary strictures and obstruction, recurrent cholangitis, choledocholithiasis, secondary biliary cirrhosis, and cholangiocarcinoma. Diagnosis suspected in patient from high risk area with unexplained biliary stricturing/cholangitis, and confirmed on isolation of eggs in stool or duodenal aspirate. Treatment with praziquantel or albendazole, but biliary lesions may persist.

Clostridial infections of the GI tract

For *C. botulinum* see botulism.

Pseudomembranous colitis (PMC): synonymous with
***Clostridium difficile* colitis**

- *C. difficile* was discovered in 1935 but only associated with antibiotic-associated diarrhea in 1978. It is a Gram-positive obligate anaerobe that can form spores, which facilitates antibiotic resistance. Can be found in the stools of healthy newborns, but seldom part of the normal commensal flora. Colonization normally follows antibiotic ingestion, cancer chemotherapy, or infection by other pathogens (*Salmonella, Shigella*).
- GI damage depends on two exotoxins, A and B. They are cytotoxic, destroying actin filaments making up the cell skeleton. Serum antibodies to toxins are common in the general population, although it is not clear if they confer protective immunity.

- Asymptomatic carriage is rare in healthy adults but not in hospital patients (7% positive on admission to hospital, rising during stay, but only 30% of these develop diarrhea).

Risk factors

- Antibiotics. First seen with clindamycin, but amoxycillin and the cephalosporins are now most frequently implicated.
- Other risk factors are extremes of age, recent GI surgery, malignancy, and prolonged hospital stay.

Clinical features

- Diarrhea and abdominal cramps usually occur within the first week but can be delayed up to six weeks.
- Nausea, fever, and dehydration can accompany severe colitis.
- Abdominal examination may reveal distension and tenderness.
- Sigmoidoscopy (not simple proctoscopy; the rectum is spared of pseudomembranes in 30%) reveals characteristic yellow-white raised plaques, 2–5 mm diameter. Biopsy reveals a characteristic "summit lesion," an outpouring of pus from a microulceration of the surface epithelium.
- Fulminant *C. difficile* colitis can present acutely in the previously well or develop during the course of milder infection. Look for fever, tachycardia, tenderness, guarding, and reduced bowel sounds. Plain radiograph may show <u>toxic megacolon</u>; the bowel wall may appear very thick on CT scanning.
- *C. difficile* infection can complicate <u>ulcerative colitis</u>: a 5–25% incidence of toxin-positive stools has been reported, not always after antibiotic exposure. Always get a stool for *C. difficile* toxin in patients with relapses of IBD.

Diagnosis

- Stool culture is sensitive but needs anaerobic culture facilities, takes two to five days, and reveals toxigenic and nontoxigenic strains.
- Same-day enzyme immunoassays are available for toxins A and B.

Management

- Oral <u>METRONIDAZOLE</u> 400 mg tds is recommended as first-line therapy, but some clinicians feel this is less effective than vancomycin 125 mg qds, and this author recommends oral vancomycin as first-line treatment for severe or fulminant PMC.
- Relapse occurs in 20% of successfully treated patients. Options include withholding further antibiotics to allow normal flora to re-establish, giving probiotics (*Saccharomyces boulardi* reduces *C. difficile* recurrence rate) or a 14 day course of vancomycin followed by a course of anion-binding resin such as cholestyramine.
- There is no proven benefit in treating asymptomatic carriers.

Necrotizing enterocolitis

A severe and fulminating colitis classically occurring in neonates (although the association here with *Clostridium* is not proven) but in adults associated with gas gangrene of the bowel wall.

Clostridium perfringens
- A food-borne pathogen usually producing diarrhea and vomiting due to enterotoxin produced by *C. perfringens* type A. 90% of cases caused by meat or poultry cooked adequately but then left to stand for four to twenty-four hours and then served cold or poorly rewarmed. Symptoms include cramps and diarrhea and are usually short-lived (less than 24 h): vomiting and fever are unusual. Fatalities are very rare.
- In sporadic outbreaks, especially in Papua New Guinea, the disease is called pig bel, resulting from feasting on poorly cooked pork contaminated with *C. perfringens* type C. A vaccine can prevent disease. Treatment includes high-dose benzylpenicillin.

Coccidia

Intracellular protozoan pathogens. Genera *Cryptosporidium, Cyclospora, Isospora* can cause acute self-limiting diarrheal illness in immunocompetent hosts and severe chronic diarrhea in the immunosuppressed. They all replicate in the enterocyte and can also shed cysts or spores that are excreted in the stool.

Cryptosporidium parvum
- Responsible for several large water-borne outbreaks of diarrhea disease. In developed countries, 15– 30% of people are seropositive (higher in developing countries). Common cause of diarrhea in AIDS and other immunosuppressed states.
- Mean incubation period 9 days; mean duration of disease 12 days. Watery but not bloody diarrhea, abdominal cramps, mucus PR. Extraintestinal manifestations rare in the immunocompetent, but <u>cholecystitis</u> in 10% AIDS patients, and has been implicated as cause of HIV cholangiopathy (see <u>HIV and the liver</u>). Diagnosed by finding oocytes in stool samples.
- ***Treatment.*** Antibiotics are not effective. Supportive treatment with fluid replacement is the main therapy. May resolve with immune reconstitution associated with HAART for HIV.

Cyclospora cayetanensis
- Discovered in the 1990s, Cyclospora appears a relatively common cause of diarrhea in patients with AIDS in developing countries but is rare in developed countries, although sporadic outbreaks have been reported. The disease is self-limiting in immunocompetent hosts. Diagnosis is by stool microscopy, which reveals 8–10 μm spheres. Treatment with co-trimoxazole is effective.

Isospora belli
- Responsible for 15% cases of diarrhea in AIDS patients in developing countries. Rare in immunocompetent people. Can cause eosinophilia. Sensitive to co-trimoxazole.

Box 7.2 Causes of cobalamin (vitamin B12) deficiency

- Inadequate dietary intake
  - Vegans
  - Alcoholics
- Inadequate release of food-bound cobalamin
  - Achlorhydria
  - PROTON PUMP INHIBITORS
- Loss of active intrinsic factor (IF)
  - Pernicious anemia
  - Gastrectomy
  - Congenital lack/abnormality of IF
- Proximal small-bowel disease and pancreatic disease
  - Pancreatic insufficiency
  - Gastrinoma
  - Tropical sprue
  - Small-bowel bacterial overgrowth
  - Fish tapeworm diphyllobothrium latum (rare)
- Ileal disorders
  - Mainly loss of absorptive mucosa through surgery or mucosal disease
  - Crohn's disease
  - TB (see TB and the GI tract)
  - Lymphoma
  - Dysfunctionnal uptake and use of cobalamin by cells; R binder deficiency, transcobalamin II deficiency, some drugs (colchicine)
- Miscellaneous (rarely lead to clinical anemia)
  - Pregnancy
  - Thyrotoxicosis
  - Erythroid hyperplasia
- Drugs
  - PAS
  - Colchicine
  - Neomycin
  - Metformin

Cryptosporidium

See: Coccidia.

Cytomegalovirus (CMV)

50–80% people are seropositive for CMV. Primary infection in immuno-competent hosts causes few or no symptoms.

Immunosuppression can lead to CMV retinitis, pneumonitis, colitis, and esophagitis. CMV is third commonest pathogen in AIDS after pneumocystis and candida (see HIV and the gut).

CMV colitis

Occurs in 2–15% of patients with solid organ transplants (average time is five to seven months after transplant) and 3–5% patients with HIV/AIDS. It is rare in immunocompetent hosts but can complicate ulcerative colitis, especially in patients receiving steroids. Patients with steroid-dependent colitis who present with refractory disease should be assessed for CMV infection, as this is increasingly being recognized as prevalent.

Diagnosis. Sigmoidoscopy or colonoscopy allows mucosal visualization and biopsy. Histology may reveal inclusion bodies and immunohistochemistry may show CMV antigen.

CMV esophagitis

Unknown in healthy hosts, Found in 10–25% patients with AIDS undergoing upper GI endoscopy. Symptoms include odynophagia, nausea, vomiting, fever, diarrhea, weight loss, chest pain. Diagnosis usually involves upper GI endoscopy and biopsy: appearances are classically of large shallow ulcers.

Therapy. Intravenous GANCICLOVIR for three weeks.

Dysentery

A clinical term: bloody mucoid diarrhea, tenesmus, fever, cramps, and polymorphs in the feces. It implies an invasive pathogen affecting the large bowel, commonly *Shigella*, enteroinvasive or enterohemorrhagic *E. coli*, or amoebiasis (note: amoebiasis does not give leucocytes in the stool). See Acute diarrhea.

Escherichia coli

A major component of the normal intestinal microflora. There are six types of pathogens.
- **Enteropathogenic *E. coli* (EPEC)**. Produces watery diarrhea in children and neonates. Virulence is via localized adherence to enterocytes. Infection is usually self-limiting.

- **Enterotoxigenic *E. coli* (ETEC)**. Affects children in developing countries and travelers. Bacteria bind to enterocytes, produce heat labile or heat stable toxin leading to watery diarrhea that can be mild or severe. Antibiotics usually not needed, although effective therapy given early (quinolone, septrin, tetracycline) can shorten duration of diarrhea.
- **Enteroinvasive *E. coli* (EIEC)**. Rare cause of dysentery. Resembles *Shigella*.
- **Enterohemorrhagic *E. coli* (EHEC):** An important invasive pathogen responsible for 15–35% of hemorrhagic colitis: *E. coli* 0157 associated with <u>hemolytic–uremic syndrome</u> (especially in children) and thrombotic thrombocytopenic purpura. Commonest vehicle is hamburger meat. Incubation period 1–14 d, can produce marked colitis. AXR can show submucosal edema (thumbprinting). Laboratory studies can reveal *E. coli* 0157 serotypes or characteristic shigalike toxins (Stx I and II). **Antibiotics do not help and may increase risk of HUS**.
- **Entero-aggregatory *E. coli* (EAggEC)**. Pathogenicity uncertain but may be associated with diarrhea in HIV-positive people who seem to respond to ciprofloxacin.
- **Diffusely adhering *E. coli* (DAEC)**. Pathogenicity uncertain, virulence factors unknown.

Flukes (flatworms, trematodes)

The three common **intestinal flukes** are *Fasciolopsis*, *Heterophyes*, and *Echinostoma*. They tend to be geographically restricted (Asia, Indonesia). People get infected by eating fish or freshwater plants infected with metacercariae. *Fasciolopsis* can be up to 7.5 cm long; *Heterophyes* and *Echinostoma* are only a few mm long. Symptoms are often minimal but may include abdominal cramps, and mild diarrhea. Diagnosis in all cases involves finding eggs in the stool. Treatment with praziquantel, 25 mg/kg every 8 hrs for 1 day.

   Liver flukes include <u>*Clonorchis*</u>, *Opisthorcis*, *Fasciola*.
- *Clonorchis* and *Opisthorcis* are endemic to Southeast Asia (one species found in Russia/Ukraine). Infection occurs by eating metacercariae in undercooked fish. The worms grow into adults in the biliary tree and can cause <u>cholangitis</u>, <u>biliary strictures</u>, and <u>liver abscesses</u>. The most important complication is <u>cholangiocarcinoma</u>.
- *Fasciola* is similar to <u>*Clonorchis*</u> and *Opisthorchis* but has a worldwide distribution, is larger (up to 7 cm long), and is frequently asymptomatic. They migrate from the intestine into the liver across the peritoneal cavity and can cause abdominal pain and hepatomegaly in this phase. They can cause intermittent biliary obstruction and cholangitis. They release few eggs, so stool analysis is insensitive: diagnosis is by an ELISA test on serum. They are resistant to praziquantel, and triclabendazole is the drug of choice.

Blood flukes include <u>schistosomiasis</u>.

Giardiasis

Giardia lamblia is a protozoan with flagella and a common cause of malabsorptive diarrhea. Worldwide, infects children more than adults; infection can be waterborne, food borne, or person–person.

There is a cyst form and a motile trophozoite. Cysts can survive for weeks in cold water. If they are swallowed the cyst wall is dissolved by stomach acid and the trophozoites are released and adhere to small bowel enterocytes.

Clinical signs can include diarrhea, fatigue cramps, bloating, weight loss, and fever. The signs vary and may depend on host immune response; common variable immunodeficiency is associated with severe disease, but no increase in severity has been reported in AIDS.

Diagnosis. Stool exam is only 50% sensitive. Duodenal biopsy is better (ca. 80%) but testing stool by ELISA or direct fluorescence antibody microscopy is probably first choice.

Treatment. Tinidazole 2 g single dose or METRONIDAZOLE 250 mg tds for 5 d. In pregnancy, use paromomycin (25–35 mg/kg/day in 3 divided doses for 7 d). Treatment may fail and need higher doses of metronidazole but confirm persistent infection before retreating, look for immune deficiency (check immunoglobulins for common variable immune deficiency), and remember the high incidence of lactose intolerance after *Giardia* infection.

Helminth infection

Parasitic worms (helminths) are classified into roundworms (nematodes) tapeworms (cestodes), and flukes or flatworms (trematodes). Travel, migration, and exotic cuisine allow helminths to appear in any locale. They are complex and often well adapted to their host—so much so that light infection may cause no symptoms, only heavy infestation resulting in disease. They almost never cause diarrhea but are a potent cause of eosinophilia or eosinophilic gastroenteritis. They often induce a Th2 response (Il-4 mediated): this may limit multiplication but also impairs excessive Th1 responses. Diseases mediated by Th1 such as Crohn's disease and multiple sclerosis are rare where helminths are common; it may be that parasitic infection offers some protection against immune mediated disease.

Herpes simplex

A DNA virus, causing painful vesicles with erythematous bases in squamous epithelium of skin, mouth, esophagus. Resolution of infection is followed by latency in roots and ganglia supplying affected regions.

90% of cases of primary herpetic gingivostomatitis occur in people before puberty. Recurrent orolabial herpes simplex is common and precipitated by illness, sunlight, or stress. Topical <u>ACICLOVIR</u> speeds healing and reduces severity. Immunosuppression predisposes to infection but the symptoms may be milder (e.g., just nausea and vomiting, while immunocompetent people may have acutely painful swallowing). Also see <u>HIV and the gut</u>.

Diagnosis usually made at endoscopy. 1–3 mm vesicles appear in mid-to distal esophagus: the centers slough to form "volcano" lesions. Biopsies for diagnosis should include epithelium. Virus can be detected by culture or immunostaining within 24 hours. Treatment is with <u>ACICLOVIR</u>, although resistant strains are beginning to emerge. Complications of untreated disease include mucosal necrosis, esophageal perforation, hemorrhage, strictures, HSV pneumonia, <u>tracheo-esophageal fistulae</u>. Perianal infection can occur, especially in AIDS patients, usually with HSV type 2. This causes painful ulcers, tenesmus, and occasional bleeding. Treatment is with <u>ACICLOVIR</u> and topical anesthetics: avoid steroid ointments.

HSV can also infect the colon and is a cause of bloody diarrhea in immunocompromised patients; sigmoidoscopy shows characteristic vesicles.

Herpes zoster

Zoster can cause severe <u>esophagitis</u> in immunocompromised people (see <u>HIV and the gut</u>), although esophageal involvement is relatively mild compared with that seen in encephalitis, pneumonitis, and hepatitis). Zoster can be distinguished from simplex by culture or immunostaining but much more practically by the presence of skin lesions (rare with HSV). Gastric involvement is rare. T7 through L1 nerve involvement can cause abdominal pain before lesions appear. Sacral nerve root involvement can give constipation and pain with defecation.

Treatment with <u>ACICLOVIR</u>, and foscarnet as second-line treatment.

Hookworms

See: <u>round worms</u>.

Leptospirosis

Background

- Weil's disease refers to the 10% of infections due to spirochaete *Leptospira* that result in clinical liver disease. Endemic human infection in the tropics (30% seropositivity for exposure), but in West *L. icterohemorrhagiae* mainly carried by rats.
- Direct contact with infection in soil, water, or urine (organisms entering through skin abrasions/cuts) explains epidemiological link with sewage workers, farmhands.

Clinical features

- Incubation period of 7–14 days, followed by initial septicemic phase, with influenzalike illness, including headache, myalgia, leg pain, dyspnea. Lasts 4–7 days, and improvement associated with clearance of circulating leptospira. Second immune-mediated phase occurs after further two days, characterized by fever, meningeal irritation, iritis, skin lesions (bleeding, petechiae, purpura, ecchymosis), renal failure (acute tubular necrosis), jaundice, and hepatomegaly.
- Death (5–10%) due to renal/cardiorespiratory disease, and rarely liver failure.

Investigations

Diagnosis never made unless thought about. Careful history of possible exposure essential (e.g., caving). See <u>Recent-onset jaundice</u>.
- cBC: ↑Hb, ↓WCC, ↓platelets.
- LFTs: ↑Bili, ↑AST, ALP normal. Deranged clotting in severe disease.
- Creatine kinase elevated in > 50% with liver disease.
- Blood/CSF culture: high yield in first phase.
- Urine (dark field) microscopy positive in second phase (and for several weeks).
- ELISA for *Leptospira* IgM highly sensitive and specific, and is most widely used diagnostic test.

Management

- Effective supportive care essential (may need renal dialysis).
- Doxycycline (100 mg bd PO) highly effective if given early, or IV penicillin.

Listeria monocytogenes

Gram-positive bacteria. Can cause outbreaks of disease. Sources include raw or unpasteurized milk or cheese and prepackaged meats. Immunocompetent people can develop gastroenteritis with fever, headache, pain, nausea, and diarrhea. This is usually not accompanied by bacteremia, whereas listeriosis is a systemic disease that can attack immunocompromised patients, neonates, and pregnant women—it is often associated with bacteremia that can seed heart valves, meninges, or other organs. Treatment varies, depending on clinical syndrome. Usually ampicillin in combination with gentamicin.

Microsporidia

Obligate intracellular protozoan parasites that can cause disease in the immunocompromised patient. Commonest is *Enterocytozoon bieneusi* which infects small intestine and causes severe diarrhea. Diagnosis is best made by PCR from feces or biopsies. Spores can be detected in stool studies with special staining, so alert the laboratory.

Nematodes

See: roundworm (nematode) infection.

Parasitic infection

Parasites of the GI tract are classified into worms or helminths (see roundworms, tapeworms, and flukes or flatworms) and protozoal infections (see amoebiasis, giardiasis, coccidia and trypanosomiasis).

Pseudomonas

- Can affect every portion of the GI tract. Most commonly affects very young children and adults with hematological malignancies and chemotherapy-induced neutropenia. Colonization of the GI tract is an important portal of entry for pseudomonal bacteremia in patients who are neutropenic. Spectrum of disease can range from very mild symptoms to severe necrotizing enterocolitis with significant morbidity and mortality.
- Epidemics of pseudomonal diarrhea can occur in nurseries. Young infants may present with irritability, vomiting, diarrhea, and dehydration.
- The infection can cause enteritis, with patients presenting with prostration, headache, fever, and diarrhea (Shanghai fever).
- *Pseudomonas* typhlitis typically presents in patients with neutropenia resulting from acute leukemia, with a sudden onset of fever, abdominal distension, and worsening abdominal pain.

Protozoa

See: amoebiasis, giardiasis, coccidia, microsporidia, and trypanosomiasis.

Rotavirus

See: Emergencies: Acute diarrhea.

Roundworm (nematode) infection

Think of four groups:

Infection confined to human GI tract

Organisms include *Tricuris* (whipworm), *Enterobius* (pinworm), *Capillaria* (important in Phillipines and Far East), and *Tricostrongylus* (human infection most prevalent in Middle East and Asia). Distribution is worldwide but commonest in areas of poor sanitation. Humans ingest the eggs; the larvae penetrate the intestinal mucosa and mature into adults that are confined to the gut. Heavy tricuris infestation can cause diarrhea and rectal prolapse. Eosinophilia is common. Pinworm infestation is common in developed countries. Eggs are laid on the peri-anal skin, which causes intense pruritus.

Diagnosis is by finding eggs in the stool or worms attached to the mucosa: for pinworms, tape applied to the peri-anal area and then examined under the micsroscope may reveal eggs. Treatment is with albendazole or mebendazole. **Note.** *Tricuris* induces a strong Th2 response and minimizes Th1 response. This has led to experimental administration of the pig whipworm to patients with inflammatory bowel disease; initial results are promising.

Infection begins in the GI tract; larvae invade and reach the lungs, migrate to pharynx, are swallowed, and mature in the gut

Adult *Ascaris* can be 10–25 cm long. Infection is common (1.2 billion worldwide; only cold dry climates are spared). Clinical features can result from migration of larvae through the lung (bronchospasm, bronchiolar inflammation, urticaria, or other manifestations of hypersensitivity) or in heavy infections, by blocking the gut or biliary tree. Diagnosis is by finding eggs in stool. Treatment is with albendazole or mebendazole.

Larvae invade the skin, migrate to the lungs, then are swallowed and mature in the gut

Hookworms (*Ankylostoma, Necator*) and <u>Stronglyoides</u>.

Hookworms secrete an anticoagulant and change their location often: they are a significant cause of iron deficiency anemia. Spread is facilitated by walking barefoot and using human feces as manure. Clinical features include a rash at the site of penetration and sometimes pulmonary hypersensitivity reactions. Iron deficiency anemia and low albumin can occur. Eosinophilia is common. Diagnosis is by finding eggs in stool and treatment is with albendazole or mebendazole.

See separate entry for <u>Strongyloides</u>.

Intestinal nematodes of animals that can infect humans

Trichinella, cutaneous larva migrans caused by *Ancylostoma*, visceral larva migrans caused by *Toxocara*, and anisakiasis.

Trichinosis caused by *Trichinella* results from eating poorly cooked infected meat. Larvae burrow into the gut wall and migrate to skeletal muscle; extraocular muscles are often affected. Diagnosis is serological or rarely by muscle biopsy: Creatine kinase (CK) is raised in 50%. Treat with albendazole or mebendazole.

Cutaneous larva migrans is a serpiginous dermatitis that is itchy and can be papulovesicular. Common in tropical and subtropical Africa, Caribbean, and Latin America. Hookworms of dogs and cats burrow through the skin. Treatment is with oral ivermectin or albendazole.

Visceral larva migrans results from ingestion of eggs of *Toxocara* living in dogs or cats. Larvae penetrate the intestine but cannot complete their life cycle in humans and wander through various organs. Clinical course is very variable; the classical triad is eosinophilia, hepatomegaly, and hypergammaglobulinemia. There is an ELISA used to detect anti-*Toxocara* antibodies. Treatment is diethylcarbamazine or albendazole.

Anisakiasis is caused by nematode pathogens of fish and occurs if contaminated fish or squid are eaten raw or undercooked. Mucosal invasion of the stomach can cause severe gastritis or profuse hemorrhage within 12–24 h of ingestion.

Salmonella

A group of Gram-negative bacilli, causing food-borne infection transmitted by "flies, fingers, food, feces, and fomites." Recent pandemics in Western countries are especially due to infection of commercial eggs and poultry.

Salmonella penetrate the ileum and the colon, with hematogenous spread to other organs. There are five clinical syndromes of disease (Box 7.3).

Salmonella gastroenteritis. Incubation period usually 6–48 hours. Symptoms include nausea and vomiting, cramps, and diarrhea. Diarrhea usually lasts three to four days and can vary from a few loose stools to dysentery. Fever in 50%. Pain is central or right lower quadrant. 2–6 per 1,000 affected become chronic carriers.

Risk increased by hemolytic anemia, leukemias, lymphoma, cancer, steroids, chemotherapy, gastric surgery or acid suppression, schistosomiasis.

Treatment. Most patients with uncomplicated salmonella should not have antibiotics (high rate of associated relapse and emergence of resistant strains). Indications for treatment include associated malignancy or immunosuppression, cardiovascular abnormalities, and presence of orthopedic prostheses. Amoxicillin, co-trimoxazole, or a quinolone, such as CIPROFLOXACIN, are usual antibiotics, but there is some evidence of increasing drug resistance.

Box 7.3 Clinical syndromes of *Salmonella* infection

- **Gastroenteritis**—seen in 75% of infections
- **Bacteremia**—with or without gastroenteritis, associated with endocarditis and arteritis—10% of cases
- **Typhoid or enteric fever**—about 10% cases
- **Localized infection** (bones, joints, meninges)—5%
- **Carrier state** in asymptomatic people

Sarcoidosis

Inflammatory multisystem disease of uncertain origin. Within the GI system it particularly affects the liver, and sarcoid is one of important causes of <u>hepatic granulomas</u>.

Clinical features
- Often asymptomatic, with incidental liver function test abnormalities in patients with symptomatic lung, skin, or eye disease.
- Hepatomegaly, fever, right upper quadrant discomfort, in association with <u>hepatic granulomas</u> may occur.
- Rare presentations include severe intrahepatic cholestasis; <u>portal hypertension</u> due to cirrhosis/granulomas; and extrahepatic biliary obstruction due to portal lymph nodes, bile duct inflammation, and pancreatic sarcoid with distal <u>biliary stricture</u>.

Investigation
- Liver function tests often show. ↑ALP/GGT and mild ↑AST/ALT. When previous diagnosis of sarcoid not made, elevated serum angiotensin converting enzyme (SACE) and lung changes (e.g., bilateral hilar lymphadenopathy) may aid diagnosis.
- CT or U/S findings nonspecific, but granulomas may occasionally coalesce to form 0.5–3 cm nodules.
- <u>Liver biopsy</u> shows noncaseating granulomas in > 80%. Cirrhosis on biopsy has been reported in 6%.

Management
- <u>URSODEOXYCHOLIC ACID</u> may improve symptoms in intrahepatic cholestasis.
- Oral <u>CORTICOSTEROID</u> therapy induces clinical and biochemical improvement in patients with granulomatous hepatitis on biopsy. Duration of use uncertain, as relapse rate high if only short-term treatment given.
- Immunosuppression less effective in established cirrhosis and portal hypertension, and <u>liver transplantation</u> may rarely need considering.

Schistosomiasis

Epidemiology + pathogenesis
- Schistosomes are blood flukes, with which 200 million people are chronically infected. Endemic areas include Africa, S. America, Far East, and S.E. Asia.
- Hepatosplenic schistosomiasis caused by *S. mansoni*, *S. japonicum* and *S. mekongi* (not *S. hematobium*, which causes urinary schistosomiasis).
- In life cycle, eggs excreted into water in feces, from where free-swimming miracidia infect freshwater snail, and develop into cercariae. These infect man through intact skin, enter the circulation, and mature into 1–2 cm adult worms within the portal venous system.

Proportion of eggs produced may be retained within tissues, inducing a granulomatous inflammatory response that leads to <u>portal hypertension</u> ("presinusoidal") but not cirrhosis.

Clinical features

- Acute schistosomiasis (Katayama fever) develops 3–6 weeks after primary infection, and coincides with egg laying. Fever, malaise, abdominal pain, and diarrhea, which may last for several weeks. Associated hepatosplenomegaly may be found.
- Only small proportion of chronically infected people suffer significant clinical problems. Features are primarily due to <u>portal hypertension</u>, with varices, splenomegaly, and ascites. Stigmata of chronic liver disease and liver failure are rare, and as a result bleeding from gastro-esophageal varices carries better outcome than in those with cirrhosis. Recurrent abdominal pain, bloody diarrhea, and inflammatory colonic polyposis may also occur in chronic infection.

Investigation

- Peripheral eosinophilia characteristic of acute infection.
- Raised cholestatic liver tests (ALP, GGT) often seen.
- Stool analysis for ova often negative in acute infection. Yield for identifying ova improved by repeat stool samples and from biopsies at sigmoidoscopy.
- Schistosomal ELISA confirms exposure (and if negative reliably excludes infection), but not useful in distinguishing past from ongoing infection.
- <u>Liver biopsy</u> may show characteristic periportal fibrosis.
- Portal venous fibrosis may be seen on <u>CT scanning</u>.

Management

- Antischistosomal treatment (e.g., praziquantel 40 mg/kg/bid PO for one day) clears infection in 60–95% of cases, with reduction in egg burden in the others. It may prevent progression of chronic infection, but does not reverse portal hypertension.
- <u>Portal hypertension</u> may require standard management of its complications (e.g., primary/secondary prophylaxis).

Shigella

An important cause of bacterial dysentery and <u>food poisoning</u>. The organism attacks the colon and terminal ileum; invasion beyond the intestinal mucosa and bacteremia are rare. Four subgroups: *S. dysenteriae,* (most severe) *S. flexneri, S. boydii, S. sonnei* (mildest).

Clinical features include lower abdominal pain, rectal discomfort, and diarrhea (may be bloody). Fever present in 40%. Complications include intestinal perforation and arthritis (usually HLA-B27-associated—see <u>Reiter's syndrome</u>). Infection tends to be milder in children (one to three days) than in adults (approximately seven days).

Diagnosis. Send stool for culture and sensitivity. Sigmoidoscopy shows a colitis and rectal biopsy may help in suggesting an infective cause rather than ulcerative colitis.

Treatment. Avoid opiate analgesics. Antibiotics are often not needed but are reasonable treatment if the diarrhea is persisting by the time of positive stool cultures. Ampicillin and co-trimoxazole are most used, but resistance has increased recently. Quinolone (e.g., <u>CIPROFLOXACIN</u>) resistance is < 1%.

Strongyloides

Strongyloides stercoralis is one of the most important intestinal nematode infections. Endemic in tropical areas, but may persist for decades following exposure, due to autoinfection. Adult worms (3 mm long) usually reside in duodenum/jejunum. Eggs may hatch in stool prior to defecation, and larvae may then penetrate bowel wall, circulate to lung, and mature into more adults. See <u>roundworms</u>.

Clinical features
- Local rash (cutaneous larva migrans) due to skin penetration by larvae.
- Chronic intestinal infection may be asymptomatic, or associated with abdominal discomfort, bloating, bulky loose stools linked to small bowel infection (i.e., similar to <u>giardiasis</u>).
- Heavy infestation (e.g., associated with immunosuppression) may cause asthma, pulmonary hemorrhage, profuse diarrhea, bowel- wall thickening, and fatal Gram-negative sepsis.

Investigations
- CBC: eosinophilia in 50%.
- Stool microscopy may show larvae or eggs (but only 25% sensitivity, and always negative in early infection).
- Serological test using ELISA available.
- Endoscopy: subtotal villous atrophy, lymphocytic infiltrate, eggs, and larvae in submucosa may be seen on low duodenal histology.

Management
Ivermectin 150 µg/kg PO × 1 dose, or thiabendazole 50 mg/kg/day for two days (extended to 10 days if hyperinfection) are effective.

Tapeworms (cestodes)

Fish tapeworm. *Diphyllobothrium latum* is acquired by people eating raw or undercooked fresh water fish. Disease is endemic in northern Europe, Russia, and Alaska. Worm is not invasive and causes no direct symptoms. It absorbs nutrients through its surface including cobalamin and can cause vitamin B12 deficiency. Diagnosis made by finding eggs in stool. Treatment with praziquantel (single dose, 10 mg/kg) or albendazole 400 mg/day for three days.

Beef and pork tapeworms. Colonization occurs by eating raw or undercooked meat infested with cysticerci of *Taenia saginata* or *T. solium*. 50 million people are affected in areas where livestock are exposed to untreated human waste and humans eat raw or undercooked meat. Most people are asymptomatic. Most feared complication is cysticercosis, which occurs when people consume *T. solium* eggs. These release oncospheres that penetrate the intestinal wall and produce inflammation in the brain, spinal cord, eye, and heart. Diagnosis is by finding eggs or proglottids in stool. Treatment is with praziquantel (single dose, 10 mg/kg) or albendazole 400 mg/d for three days.

Other tapeworms. The commonest tapeworm affecting humans is the dwarf tapeworm or *Hymenolepis nana*, which can be transmitted from person to person without an intermediate host.

Traveler's diarrhea

See: Acute diarrhea

Trematodes

See: flukes (flatworms, trematodes).

Trypanosomiasis

Trypanosoma cruzi is endemic in central Brazil, Venezuela, and Argentina, and spread among humans by the reduviid bugs of the *Triatominae* group. The name reduviid comes from the Latin reduvia, meaning hangnail, and relates to the curved, powerful beaks adapted to suck blood from mammals. The bugs defecate when biting and the parasite is introduced when the bite is scratched. Chronic disease results from widespread destruction of autonomic ganglion cells in the heart, gut, respiratory tract, and urinary tract. It is thought that autoimmune damage occurs to cardiac or nerve epitopes cross-reacting with *T. cruzi* antigens. Resulting cardiac arrhythmias can be fatal. GI involvement can produce megaduodenum or <u>megacolon</u> as well as megaesophagus, which helps to distinguish the disease from idiopathic <u>achalasia.</u> Small bowel dilatation and lack of peristalsis can also be found.

Diagnosis can be made by demonstration of trypanosome forms on blood smears but is more usually made by a serological complement fixation test.

Treatment of the infection uses the drugs nifurtimox and benznidazole; treatment of the achalasia syndrome in Chagas's disease is similar to that of idiopathic <u>achalasia.</u>

Tuberculosis and the GI tract

Historically related to the severity of pulmonary involvement, especially pulmonary cavitation and positive sputum smears (increased risk of swallowed organisms). In modern series, chest X-ray is unremarkable in most patients seen with intestinal TB.

Location and pathology. Can affect any part of the GI tract, including gut lumen, liver (see <u>hepatic granulomas</u>), and pancreas (mass may mimic pancreatitis or tumor). Ileocecal area and jejunum are the commonest sites affected. Incompetence of the ileocecal valve (due to disease on either side), said to distinguish TB from <u>Crohn's disease</u>. Key pathological features are thickening of the bowel wall, transmural granulomas (caseation is often seen in regional lymph nodes but not always in mucosal granulomas), mesenteric lymphadenopathy, serosal tubercles easily visible on laparotomy or laparoscopy but not on <u>CT scanning</u>.

Clinical features. Abdominal pain in 90%. Weight loss, fever, altered bowel habit can occur. Two-thirds have a mass in the right iliac fossa. Intestinal obstruction is commoner than perforation.

Diagnosis. Often delayed and difficult. Acid-fast bacilli are seen in a minority of cases. The organism can be cultured from infected tissues but takes 6–12 weeks; PCR can help. A positive tuberculin skin test does not always mean active disease, and if the immune response is impaired (old people, those with substantial weight loss/malabsorption, HIV positive), skin testing can be negative in active disease. Laparoscopy can be useful in allowing biopsy of serosal nodules. Differential diagnosis includes <u>Crohn's disease</u>,

Yersinia infection, cecal involvement with cancer or amebiasis. Syphilis and lymphogranuloma vernereum are quoted but now vanishingly rare.

Treatment. No controlled studies but three-drug regimen for 12 months recommended.

Weil's disease

See: leptospirosis.

Whipworm

- *Trichuris trichiura* is a roundworm of the phylum *Nematoda*. The adult worm usually reaches 3–5 cm in length and has a lifespan of one to three years. Estimated worldwide infection rate of 800 million.
- Organism spread via the fecal–oral route, and humans are only hosts. Embryonated (mature) eggs are ingested.
- Usually asymptomatic, but heavy worm infestation may result in lower abdominal discomfort, flatulence, and altered bowel habit.
- *Trichuris* dysentery syndrome characterized by bloody diarrhea, tenesmus, and anemia, but is rare.
- Diagnosis made by identifying *T. trichiura* eggs on stool microscopy.
- Treatment with mebendazole 100 mg bid for three days.

Yersinia

A genus of Gram-negative rods. *Yersinia pestis* is responsible for plague—a disease with an important role in human history. Other species (e.g., *Yersinia enterocolitica*) produce a self-limiting gastroenteritis.

Y. enterocolitica causes damage by invading epithelium overlying Peyer's patches, (especially in the terminal ileum) then spreading to the lamina propria.

Epidemics relate to consumption of contaminated milk and ice cream. Rare (one culture-confirmed case per 100,000 people per year in the United States). Two-thirds of cases are of enterocolitis; children under five are most commonly affected. Associated mesenteric adenitis is common and the condition may be confused with appendicitis; ultrasound can be helpful in separating these conditions.

In adults, erythema nodosum, erythema multiforme, and reactive polyarthritis can occur, usually one to two weeks after onset of diarrhea.

Diagnosis. Antigens can be found in mucosal biopsies. Specific IgA antibodies may be found in the blood. *Y. enterocolitica* may be grown in culture.

Treatment. Although the disease is usually diagnosed late, when antibiotics probably do not alter the course of the gastrointestinal infection, treatment with chloramphenicol, septrin, or a quinolone is indicated in severe infections.

Intestinal manifestations of systemic disease

Acromegaly and GI tract

- Increased risk of colonic polyps and <u>colon cancer</u> in acromegaly: precise extent of risk unclear. A screening colonoscopy at diagnosis of acromegaly is recommended, repeated every five years (three years if increased risk—adenoma at first colonoscopy or increased IGF-1 levels). Evidence for this based on single centrer experience showing 13–14 times increased risk of colon cancer, particularly right-sided.[1] Larger studies suggest two to three times the risk over controls.
- Colonoscopy often difficult due to long redundant colon. Conventional <u>bowel preparation</u> is less effective in acromegalics, and double quantities, preferably of osmotically active polyethylene glycol-based solutions, are suggested.
- Clinical enlargement of spleen, liver, or kidneys is unusual and warrants further investigation. Other GI complications include macroglossia and those relating to the use of the somatostation analogue <u>OCTREOTIDE</u> (used because it suppresses growth hormone secretion and can shrink a proportion of pituitary tumors because of their high somatostatin receptor density).

Acute intermittent porphyria

See: <u>porphyrias</u>.

Alcohol dependency

Epidemiology

Alcohol is the third leading cause of preventable death in the United States (behind smoking and obesity). Lifetime prevalence of dependency approximately 10% in men, 4% in women in the United States.

Clinical features

As well as <u>alcohol-related liver disease</u>, most other systems damaged: gastrointestinal (<u>esophagitis</u>, <u>gastritis</u>, <u>acute</u> and <u>chronic pancreatitis</u>); neurological (cortical atrophy/dementia, <u>Wernicke's encephalopathy</u>, peripheral neuropathy); endocrine (pseudo-Cushing's, diabetes mellitus, hypoglycemia, alcoholic ketodacidosis, hypoandrogenization); cardiovascular (dilated cardiomyopathy, conduction defects). Important cause of malnutrition, and increased risk of range of malignancies (e.g., <u>pancreatic</u>/<u>esophageal</u>/<u>gastric cancer</u>, <u>hepatocellular</u>, bladder carcinoma).

Assessment

- Dependency is not defined by a given quantity of alcohol consumed.
- On examination, features of chronic liver disease may be present.
- Although blood tests may suggest alcohol excess ($\uparrow$AST> ALT, $\uparrow$GGT, $\uparrow$MCV, $\downarrow$platelets), at least three of the eight DSM-IV criteria for alcohol dependency should be met (see Box 8.1).

Management

Many physicians have a nihilistic view toward the patient with alcohol dependency, but a number of interventions are of benefit. Aim of treatment is to stop alcohol, or reduce to manageable levels (complete cessation is usually the most effective goal in the patient with dependency).

- Psychological assessment and support is the cornerstone of treating dependency. First step involves an unequivocal clarification of the problems being caused by alcohol, and an assessment of the patient's readiness for change.
- Specialist alcohol-support agencies are available (e.g., Alcoholics Anonymous [AA]), and the patient should be given clear details of how to access services.
- Range of medications have been used to maintain abstinence in conjunction with psychological input, including disulfuram (which causes nausea and vomiting with coincident alcohol), and acamprosate (stimulates GABA transmission, and maintains abstinence in 12–18% of patients, compared with 5–7% on placebo).
- In the patient with severe physical dependency (e.g., marked withdrawal symptoms), who is committed to stopping, admission to hospital for acute detoxification may be indicated, and alcohol withdrawal pre-empted and treated prophylactically.

Box 8.1 Criteria for alcohol dependency

- Continued drinking despite physical or psychological consequences caused or exacerbated by alcohol
- Neglect of other activities
- Inordinate time spent drinking or recovering
- Drinking more or over a longer period than intended
- Inability to control drinking
- Tolerance (defined as increased amounts needed for effect)
- Withdrawal symptoms on cessation of alcohol
- Drinking to relieve or avoid withdrawal symptoms

Box 8.2 CAGE questionnaire is also a useful screening tool for problem drinking

1. Have you ever felt the need to **C**ut down on your drinking?
2. Have people **A**nnoyed you by criticizing your drinking?
3. Have you ever felt bad or **G**uilty about your drinking?
4. Have you ever had a drink first thing in the morning to steady your nerves or hangover (**E**ye-opener)?

1 Jenkins, PJ and Fairclough, PD. (2001). *Clin. Endocrinol.* 55: 727

Alcohol withdrawal and delirium tremens (DT)

Abrupt cessation of alcohol in patient with history of chronic excess (see alcohol dependency, alcoholic liver disease) may lead to clinical features that, in their severest form (DT occurs in 5% with alcohol withdrawal), may carry mortality of 5–35%. On stopping alcohol, a decrease in the inhibitory neurotransmitter GABA results in unopposed increase in sympathetic activity.

Clinical features

- Alcohol withdrawal symptoms may develop < 8 hours since last drink (usually peaking at 48–72 hours)—confusion, hallucinations (auditory, visual, or olfactory), agitation, insomnia, nausea, vomiting. Generalized epileptic fits may occur. Signs of sympathetic drive: ↑HR, ↑BP (systolic > 160 mmHg, diastolic > 100 mmHg), sweating, tremor, dilated pupils, fever.
- Delirium tremens signs and symptoms include all the above, but to a greater severity. Neuropsychiatric manifestations prominent. > 20% mortality if untreated; 5% with treatment. Death is often due to complications of hyperthermia, electrolyte imbalance, volume depletion, infection, hypertensive crisis, or cardiovascular collapse.

Diagnosis

Largely clinical diagnoses. Always consider in any recently admitted agitated, confused inpatient. Important differential diagnoses include drug intoxication (alcohol or other drugs), Wernicke-Korsakoff's syndrome, hepatic encephalopathy, or intracranial hematoma.

Investigation

- Bloods:
  - CBC: ↑WCC, ↑MCV, ↓platelets may be seen.
  - Clotting: ↑PT/APPT suggests significantly impaired liver function.
  - Electrolytes, LFTs: dehydration common; abnormal liver function tests not a prerequisite for alcohol withdrawal; Mg^{2+} levels often decrease.
  - Glucose: seizures may occur secondary to hypoglycemia.
  - Detectable alcohol during "withdrawal" suggests another diagnosis.
  - Measure serum anticonvulsant levels if patient taking these (often the case in alcoholics).
- EKG: excludes other causes of tachycardia (e.g., AF common).
- CT brain: in any patients with history of head injury, atypical presentation, focal neurology, or prolonged postictal phase.
- CXR, and cultures (e.g., blood, urine, sputum) if any sign of sepsis.

Management

- Manage patient in calm, safe environment. Monitor vital signs (HR, BP, temperature).
- Peripheral IV cannula. Give fluids (e.g., 5% dextrose 1 l over eight hours).
- Thiamine 100 mg IV/PO/IM initially, then 100 mg PO daily. Magnesium sulphate 1 g IM/IV (note IM injection is painful) every six hours for 24 hours if required.
- Benzodiazepines of proven benefit (e.g., lorazepam 1 mg = diazepam 5 mg = chlordiazepoxide 25 mg), but no universally agreed protocol. Shorter acting lorazepam favored in liver disease, and midazolam increasingly used.
- Mild–moderate alcohol withdrawal:
  - "Symptom triggered" regimens (e.g., Chlordiazepoxide 50–100 mg PO every two hours until symptoms controlled, then prn) give better control and shorter treatment duration than "fixed-schedules.."
  - "Fixed-schedule" regimen shown in Table 8.1.
- Severe withdrawal/DTs:
  - Lorazepam 1–4 mg IV every one to three hours (interval dosing). Onset of action occurs two to five minutes after IV injection, but peak plasma levels one to six hours. Close monitoring for respiratory depression essential. Adjust dosage and frequency to patient response (aim for calm, but awake). Dosage not to exceed 240 mg/24 hours.
  - Haloperidol given in addition if severely agitated. 3 mg IV, with doubling of successive doses every 30 minutes until calm.
- Other drugs for withdrawal (e.g., barbiturates, propofol, carbamazepine, clonidine) should not be used as first-line therapy.

Table 8.1 "Fixed schedule" chlordiazepoxide oral regimen for alcohol withdrawal

	Dose	Frequency
Day 1	50 mg	every 4 hours
Day 2	50 mg	every 6 hours
Day 3	25 mg	every 4 hours
Day 4	25 mg	every 6 hours

Amyloidosis

Group of diseases characterized by extracellular deposition of abnormal fibrillar proteins. Classification is by capital A for amyloid followed by an abbreviation for a fibril protein.

- **Light chain (AL) amyloidosis** involves clonal excess of immunoglobulin light chains and can manifest as multiple myeloma. GI manifestations include macroglossia, GI bleeding, and motility problems. Management is with hematological chemotherapy.
- **In reactive systemic (AA) amyloid** the precursor protein is the acute phase reactant serum amyloid A. It occurs in less than 2% of patients with Crohn's and is very rare in UC. Presentation is usually with nephrotic syndrome but the liver and spleen may also be affected.
- Familial Mediterranean fever also involves AA protein; in this disease colchicine has been shown to prevent renal failure from amyloid deposition.
- Gastroenterologists are sometimes called to help make the diagnosis of amyloid; rectal and duodenal biopsies are positive in over 80% of cases if submucosa is present in the biopsy.

Angio-edema

Hereditary angio-edema is an autosomal dominant disorder caused by a deficiency of C1 esterase inhibitor, a regulator of the activated first component of complement. Pathogenesis not fully understood, but kinin release may mediate increased vascular permeability.

Clinical features include recurrent edema of skin and mucous membranes. Although there can be tingling or burning at the onset, the lesions are painless and, unlike urticaria, pruritus is absent. Onset is usually in childhood and a family history is usually present. Attacks may be precipitated by local trauma, dental extractions, or surgery. Laryngeal edema can cause airway obstruction. Gastrointestinal involvement includes colicky pain, diarrhea, and vomiting. Fluid loss can lead to hypotension and shock: fever and leucocytosis are absent, bowel sounds may be increased, and there is no peritonism.

Diagnosis involves finding reduced C4 levels and a reduction in C1 esterase inhibitor.

Treatment. Anabolic steroids such as danazol and stanozolol can prevent attacks, but may have other actions than simply raising levels of C1 esterase inhibitor since patients often respond to low doses that are insufficient to raise complement levels. Doses are tailored to clinical rather than biological response. In known cases, premedication with C1 esterase inhibitor concentrates should be considered before interventional procedures such as upper GI endoscopy.

Anorexia nervosa

An eating disorder characterized by a distorted body image, an inability to interpret hunger and satiety, and a paralyzing sense of ineffectiveness (also see bulimia).

Etiology and pathogenesis

Not a true loss of appetite, rather a preoccupation with food and eating. Recently reported incidence of 30–150 per 100,000 in 16–25 year old women, making it the third commonest illness in the age group after obesity and asthma. Role of psychosocial factors is much studied and outside our scope here.

Clinical features include hypothermia, bradycardia, hypotension, acrocyanosis, carotinaemia giving a yellow appearance to face and hair, thin hair (lanugo) over face, arms, and back, and amenorrhea.

Investigation may reveal hypokalemia, hyponatremia, and "sick euthyroid" indices (low free thyroxine with a normal TSH).

Complications Arrhythmias, effects on bone mineralization/osteoporosis, and depressed menstruation and reproductive function. Gastrointestinal complications include constipation, pancreatitis, esophagitis, peptic ulceration, abnormal liver function tests (and biochemical hepatitis), malabsorption, and reduced taste.

Treatment is difficult and centers on an interlocking approach to the psychological, nutritional, and medical problems. Sadly, while early mortality remains around 5%, late mortality can be as high as 20%, with suicide, arrhythmias, and infections the leading causes of death.

Autonomic neuropathy

Etiology

Autonomic neuropathy affecting the gastrointestinal tract occurs as a complication of diabetes mellitus and Parkinsons's disease. Less common causes include rare types of amyloid, Fabry's disease, and porphyria.

Clinical features

Symptoms relate to postural hypotension and genitourinary involvement (impotence, loss of morning erections, urinary urgency). Gut stasis can give rise to bacterial overgrowth, which can produce diarrhea and malabsorption. Nausea, vomiting, abdominal pain, and distension can all occur as a presenting problem.

Examination

In the gastrointestinal system, test for a succussion splash suggestive of gastroparesis, and look for fecal impaction.

Investigations

Autonomic function tests may help. Endoscopy is a poor test for motility: better to get a video swallow, barium meal, or gastric emptying study. Colonic motility can be assessed using a shapes test where clearance of differently shaped radio-opaque markers is assessed on sequential plain abdominal X-rays.

Treatment

Small frequent meals and avoiding anticholinergics, narcotics, and sympathomimetics. Gastric pacing, via an implantable electrical stimulator, can be used in patients with gastroparesis refractory to medical therapy.

Behçet's syndrome

After H. Behçet, Turkish dermatologist, died 1948.

- Vasculitis affecting several organ systems. Said to occur along the old silk road from the Middle East to Japan: Incidence is highest in Turkey (370 cases per 100,000), Iran (16–100 per 100,000), Saudi Arabia and Japan (13 per 1,000,000). Onset typically in third and fourth decades, more common in males in Middle East but females in Far East.
- Pathophysiology unknown, the basic lesion is a vasculitis. Neutrophil function is abnormal (enhanced neutrophil–endothelial cell adhesion, positive pathergy test).
- Diagnostic criteria include: oral aphthous ulcers (which are recurrent, painful, and nonscarring) plus two of: genital ulcers, uveitis (anterior or posterior), pustular vasculitis, synovitis, menigoencephalitis, and exclusion of patients with IBD, SLE, Reiter's, and herpes. Aphthoid ulcers may occur anywhere in the GI tract, most commonly in the ileo-cecal region, but also right colon and esophagus.
- GI lesions are usually treated with steroids, 5-ASA, or thalidomide: colchicine and azathioprine are used for systemic manifestations.

Beriberi

Clinical manifestation of <u>vitamin B1</u> (thiamine) deficiency. Cause is inadequate intake (including diets high in polished rice, which contains thiaminase; also alcoholics). Affects cardiovascular system (wet beriberi: sodium retention, edema, high output left ventricular failure) and nervous system (dry beriberi: motor and sensory neuropathy and Wernicke–Korsakoff psychosis). Associated with reduced red-cell transketolase, which requires thiamine as a cofactor. Those with <u>alcoholic liver disease</u> have reduced capacity to absorb thiamine so always give thiamine supplements.

Body mass index (BMI)

Also known as the Quetelet index. Defined as body weight (kg) divided by height (m) squared (see BMI chart in Appendix 2). It correlates well with obesity but is not a direct measure of adiposity. The World Health Organization definitions of body weight categories are shown in the table opposite. See obesity surgery.

Table 8.2 Body weight categories

Category	Body mass index (kg/m^2)
Underweight	< 19
Normal weight	19–24.9
Mild overweight	25–29.9
Moderate overweight	30–39.9
Severe overweight	> 40

Bulimia

Initially used to describe a syndrome of gluttonous overeating and induced vomiting; more recently applied to the psychiatric diagnosis of **bulimia nervosa**, which centers on a maladaptive behavior employed to control calorie consumption and promote weight loss. As with anorexia nervosa, incidence has increased in recent years; it is more common than anorexia and estimated to affect 2–5% of school- and college-age females. Hallmark personality features are loss of control, low self-esteem, and guilt. Most bulimic individuals are of normal weight and perceive their eating behavior as problematic, often seeking medical help (unlike the patient with anorexia nervosa). Important physical signs are salivary gland hypertrophy, dental enamel erosion, excoriations on knuckles (caused by digitally induced vomiting), and chronic sore throat. Medical complications can include electrolyte disturbances (hypokalemia, hypomagnesemia, hypoglycemia, hyperprolactinemia) as well as esophagitis, pancreatitis, abdominal pain, constipation, and cathartic colon.

Carcinoid

Tumors arising from enterochromaffin cells (derived from neural crest cells: also called APUD cells (**A**mine **P**recursor **U**ptake and **D**ecarboxylation) at the base of intestinal crypts. GI carcinoids account for 95% of all carcinoids and about 1.5% of all GI tumors. They secrete a range of hormones, including 5-HT (serotonin—metabolized in the liver by monoamine oxidase into 5-hydroxy-indole-acetic acid (5-HIAA) and excreted in the urine), ACTH, histamine, bradykinin, and kallikrein.

Clinical features
Most patients are asymptomatic but can present with pain, obstruction (20%), weight loss (15%), palpable mass (15%), or perforation of hemorrhage (rare).

Carcinoid syndrome arises when the hormonal load exceeds the capacity of the monoamine oxidase in the liver and lung to metabolize serotonin—most patients with carcinoid syndrome have liver metastases from a bowel carcinoid.

Clinical features of carcinoid syndrome include diarrhea and abdominal cramps (70%), flushing of skin and telangiectasia, right-sided heart failure from right-sided endocardial fibrosis leading to tricuspid regurgitation, and pulmonary valve stenosis.

Carcinoids at different sites of the GI tract can behave rather differently:

- **Foregut carcinoids** are rare: tumors are usually slow growing and benign. Gastric carcinoids have been classified into type I (small benign tumors associated with chronic atrophic gastritis and hypergastrinemia), type II (large, polypoid lesions, prone to metastases, and associated with multiple endocrine neoplasia type 1 (MEN-1) and Zollinger–Ellison syndrome (see gastrinoma), and type III (large, solitary, sporadic tumors not associated with raised gastrin levels).
- **Midgut carcinoid.** Most commonly occurring tumor of the small bowel. Ileum is commonest affected site (90%). Tumors may be multiple, and liver metastases occur in 25%.
- **Hindgut carcinoid.** Colonic carcinoids account for 0.3% of colon tumors. 75% occur in the ascending colon. A carcinoid may be an incidental finding on examination of a removed appendix, usually in patients aged 20–40 years. In patients with a tumor at the base of the appendix or if the tumor is larger than 2 cm, a right hemicolectomy is indicated. In patients with carcinoid at the appendix tip, appendicectomy alone is adequate.

Differential diagnoses include pancreatic endocrine tumors, or rare abdominal tumors such as desmoids.

Investigations Elevated hormone output demonstrated with gut hormone screen (e.g., ↑ chromogranin A), and 24-hour urine collection for 5-HIAA (note: may be falsely ↑ by bananas, avocado, pineapple, walnuts, coffee, and chocolate). Ultrasound is not specific, but may lead to more appropriate investigation. CT scanning is better at providing anatomical information, and endoscopic ultrasound and angiography may be necessary. Barium studies are of low yield. The most promising techniques include octreotide and MIBG (metaiodobenzylguanidine) scanning. PET scanning increasingly used to identify metastatic lesions.

Management Surgical cure may be possible for isolated lesions (or limited liver metastases). For those with carcinoid syndrome OCTREOTIDE may effectively control hormone release, but other symptomatic approaches may also be necessary (e.g., loperamide for diarrhea). Palliative approaches to reduce tumor load include hepatic artery embolization for large hepatic metastases; INTERFERON-ALPHA; chemotherapy (e.g., streptozocin, 5-fluorouracil, and doxorubicin); radio-isotope iodine (I^{131}) MIBG or octreotide therapy. Carcinoid tumors are generally slowly progressive (> 80% five-year survival in surgically treated patients, and even in those with metastatic disease, median survival > two years). Also see pancreatic endocrine tumors.

Chronic granulomatous disease (CGD)

Rare genetic immune deficiency in which phagocytes are unable to kill bacteria and fungi as a result of defects in the electron transport chain underlying the respiratory burst. It is classified according to mode of inheritance and component of reduced NADPH oxidase affected. 65% are X-linked, the remainder are autosomal recessive.

GI involvement is common (30% of all cases; more common in X-linked patients) and involves an abnormal inflammatory response with persistent tissue granuloma formation (presumed due to inadequate clearance of bacterial or fungal antigens).

Clinical features

In most patients, GI involvement is granulomatous or ulcerative involving the colon. Symptoms include abdominal pain, diarrhea (which may be bloody), and nausea and vomiting. In many cases the phenotype is clinically and radiologically indistinguishable from inflammatory bowel disease; the patchy distribution and presence of granulomas are more suggestive of Crohn's disease than ulcerative colitis. There is a high frequency of pyloric obstruction. Clinical similarity offers a tantalizing clue about possible pathogenic mechanisms in inflammatory bowel disease. Recently reported association in Crohn's disease of mutations in NOD-2, which is involved in recognition of the bacterial product MDP, suggests that failure to deal adequately with bacterial infection could be common to CGD and Crohn's disease.

Management

Treatment of GI involvement in CGD is not well defined and usually involves CORTICOSTEROIDS. Treatment with gamma-interferon reduces serious infections but does not seem to aggravate GI inflammation in CGD.

The prognosis is poor: mean age of death in patients with GI involvement is 14 years.

Cronkite–Canada syndrome

Reported in 1955, it is a noninherited syndrome occurring in middle-age or older people. It consists of diffuse polyposis, dystrophic changes of fingernails, alopecia, cutaneous hyperpigmentation, and a malabsorption syndrome with diarrhea, weight loss, and abdominal pain.

The malabsorption is progressive and the prognosis poor. Bacterial overgrowth can be a complicating factor.

Cystic fibrosis (CF) and the GI tract

Epidemiology + pathogenesis

Autosomal recessive condition, with disease prevalence of 1:3,000 of northern European ancestry and gene carriage in 1:25. CF results from mutations in gene for the cystic fibrosis transmembrane conductance regulator (CFTR), a cAMP-activated chloride channel found in secretory epithelia. Disease involves major complications of pulmonary and GI system, due to production of dehydrated protein-rich secretions.

Clinical features

- GI tract complications increasingly common, due in part to improved management of pulmonary complications and longer life expectancy (median 30 years).
- CF is the commonest cause of exocrine <u>pancreatic insufficiency</u> in childhood (occurs in 90–95% of children with CF), and severity of pancreatic disease parallels lung involvement. Presents with failure to thrive, steatorrhea, colicky abdominal pain. Predisposes to malabsorption of fat-soluble <u>vitamins</u> A, D, E, and K. Diabetes mellitus in 8–12% of patients >25 years.
- Bile duct plugging due to secretions may lead to indolent development of secondary biliary cirrhosis and <u>portal hypertension</u>. Hepatic congestion due to pulmonary hypertension/right heart failure. <u>Fatty liver</u> in 20%; <u>gallstones</u> in 15% of young adults with CF.
- CF may result in meconium ileus at birth (12% of neonates with CF) and in distal intestinal obstruction syndrome (DIOS) later. Intestinal obstruction, intussusception, rectal prolapse may occur. Excessive <u>PANCREATIC ENZYME SUPPLEMENTS</u> associated with colonic strictures (fibrosing colonopathy).

Investigations

- Diagnosis usually made in infancy, based on typical pulmonary ± GI tract manifestations, a family history, and positive results on sweat test. Confirmation by genetic testing in most cases.
- Investigation of GI complications dependent on specific presentation.
- Check vitamin A, E, D, K levels.

Box 8.3 **CF mutations and pancreatitis**

Recent observations suggest that heterozygosity for CFTR may be linked to recurrent <u>acute pancreatitis</u> and idiopathic <u>chronic pancreatitis</u>. Few of these patients have any evidence of pulmonary disease or abnormal sweat tests.

Management

- Multidisciplinary approach to care, with expert nutritional support.
- Vitamin supplements for vitamin deficiencies.
- <u>PANCREATIC ENZYME SUPPLEMENTS</u> for exocrine insufficiency
- Lung and <u>liver transplantation</u> has been successful.
- Gene therapy remains the ultimate goal for treatment of CF.

Dermatitis herpetiformis

An intensely pruritic papulovesicular rash that is usually symmetrically distributed on the extensor surfaces of the elbows as well as the on the buttocks, knees, sacrum, face, neck, and trunk. Very closely associated with <u>celiac disease</u>; nearly 100% have abnormal jejunal mucosa. Characterized by IgA at the dermo-epidermal junction away from sites of blistering. Pathogenesis unknown. Treatment involves dapsone 1 2 mg/kg, which is effective in treating the skin lesions and the pruritus. All patients should go on gluten-free diet.

Diabetes and the GI tract

Altered gut motility due to <u>autonomic neuropathy</u> can result in:

- **Diabetic gastroparesis.** Delayed gastric emptying on scintigraphy is found in up to 50% of unselected patients. About 25% of insulin-dependent diabetics with peripheral neuropathy report nausea, vomiting, anorexia, and heartburn. Suspect the diagnosis in a patient with appropriate symptoms and a negative endoscopy or barium study. Pathophysiology is complex and may involve impaired visceral sensation, gastric smooth muscle degeneration, a local myopathic effect of hyperglycemia, or altered secretion of gut hormones. Management centers on small frequent meals, tight control of blood sugar, and <u>PROKINETICS</u> such as metoclopramide or erythromycin. Domperidone is another agent which has been shown to be affective but is not available in the United States. Jejunostomy feeding tubes may occasionally be needed especially if the disease is localized to the proximal small intestine. External electrical pacing has been suggested to improve gastric emptying but is not widely used.
- **Diabetic diarrhea.** This occurs in association with long-standing insulin-dependent diabetes and is associated with <u>autonomic neuropathy</u> and occasionally fecal incontinence. It may also be associated with <u>bacterial overgrowth</u>. In some patients exocrine

pancreatic insufficiency may contribute to the pathogenesis. Management is with anti-diarrheal agents such as loperamide or codeine. If exocrine pancreatic insufficiency is the problem then management with pancreatic enzyme supplements is the treatment of choice. OCTREOTIDE has been useful in selected patients.

Fatty liver. Abdominal ultrasound will often include a report of "fatty liver," reflecting the accumulation of lipid in hepatocytes. This occurs as part of a **metabolic syndrome** incorporating obesity, hypertension, and diabetes. A proportion of patients with nonalcoholic fatty liver disease (NAFLD) will have steatohepatitis, which may progress to fibrosis and cirrhosis and is not the benign process it was once considered to be. Recent studies indicate that diet and exercise may prevent and reverse fat deposition in the liver.

Down syndrome and GI tract

Trisomy 21 affects 1:650 live births in the United States and is increased in mothers older than 35, and is characterized by a wide range of phenotypic abnormalities, including short stature, learning difficulties, wide epicanthic folds, and macroglossia. GI problems can be subdivided into the following.

Embryological. Imperforate anus; duodenal/jejunal atresia; Hirschsprung's disease (2% of cases).

Motility. Feeding problems; constipation, gastro-esophageal reflux.

Immunological
- Celiac disease: affects > 5% of people with DS (> 40-fold increase over nonDS population).
- Autoimmune hepatitis: probable increased frequency.
- Hepatitis B and associated autoimmune thyroiditis: increased rate of HBV infection may relate to history of institutional living, but high frequency of chronicity probably due to inherent immune defects in DS.

Ehlers–Danlos disease

After Edward Ehlers, a Danish dermatologist, in 1901 and Henri Danlos, a French physician, in 1908.

A group of 10 rare (frequency approx. 1 in 400,000) inherited disorders of collagen metabolism resulting in a decrease in the tensile strength and integrity of the skin, joints, and blood vessels. The classical types I and II involve defects in type V collagen. The most relevant to gastroenterologists is type IV, involving a defect in type III collagen (chromosome locus 2q31), which can present with spontaneous rupture of the bowel or medium-sized arteries. Patients have prominent venous marking easily visible through the skin. It is the only type with increased mortality (median life expectancy 50 years).

Elderly and the GI tract

GI disease is generally more common in the elderly than the young (e.g., colonic <u>diverticula</u> in > 50% people > 60 years). In most cases the patient's age has little effect over their management. A number of interlinked factors contribute to the high rate of GI symptoms in the elderly.

Malignancy. All the major GI tract cancers increase in prevalence with age, with steep increases after the age of 60 (e.g., <u>gastric</u>, <u>esophageal</u>, <u>pancreatic</u>, <u>colonic cancer</u>).

Comorbidity. E.g., <u>Parkinson's disease</u> (leads to constipation *per se* and secondary to anticholinergic drugs); motor neuron disease (dysphagia—see <u>Mouth and swallowing problems</u>); Alzheimer's disease (poor nutrition, <u>fecal incontinence</u>).

Drug effects. Motility disorders, especially constipation, promoted by wide range of drugs: e.g., diuretics, **ANTICHOLINERGICS**, antidepressants, opiate analgesics. NSAIDs for joint pain/disease contribute to <u>peptic ulceration</u>.

Immobility. Leads to GI motility problems due to range of reasons, including embarrassment at needing assistance, associated depression, and antiphysiological posture for defecation of being supine/semi-supine. Supine position may also encourage gastro esophageal reflux.

Nutrition. Malnutrition is prevalent in the elderly, particularly if hospitalized, socially isolated, or with mental//physical health problems. There are difficult ethical considerations surrounding the use of artificial feeding in those with severe dementia and inadequate nutrition.

Specific considerations

Constipation

- 25% prevalence of constipation/straining in elderly living at home (increases to 50% in those in hospital/institutional care).
- Fecal impaction and incontinence in >10% of those >75 years.
- Poor fluid intake, immobility, and drugs all contribute.
- Laxatives used regularly by 20–30% of people > 65 years.
- In hospital patients, stimulant/osmotic <u>LAXATIVES</u> more effective than fiber, which may encourage fecal impaction in immobile patients.

Dyspepsia. Common practice of performing endoscopy in all elderly patients with new-onset dyspepsia recently challenged by NICE guidelines. These advise that endoscopy should not be 'age-dependent', and that endoscopy for dyspepsia should be reserved for those with alarm symptoms (see <u>Dyspepsia and reflux</u>).

Acute abdominal pain. In elderly, the development of peritoneal signs after perforation of a viscus or similar intrabdominal event (e.g., <u>intestinal ischemia</u>) may be impaired, leading to usual presentation being masked, and hence late diagnosis.

Gallstones. ERCP with sphincterotomy and stone extraction, without subsequent cholecystectomy, has been advocated for elderly patients with choledocholithiasis. However, > 40% will get further biliary problems within two years with this approach. Although cholecystectomy is safe in the elderly, long-term endobiliary plastic stenting may be appropriate if cholecystectomy/ bile duct clearance not possible. Treatment with the gallstone dissolution agent Ursadiol (300 mg po bid) is a suitable treatment alternative for elderly individuals who cannot undergo cholecystectomy. Therapy is life long and works best for single, medium-size stones (3–9 mm).

Endometriosis affecting the GI tract

Endometrial tissue outside the uterus may occur, usually without symptoms, in 15% of menstruating women. In women undergoing surgery for endometriosis, 30% have intestinal involvement, usually of the rectosigmoid colon. Penetration of endometriomas into the bowel can cause partial obstruction with pain and constipation. Intestinal bleeding is rare: endometrial deposits do not usually invade the mucosa but are associated with muscular hypertrophy and fibrosis. Less than half of patients show cyclical symptoms associated with menses, but nearly all women with intestinal involvement have associated features of pelvic endometriosis.

Diagnosis can be difficult. Rectal biopsy is normal unless there is associated rectal bleeding. CT and MRI are usually nonspecific because of the small size of endometrial deposits. Endorectal ultrasound may be useful but experience is limited. Laparoscopy can be diagnostic and allows tissue diagnosis.

Differential diagnosis includes irritable bowel syndrome, Crohn's disease, and even colon cancer. Diverticular disease usually occurs in older women and radiation-induced stricturing should be diagnosed from the history. Malignant degeneration of extra-ovarian endometriosis is rare but documented. Very rarely mucosal involvement by endometrial tissue can simulate adenomatous polyps.

Treatment. If medical treatment with hormonal control fails, surgical resection is usually recommended. If ovarian function is preserved, recurrence of symptoms is substantial.

Eosinophilia and the GI tract

The differential diagnosis of a peripheral blood eosinophilia in association with GI symptoms includes:
- **Drugs** (aspirin, sulphonamides, penicillin, cephalosporins, azathioprine, carbamazepine).
- **Vasculitis** (e.g., Churg–Strauss syndrome).
- **Lymphoma.**
- **Connective tissue disorders** (scleroderma/dermatomyositis).

- **Addison's disease.**
- **Parasites** are an important cause. Invasive helminths are classically the causal group. Hook worm (see <u>roundworms</u>) and pinworms may cause eosinophilic infiltration. *Giardia* can cause eosinophilic infiltration of the jejunum without peripheral blood eosinophilia. People who eat raw fish may be infected with anisakis. <u>Schistosomiasis</u>, *ascaris*, *tricuris* can cause eosinophilia and abdominal pain *Fasciola* can cause right upper quadrant pain, fever, hepatomegaly.
- **Asthma and allergic rhinitis** are common and can cause peripheral eosinophilia.
- <u>Eosinophilic gastroenteritis</u> (see below).

Eosinophilic gastroenteritis

Rare disease, usually presenting at age 30–50 years with following diagnostic criteria:

- Presence of GI symptoms.
- Eosinophilic infiltrate of one or more areas of the GI tract on biopsy.
- Absence of involvement of organs outside the GI tract.
- Absence of parasitic infestation or other cause of peripheral blood eosinophilia.

Pathogenesis is poorly understood but involves damage to the gut wall through degranulation of eosinophil granules. The trigger for this is unknown but may involve type-1 allergy or parasitic causes.

Clinical features. Stomach and small intestine are most commonly affected but any part of the GI tract may be involved. Most commonly, the disease affects mucosa and submucosa, and this leads to colicky pain, nausea, vomiting, diarrhea, and weight loss. If the muscle layer is mainly affected, presentation can be with pyloric or upper GI obstruction. Very rarely serosal disease can cause eosinophilic ascites.

Investigation. 80% have a peripheral blood eosinophilia. Serum iron and albumin may be low. The IgE may be raised, especially in children. Stool studies are necessary to exclude parasitic infestation. Histological samples from affected areas are needed for diagnosis.

Treatment

- If there is no muscle or serosal involvement, dietary manipulation is reasonable, especially if there is a history suggestive of food intolerance. Children often respond well to diet—milk protein is the most often implicated allergen.
- If there is a history of travel or residence in high-risk areas, a trial of antiparasitic therapy, such as mebendazole 100 mg bid for three days is reasonable.
- <u>CROMOGLYCATE</u> (200 mg tds–qds) is often tried; it stabilizes mast cells and can reduce antigen absorption by the small intestine.

- CORTICOSTEROIDS are used in patients who fail to respond to the above measures or in those with obstructive symptoms or eosinophilic ascites. 90% of patients respond to oral steroids in a dose of 20–40 mg/day. The dose can be tapered over several weeks and 30–50% will relapse on stopping steroids. Use second-line immunosuppressives because steroid-sparing agents in patients who are steroid-dependent has not been examined systematically.

Box 8.4 Eosinophils in the GI tract

- Eosinophilic infiltration of the GI tract by itself does not indicate eosinophilic gastroenteritis. The diagnosis requires full thickness infiltration of the gastrointestinal mucosa and exclusion of known causes including drugs and parasites.
- Causes include:
  • IgE-mediated food allergy
  • Gastro-esophageal reflux disease
  • Allergic colitis and inflammatory bowel disease
  • Cow's milk allergy
  • Gastric cancer
  • Hypereosinophilic syndrome

Erythema nodosum (EN)

Red, well demarcated, raised 1–6 cm lesions usually limited to the extensor aspects of the lower legs. Wide range of causes, including infection (e.g., Streptococcus, Campylobacter, TB, Yersinia, fungal infection), drugs (e.g., sulphonamides), sarcoidosis, Behçet's syndrome. EN occurs in approximately 2% of patients with IBD (Crohn's disease > ulcerative colitis), and usually parallels disease activity. Histology of lesions shows a panniculitis. Individual lesions usually spontaneously resolve in six weeks, but others may occur. Nonsteroidal anti-inflammatories may help, as may control of underlying activity of IBD.

Fabry's disease

An X-linked disorder of glycolipid metabolism due to deficiency or absence of α-galactosidase A. Sphingolipid deposition occurs in all tissues. GI manifestations include impaired motility leading to recurrent cramping abdominal pain, and watery stools. Bacterial overgrowth and delayed gastric emptying can occur. Electron microscopy show lipid-filled vacuoles in ganglion cells of Meissner's plexus and endothelial cells: lipid deposition in small vessels can lead to vasculitis and thrombosis. Mucosal enterocytes are normal.

Familial mediterranean fever

Epidemiology + pathogenesis

Autosomal recessive disease, affecting up to 1:200 in high-prevalence populations (e.g., Sephardic Jews, Armenians). Mutations of MEFV gene on chromosome 16 encode for Pyrin, expressed in neutrophils.

Clinical features

Symptoms begin at < 20 years in > 95% of cases. Recurrent episodes of fever, peritonitis (mimicking acute abdomen), pleurisy, arthritis, and rash. Episodes last 24–72 hours. Amyloid A deposition may lead to renal failure. Presentation to gastroenterologists with unexplained recurrent attacks of pain (often with "negative" laparotomies). See Acute abdominal pain.

Investigations

Diagnosis never made unless considered!
- ↑ Acute phase response (ESR, CRP) and neutrophilia.
- ↑ IgD in 13%.

Genetic analysis for common MEFV mutations allows definitive diagnosis, so less role for "trial of colchicine."

Management

Colchicine 600 µg BID orally markedly effective in > 95% of cases, and may prevent development of amyloidosis.

Felty's syndrome

First five cases described in 1924 by American physician Augustus Felty in *Johns Hopkins Medical Bulletin*.

The clinical combination of rheumatoid arthritis, splenomegaly, and leucopenia. Occasional relevance to gastroenterologists as > 50% have abnormal liver histology ranging from portal fibrosis to nodular regenerative hyperplasia. This can cause portal hypertension and variceal bleeding.

Graft versus host disease (GvHD)

- Can affect any part of the GI tract. Most common after bone marrow transplants, it is caused by "foreign" (allogeneic) immune cells.
- Acute GvHD occurs during posttransplant days 21–100; chronic GvHD occurs after day 100. Usually affects small and large intestine, less commonly the stomach and esophagus.
- Gastric involvement often causes nausea, vomiting, upper abdominal pain. Endoscopy and gastric biopsies are necessary. Histology shows necrosis of single cells in large and small intestinal crypts.

- Jaundice due to cholestasis is a feature of severe acute GvHD.
  <u>Liver biopsy</u> may show bile duct damage and eventually ductopenia.
  Hepatocellular necrosis is rare.
- Acute GvHD is treated with high-dose <u>CORTICOSTEROIDS</u>.
  First-line treatment of chronic GvHD is with <u>CYCLOSPORIN</u> and
  <u>CORTICOSTEROIDS</u>; but further treatment is ineffective and difficult.

Gut hormone profile

- Measurement of serum gut hormones (see Table 8.3) can be an
  invaluable part of investigation of patients with suspected <u>carcinoid</u> and
  <u>neuroendocrine/pancreatic endocrine tumors</u>. However, completely
  invalid results may be obtained if sample is not taken and handled
  correctly.
- <u>Serum chromogranin A</u> correlates quite well with tumor burden in
  neuroendocrine tumors, but may also be elevated in prostatic cancer.

Patient preparation
- <u>H2 RECEPTOR ANTAGONISTS</u> blockers should be stopped for 72 h,
  and <u>PROTON PUMP INHIBITORS</u> for 12 weeks, before blood is taken.
- After an overnight fast, take blood (10 ml) using a syringe and needle.

Sample preparation
- Inform the analyzing laboratory that you are taking the sample and
  when. Inform lab of patient's serum calcium and urea, list all drugs
  currently administered, clinical question, and details of any gastric
  surgery (also see <u>gastrinoma</u>).
- Transfer 10 ml of blood into a heparin tube (containing aprotinin,
  0.2 ml, 2000 kIU). Mix by inversion. Place on ice and transfer
  immediately to the laboratory. Plasma separated in a refrigerated
  centrifuge and frozen at −20°C within 15 min of venepuncture, for
  subsequent analysis.

Table 8.3 Gut hormone profile

Hormone	Normal range	Disease association
Chromogranin A	0–38 ng/l	<u>Carcinoid</u>
Gastrin	0–40 pmol/l	<u>Gastrinoma</u>
Vasoactive intestinal polypeptide (VIP)	0–30 pmol/l	<u>VIPoma</u>
Somatostatin	0–150 pmol/l	Somatostatinoma
Pancreatic polypeptide (PP)	0–300 pmol/l	
Neurotensin	0–100 pmol/l	

Hemolytic–uremic syndrome (HUS)

- Acquired and inherited forms exist, but particular interest for gastroenterologists is in the association (in 90% of cases) with verocytotoxin-producing _E. coli_ (VTEC), and the commonest strain _E. coli_ 0157:H7 (also see <u>food poisoning</u>). Other enteric pathogens associated with HUS including _Shigella_, <u>Salmonella</u>, **_Yersinia_**, and _Campylobacter_. _E. coli_ 0157 commonly acquired from unpasteurized milk or uncooked meat, but only 5% of these infections lead to HUS. Children < five years and elderly most susceptible to disease.
- Condition characterized by thrombocytopenia, microangiopathic hemolytic anemia, and renal failure. Usually presents with acute illness characterized by abdominal cramps, bloody diarrhea, nausea, and vomiting. <u>Acute pancreatitis</u> may rarely occur. Bruising, bleeding, CNS effects, and renal failure generally develop about a week later.
- Diagnosis made on clinical suspicion, blood results showing renal failure, hemolytic anemia and ↓ platelets, and stool culture showing _E. coli_ 0157.
- Treatment of the acute diarrheal illness with antibiotics or antidiarrheal agents has been linked to an increased risk of developing HUS. 70% with VTEC–HUS recover completely, 30% require long-term renal dialysis, and 5% die of the disease.

Henoch–Schönlein purpura

Edward Henoch, nineteenth century. German pediatrician. Should really be called Schönlein–Henoch, because it was first described by Henoch's teacher, Schönlein.

A clinical syndrome of palpable nonthrombocytopenic purpura, arthritis, glomerulonephritis together with abdominal pain. Common in children, but can occur in adults. The main lesion seems to be an IgA nephropathy but blood levels of IgA and complement are variable.

GI symptoms include pain, nausea, and vomiting. Bleeding can occur in 40%, which can be small or large intestinal in origin. Less common complications include intramural hematomas, intussusception, cholecystitis, appendicitis, bowel infarction, and peritonitis.

HIV and the gut

Background and etiology

- All areas of GI tract may be affected (also see <u>HIV and the liver</u>).
- Before development of highly active antiretroviral therapy (HAART) opportunistic infections associated with immunocompromise were major cause of GI problems. Now, drug-induced side effects and other nonopportunistic diseases are more common (see Table 8.4).

Table 8.4 Common GI problems in HIV patients and their causes

Cause	Comment
Esophageal disease (dysphagia/ odynophagia)	
Candida albicans	<u>Esophagitis</u> usually linked with oral thrush. Suggests CD4 < 200/µl
<u>Cytomegalovirus</u> (CMV)	Large deep ulcers
Idiopathic ulcers	Small aphthous ulcers. Usually when CD4 < 200/µl
<u>Herpes simplex virus</u> (HSV)	Diffuse, shallow ulcers
Kaposi's sarcoma, lymphoma	Often develops in oral cavity
Diarrhea	
Bacterial: <u>Salmonella, Shigella, Campylobacter, Clostridium difficile. Mycobacterium</u> TB (MTB)/*avium* complex (MAC) <u>Bacterial overgrowth</u>	*Salmonella, Shigella* more common in HIV patient, even on HAART. MAC most common identified GI opportunistic infection if low CD4. Acid-fast staining of biopsies.
Protozoal: *Cryptosporidium, Microsporidium, Entamoeba* (see <u>hydatid</u>)	Oocytes of *Cryptosporidium* found on fecal smears. Treatment difficult, but may improve with HAART.
Fungal: *Histoplasma, Cryptococcosis*	Diffuse colitis with histoplasmosis. Treatment with amphotericin B.
Viral: <u>Cytomegalovirus</u>, <u>Herpes simplex virus</u>, adenovirus	CMV colitis in 5–10% with AIDS. Mucosal ulceration with inclusion bodies on histology Treatment IV ganciclovir.
"AIDS enteropathy"	Chronic diarrhea in AIDS, where no cause found. Increasingly uncommon with more intensive investigation.
Drugs: e.g., protease inhibitors	Diarrhea mild/mod, no weight loss
Kaposi's sarcoma (KS), lymphoma	KS may cause ulceration and chronic diarrhea, but usually asymptomatic
<u>Pancreatic insufficiency</u>	
Anorectal disease	
Chlamydia trachomatis, Neisseria gonorrhoeae	Most common in homosexual men
<u>Herpes simplex virus</u>	Perianal ulceration and proctitis
Human papilloma virus	Cause of anal warts, linked to anal Ca
Idiopathic ulcers	Usually when CD4 < 200/µl

Clinical feature

Broad categories of presentation include:

- **Esophageal disease:** dyspepsia/dysphagia/odynophagia (pain on swallowing: suggests esophageal ulceration (e.g., cytomegalovirus [CMV], herpes simplex virus [HSV]).
- **Abdominal pain.** Any cause of this in the nonHIV patient can, of course, be the culprit in the patient with HIV. Inflammation, ulceration, perforation of any point in GI tract may be caused by range of pathogens, including CMV. Acute pancreatitis due to HAART, CMV, or infiltration by Kaposi's sarcoma.
- **Diarrhea** occurred in 90% of patients in pre-HAART era. Still common; now related to side effects of HAART (20% in patients taking protease inhibitor nelfinavir), and causes not related to opportunistic infection/malignancy.
- **Anorectal disease:** most common in homosexual men with HIV, with increased risk of anal squamous cell carcinoma related to HPV.

Investigation

- CD4 count guides investigation and differential diagnosis (opportunistic infections unlikely if CD4 > 200/μl).
- Three stool samples for microscopy and culture essential in patients with diarrhea.
- Upper GI endoscopy in esophageal disease, and colonoscopy necessary if diarrhea persistent, stool samples negative, and CD4 > 200/μl. Classic appearances may suggest diagnosis endoscopically (e.g., large deep esophageal ulcers due to CMV), but histology necessary. Vital that pathologists are provided with details re HIV status, CD4 count, and suspected diagnosis. Check with referring clinicians re special requirements (e.g., biopsies into viral culture medium).

Management

- Effective treatment depends on making a specific diagnosis.
- In patient presenting with opportunistic infection, commencement of HAART, with subsequent immune reconstitution, may negate necessity of antimicrobials for opportunistic infection (e.g., _Cryptosporidium_).
- Candidal esophagitis treated with fluconazole 100 mg daily for a week, but maintenance often required. Active CMV disease treated with two- to three-week course of ganciclovir IV. Idiopathic ulceration responds well to oral or intralesional steroids.
- Treatment of diarrhea depends on isolating cause. Enteric pathogens (e.g., _Salmonella_, _Shigella_) treated with standard antibiotics, but treatment for protozoal infections (e.g., _Cryptosporidium_) less effective, particularly if low CD4.

Hypogammaglobulinemia

See: immunoglobulin deficiency.

Immunoglobulin deficiency

Congenital causes

X-linked (Bruton) defect of B-cell maturation resulting in absence of functional antibodies. Patients present with recurrent pyogenic infection in infancy or childhood: GI infections occur in 30%, usually with *Campylobacter* or less often *Giardia*. T-cell function is normal. There is an increased risk of lymphoma and leukemia.

Selective IgA deficiency has a prevalence of 1/500 to 1/3,000. Usually sporadic, reversible deficiency has been reported after phenytoin, and penicillamine. There is little if any increased risk of GI infection. There is an association with celiac disease and pernicious anemia. TTG IgA is not helpful for the diagnosis of celiac disease in this situation.

Acquired causes

Common variable immunodeficiency (CVID) usually involved defective terminal differentiation of B cells. Patients present in second or third decades with recurrent infections. Gastrointestinal disease is identified in approximately 20% of patients and may be the presenting disorder in some. GI symtoms may mimic inflammatory bowel disease (ulcerative colitis,, or Crohn's disease) or celiac disease; *Giardia* is common. There is increased risk of bacterial overgrowth, parasitic and bacterial enteric infection. Atrophic gastritris and pernicious anemia can develop.

Intestinal ischemia

Can be acute or chronic, due to arterial disease or venous disease, and can affect small bowel, colon, or both.

Collateral circulation to stomach, duodenum, and rectum accounts for rarity of ischemic episodes affecting these organs. The splenic flexure and sigmoid colon are most at risk.

Acute mesenteric ischemia

Usually arterial, most commonly superior artery embolus, less commonly nonocclusive mesenteric ischemia or thrombosis of SMA. Venous thrombosis accounts for only 5–10% of patients with acute mesenteric ischemia. Most patients with arterial thrombosis have significant generalized arteriosclerosis. Classic symptom is rapid onset of severe periumbilical abdominal pain out of proportion to findings on physical examination. Diagnosis requires high clinical suspicion. Rapid diagnosis essential. Usually CT scan and mesenteric angiography (gold standard). Goal of treatment is to restore blood flow as quickly as possible. Surgery should not be delayed in patients with suspected perforation or infarction. Mortality approaches 60%. Refer to AGA guidelines.[1]

Colonic ischemia (ischemic colitis). The commonest form of intestinal ischemia.

Clinical features. Sudden onset cramping pain in left lower quadrant, with bloody stools, and mild to moderate abdominal tenderness. Diagnosis is made by contrast-enhanced CT scanning and careful endoscopy, if necessary. Barium studies are less sensitive than colonoscopy; the classical "thumbprinting" disappears in days as submucosal hemorrhages are resorbed and overlying mucosa sloughs. Management is conservative (fluids IV, bowel rest, broad spectrum antibiotics) if there is no sign of perforation or infarction. More than 50% resolve on conservative management. Increasing tenderness, fever, ileus suggests infarction and mandate operative intervention.

Intestinal angina (chronic mesenteric ischemia)

Uncommon, causing pain due to small-bowel ischemia as gastric blood flow increases after a meal. Clinical features: classically pain within 30 minutes of eating, resolving over 1–3 h. The best test is angiography. Therapy includes balloon angioplasty +/– stenting versus surgery.

Vasculitis of splanchnic circulation

Polyarteritis nodosa and rheumatoid arthritis can affect large vessels and any cause of systemic vasculitis can cause small vessel occlusion and segmental ischemia.

Kayser–Fleischer rings

- Greenish-brown ring around edge of iris, best seen by ophthalmologist using slit lamp. Due to deposition of copper-containing pigment in Descemet's membrane at posterior surface of cornea.
- Found in 90% of people with Wilson disease, but also rarely seen in other conditions of chronic cholestasis (e.g., primary biliary cirrhosis).

1 American Gastroenterological Association Medical Position Statement: Guidelines on Intestinal Ischemia. Gastroenterology 2000;118:951. AGA Techincal Review on Intestinal Ischemia. *Gastroenterology* 2000;118:954.

Multiple endocrine neoplasia (MEN)

MEN should be considered in all patients with <u>pancreatic endocrine tumors</u>. Three main syndromes:

- **MEN-1** (Wermer syndrome). Autosomal dominant.
  Hyperparathyroidism in >90%, pancreatic neuroendocrine tumors (NET) in 80% (mainly <u>gastrinoma</u> and insulinoma), and pituitary adenomas (usually prolactin secreting). Gene defect on chromosome 11. Pancreas demonstrates diffuse microadenomatosis, but in those with Zollinger–Ellison syndrome 80% of gastrinomas are in duodenum, not pancreas.
- **MEN-2a** (Sipple syndrome). Pheochromocytoma (20–40%) and bilateral medullary thyroid carcinoma are characteristic.
- **MEN-2b:** similar to MEN-2a, but thyroid carcinoma at younger age and more aggressive, and additional Marfanoid features and mucosal neuromas.

Neuroendocrine tumors (NET)

Background

NETs within the GI tract classified into two main groups: <u>carcinoid tumors</u> and <u>pancreatic endocrine tumors</u>. These are discussed separately, although both types arise from neuroendocrine cells, and may be histologically indistinguishable. Particular systemic syndromes are caused by hormones and biogenic amines released from cytoplasmic membrane-bound neuro-secretory granules.

Investigation

- Aimed at identifying functional activity, and site of primary/metastatic tumor.
- Histology of tumors shows small cells with regular, round nuclei, which stain positive for neuroendocrine markers, including neuron-specific enolase, synaptophysin, and chromogranin.
- "<u>Gut hormone profile</u>" usually includes serum gastrin, vasoactive intestinal polypeptide (VIP), glucagon, somatostatin.
- <u>CT scan</u>/<u>MRI</u> cross-sectional imaging required in all cases, but may fail to identify small (<3 cm) NETs. <u>Endoscopic ultrasound</u> (FNA) increasingly used to define small pancreatic lesions.
- Scintigraphic scanning with radiolabelled meta-iodobenzylguanidine (MIBG) or octreotide (Octreoscan) may identify primary or metastatic NETs (particularly carcinoid, which has higher somatostatin receptor expression than most other NETs). <u>Positron emission tomography (PET)</u> scanning has low yield in NET, in view of low metabolic turnover of tumors.

Clinical features

May be asymptomatic (e.g., incidental lesion seen on abdominal CT), or present with syndromes related to hormone release, or mass effect of primary/metastatic disease.

Management
- Referral to specialist center for multidisciplinary approach.
- Surgical cure attempted for localized disease (see <u>carcinoid</u> and <u>pancreatic endocrine tumors</u>).
- Palliative approaches to metastatic NET include systemic chemotherapy, somatostatin analogues (e.g., octreotide), and ^{131}I-MIBG if diagnostic scintigraphy positive.
- Options for liver lesions (commonest site for NET metastases) include surgical resection, embolization, radiofrequency ablation, and rarely <u>liver transplantation</u>.

Osler–Weber–Rendu syndrome

See: <u>hereditary hemorrhagic telangiectasia</u>.

Osteoporosis and metabolic bone disease

See also: <u>bone densitometry</u>.

Definitions
- Osteoporosis refers to defective bone formation, defined by WHO as T-score > −2.5 standard deviations below the average (T-score compares bone mineral density (BMD) to controls with peak BMD (i.e., young fit adults), whereas Z-score matches for age and sex).
- Osteopenia refers to less severe reduction in BMD (see Table 8.4), but affects >15% of young women, and 40% >50 years.
- Osteomalacia refers to defective bone mineralization, due to vitamin D deficiency.

At risk groups in gastroenterology/hepatology
- Chronic cholestatic liver disease (e.g., <u>primary biliary cirrhosis</u> (PBC) and <u>primary sclerosing cholangitis</u> (PSC)). 20% of patients with PBC have osteoporosis at time of referral, and 50% have severe bone loss at time of <u>liver transplantation</u>. All patients with cirrhosis appear at risk.
- <u>Celiac disease</u>. Osteoporosis in 5–10%, and osteomalacia in association with vitamin D deficiency.
- Inflammatory bowel disease (<u>Crohn's disease</u> and <u>ulcerative colitis</u>). Disease activity, malnutrition, bowel resection, drugs (e.g., prednisone) all predispose to osteoporosis, but long-term steroid therapy appears main reason for ↓BMD, with 40% increase in fracture risk over controls.
- Postgastrectomy status (e.g., Billroth I/Billroth II partial <u>gastrectomy</u>). Calcium and vitamin D malabsorption may both contribute to osteomalacia in 10–20%, osteoporosis in > 30% > 10 years post-surgery.
- <u>Chronic pancreatitis</u>. Malabsorption of fat soluble vitamins.
- Malnutrition, low BMI, eating disorders.
- Long-standing steroid use (e.g., <u>autoimmune hepatitis</u> and see drugs).
- Any cause of <u>body mass index</u> (BMI) < 19, or physical inactivity.

Investigation
- Bloods
  - Serum calcium. Usually normal in osteoporosis.
  - Parathyroid hormone (PTH). ↑ PTH, with ↓serum phosphate, and normal/↓ calcium suggests secondary hyperparathyroidism, vitamin D deficiency, and osteomalacia.
  - 25-(OH) vitamin D. Deficiency usually dietary, contributing to osteomalacia.
  - LFTs. ↑ALP in presence of normal GGT suggests ALP of bone origin (e.g., in osteomalacia). ALP isoenzymes can be performed to differentiate bone from liver.
  - Thyroid function tests.
- Plain X-rays: osteopenia may be visible on plain X-rays, but only after 30–40% bone loss has occurred.
- <u>Bone densitometry</u>. Bone mineral density (BMD) most accurately assessed by bone densitometry using dual energy X-ray absorptiometry (DEXA), usually of femoral neck and lumbar spine. If steroid use planned (e.g., prednisolone 7.5 mg/day for > 3 months) baseline DEXA and follow-up DEXA in 6–12 months should be performed. Spine measurements unreliable in elderly due to presence of osteophytes, extraskeletal calcification, and spinal deformity.

Management
- Give oral calcium supplements (e.g., calcium carbonate 1–1.5 g/day) and vitamin D 800 IU if in at risk group. If T score >−2.5 repeat DEXA in two years; if T score <−2.5 consider additional therapy:
  - Hormone replacement therapy (HRT) in postmenopausal women.
  - Bisphosphonates (e.g., alendronate 70 mg/week). May be used in conjunction with calcium, vitamin D, and HRT.
  - Parathyroid hormone supplementation reserved for severe osteoporosis and fractures, if patient is unresponsive to bisphosphonates, and in absence of secondary hyperparathyroidism.
- Avoid smoking and excess alcohol.
- In patients with chronic liver disease, <u>liver transplantation</u> is associated with further reduction in BMD over first year, then improvement.

Table 8.5 WHO diagnostic criteria for osteoporosis

Normal	BMD value within 1 standard deviation (SD) of young-adult mean (T-score at or above −1)
Osteopenia	BMD value between −1 S.D. and −2.5 SD below young-adult mean (T-score between −1 and −2.5)
Osteoporosis	BMD value at least −2.5 SD below young adult mean (T-score at or below −2.5)
Severe osteoporosis	BMD value at least −2.5 SD below young adult mean and presence of fracture

Oxalate stones

- Dietary oxalate (found in tea, chocolate, cola, vegetables) is usually precipitated out as calcium oxalate in the bowel and lost in stool.
- In conditions associated with <u>bile acid malabsorption</u>, and thus fat <u>malabsorption</u> (e.g., <u>short-bowel syndrome</u>, terminal ileal <u>Crohn's disease</u>), unabsorbed long-chain fatty acids compete with oxalate for available calcium. As a result, larger amounts of free oxalate reach the colon, are absorbed, and ultimately excreted in the kidney. Hyperoxaluria then predisposes to calcium oxalate kidney stones (> 20% of patients with short-bowel syndrome).
- Urinary oxalate should be measured in at-risk patients (no risk if colon removed).
- Management involves restricting high-oxalate foods and maintaining adequate fluid intake. If hyperoxaluria continues, oral calcium citrate may be used to enhance oxalate precipitation.

Parkinson's disease and the GI tract

Parkinson's disease can be associated **with swallowing problems** and **constipation**. See also <u>elderly and the GI tract</u>.

- **Drooling** is a result of reduced swallowing, correlates with the severity of the Parkinsonism and can be severe. Anticholinergics can dry the mouth but may lead to confusion. Irradiation of the salivary glands is effective, as is botox injection.
- **Dysphagia** occurs in 50% of patients.
  - Oropharyngeal problems arise because of poor tongue control, difficulty in bolus formation, and delayed transit to the pharynx. Food retention in the pharynx and consequent aspiration is common.
  - Esophageal dysmotility is common in manometric studies and there may be incomplete relaxation of the lower esophageal sphincter. L-dopa may help the oropharyngeal phase of swallowing but does not always lead to improved swallowing.
- **Heartburn** and documented esophageal reflux are more common in Parkinson's disease.
- **Constipation** in Parkinson's is common and results from slow intestinal transit and sometimes from outflow obstruction due to pelvic-floor problems. It can be masked by overflow incontinence. It may result from degeneration of the myenteric plexus and be aggravated by anticholinergic drugs as well as by inadequate intake of fiber and fluids.

Pellagra

Due to poor intake of niacin (vitamin B3) or reduced conversion of tryptophan to niacin. This latter reaction requires riboflavin, thiamine, and pyridoxine and is inhibited by excess intake of leucine. Pellagra is a wasting disease with dermatitis of exposed areas due to photosensitivity. Fatigue, insomnia, and apathy can lead to hallucinations and psychosis. Widespread mucosal inflammation causes glossitis, stomatitis, vaginitis, and diarrhea. Can be associated with drugs (isoniazid) or carcinoid.

Polyarteritis nodosa (PAN) and the GI tract

PAN is a necrotizing vasculitis affecting small and medium-sized arteries with aneurysmal dilatations up to 1 cm seen on angiography. Abdominal symptoms, usually pain, occur in about 50% of cases. Mesenteric vessels are abnormal in 80% cases; GI bleeding from ischemia is seen in about 6% and perforation in 5%. Acalculous cholecystitis can occur in about 15%; acute pancreatitis, appendicitis, biliary strictures have all been reported. Polyarteritis is a recognized association of hepatitis B infection.

Porphyrias

- Rate-limiting step in heme production is conversion of porphyrins (comprising four pyrole rings) to ↓ amino-laevulinic acid (ALA), and heme provides negative feedback on ↓ ALA synthase.
- Deficiency of specific enzymes (including ↓ ALA synthase) leads to porphyrin accumulation. Porphyrias classified according to site of porphyrin accumulation (see Table 8.5) and pattern of symptoms (i.e., acute (neurovisceral) and cutaneous [photosensitive]).
- **Acute intermittent porphyria and porphyria cutanea tarda** most common in GI practice.

Acute intermittent porphyria (AIP)

Autosomal dominant, incidence highest in Scandinavia (1:1,000). Symptoms, even in heterozygotes, triggered by alcohol, surgery, fasting, drugs (e.g., sulphonamides, barbiturates, and many others).

Clinical features

- Abdominal pain. Severe, usually lasts several days, poorly localized, but no signs of peritonitis (see Acute abdominal pain). Nausea, constipation. Symptom-free between episodes.
- Tachycardia, sweating, hypertension during acute episode.
- Polyneuropathy (peripheral neuropathy, mononeuritis multiplex, cranial nerve palsy), epilepsy, agitation, anxiety, paranoia.

Table 8.6 Classification of porphyrias

Hepatic	Erythropoitic
Acute intermittent porphyria	X-linked sideroblastic anemia
Porphyria cutanea tarda	Congenital erythropoietic porphyria
Hereditary coproporphyria	Erythropoietic protoporphyria
Variegate porphyria	

Diagnosis
Never made unless considered carefully.
- CBC: ↑ WBC during acute attack.
- Chem: ↓ serum Na^+ may relate to syndrome of inappropriate ADH.
- Urine prophyrins: porphobilinogen (PBG) > x 4 ULN, and uroporphyrin and coproporphyrin moderately elevated during acute attack. Check that lab routinely does PBG on urine porphyrin screen (some don't!). PBG levels usually stay ↑ between attacks.

Management
- High-carbohydrate intake (oral, NG feed, or IV glucose infusion) inhibits heme synthesis. Total parenteral nutrition rarely required.
- Stop medications that exacerbate hepatic porphyria. Stop alcohol and tobacco.
- Opiate analgesia often required (see pain control).
- Infusion of heme (e.g., Hematin) in severe attack is effective, as provides negative feedback to heme synthesis, and so ↓ production of porphyrins.
- 60–80% of patients never have another attack, provided precipitants sought and avoided.

Porphyria cutanea tarda (PCT)
- Most common type of porphyria. Most cases either familial (25%) or sporadic (75%), but also linked with other conditions (e.g., alcohol, hepatitis C, hemochromatosis). Presents as scarring blisters in sun-exposed areas (often dorsum of hands, forearms, face).
- Uroporphyrin and coproporphyrin significantly ↑ in plasma and urine.
- Dermatology opinion and skin biopsy may aid diagnosis.
- Elevated iron levels (e.g., serum ferritin) may be found.
- Sun-protection, phlebotomy, or desferrioxamine chelation for iron overload, and chloroquine may be effective.

Pyoderma gangrenosum

A papule, pustule, or nodule, most often seen on the leg but sometimes around a stoma, which progresses to an ulcer with undermined borders. Often displays pathergy (development of ulcers in response to minor trauma). Associated with both <u>ulcerative colitis</u> and <u>Crohn's disease</u>, but often not associated with intestinal disease activity and not unique to these disorders. Responds to topical steroid application, oral steroids, and <u>INFLIXIMAB</u>.

Radiation damage to the GI tract

The bowel can be damaged by radiation treatment for a range of tumors, including cervical cancer, prostate cancer, or combined chemoradiotherapy for <u>rectal cancer</u>. The effects of radiation on intestinal tissue depend on several factors.

- Rate of cell division (cell turnover is higher in the small intestine, which is, therefore, more sensitive to radiation damage).
- Presence of genes regulating apoptosis (experimentally radiation-induced apoptosis depends on the presence of p53 and is inhibited by bcl2; the higher levels of bcl2 in the colon and rectum may explain the greater tolerance to radiation compared with the small intestine).
- Ionizing radiation activates inflammatory and fibrogenic cytokines. TGFβ promotes fibrosis by stimulating collagen synthesis and chemotaxis of fibroblasts.

Epidemiology

Acute radiation enteritis is common (incidence 20–70%), usually occurs in the third week of a fractionated course, and is rarely life threatening unless there is pancytopenia and sepsis secondary to chemotherapy. It usually resolves 2–6 weeks after completion of radiotherapy.

Chronic radiation enteritis varies in incidence from 1–15% and the latency may range from 6 months to 25 years. Predisposing factors include older age, postoperative radiation, collagen vascular disease, combined chemotherapy, and poor radiation technique. Prolapse of small bowel into the pelvis after surgery exposes large volumes of bowel to radiation.

Pathology

Occlusive vasculitis and diffuse collagen deposition with fibrosis. Changes are progressive and result in mucosal ulceration, necrosis, and sometimes perforation.

Clinical features

- Fibrosis and vasculitis can lead to strictures and malabsorption.
- Fistulae and abscesses are serious complications that may need surgery.

- <u>Bacterial overgrowth may</u> be due to dilated bowel loops proximal to stricture.
- Patients with a history of pelvic irradiation can present with rectal bleeding due to mucosal friability or telangiectasia. They may have anorectal pain, tenesmus, or fecal urgency. Chronic inflammation can lead to reduced rectal capacity and diarrhea.

Diagnosis

Not always straightforward.

- Analysis of the treatment plan and dose distribution may show areas of high dose, and lesions found on imaging or endoscopy are usually localized to these areas.
- Recurrence of cancer often needs exclusion because the manifestations of chronic radiation colitis are nonspecific. Mucosal ulceration and thickening of small-bowel loops are radiological signs of radiation damage. Imaging requires adequate luminal distension: CT <u>enteroclysis</u> with infusion of contrast through a naso-enteric tube is probably the best single investigation, with good sensitivity and specificity for diagnosing recurrent tumor and low-grade or intermittent obstruction. It can also help in suggesting the source of occult bleeding.
- Colonoscopy is helpful if there is rectal bleeding and can help in diagnosing the cause of stricturing as well as looking for recurrent or further new primary tumors.

Management

- Be as conservative as possible: surgery is difficult and associated with high morbidity rate. Management of pelvic fistulae is complex and requires diversion before corrective surgery.
- Diarrhea can result from fast transit time, <u>bile acid malabsorption</u>, and <u>lactose intolerance</u>. Loperamide can help.
- Antibiotics can help if there is <u>bacterial overgrowth</u>.
- <u>Laser</u> therapy or <u>argon plasma coagulation</u> (APC) can control rectal bleeding due to radiation proctitis, and recent reports suggest that <u>SUCRALFATE</u> enemas or local formalin treatment (given under general anesthetic) may be of help.
- Hyperbaric oxygen stimulates new blood vessel formation and is being evaluated. Small-bowel transplantation might offer hope to a small number of pediatric patients with radiation enteritis.

Prevention is the best treatment.

- Surgical fixing of small-bowel loops out of the pelvis and any radiation field is possible by placing a biodegradable mesh that supports the small intestine out of the pelvis.
- Pharmacological agents conferring protection against the effects of ionizing radiation (e.g., amifostine) are attractive but unproven.

Refeeding syndrome

- Insulin secretion is reduced in starvation due to reduced carbohydrate intake: fat and protein are catabolized to produce energy. This results in intracellular loss of electrolytes, especially phosphate.
- Feeding results in increased insulin, which stimulates cellular uptake of phosphate. This usually occurs within four days of refeeding. Serum phosphate below 1 mg/dl can produce clinical features of rhabdomyolysis, leucocyte dysfunction, respiratory failure, cardiac failure, hypotension, muscle weakness, arrhythmias, and seizures.
- Refeeding syndrome can occur with parenteral or enteral feeding: patients with <u>anorexia</u>, cancer, <u>alcohol dependency</u> and patients who have commenced <u>PEG</u> feeding after prolonged neurological dysphagia are at risk.

Treatment involves intravenous phosphate: give 2.5 mg/kg over six hours. The plasma phosphate should be monitored every six hours and the patient should be switched to oral phosphate replacement when the plasma phosphate is 2–2.5 mg/dl.

Acute vitamin and mineral deficiencies can be precipitated by feeding without appropriate micronutrients. Folate deficiency can result in megaloblastosis and thrombocytopenia: vitamin B12 deficiency can result in lactic acidosis.

Reiter's syndrome

Hans Reiter, 1916. A triad of arthritis, urethritis, and conjunctivitis occurring after bacillary dysentery or venereal disease. Urethritis can be mild or absent and periostitis, tendonitis, and plantar fasciitis can accompany arthritis.

- Commonest in males aged 20–40 years who are HLA-B27 positive (see box). Complicates 1–2% of cases of <u>Shigella</u>; also reported after *Salmonella*, *Yersinia*, and *Campylobacter* infection.
- Presentation is usually with symmetrical lower limb arthropathy two to four weeks after bacterial dysentery. Antibiotic therapy usually not indicated as the enteric infection has resolved. The arthritis tends to be chronic and relapsing: treatment involves symptomatic relief and nonsteroidals.

Box 8.5 **HLA B27 and enteric arthropathy**

- <u>Reiter's syndrome</u>. 80% are positive for HLAB27: conversely about 20% of HLA-B27 patients will develop Reiter's after bacillary dysentery
- Ankylosing spondylitis and <u>ulcerative colitis</u>
- Sacroiliitis complicating <u>Whipple's disease</u>
- <u>Behçet's syndrome</u>

Rheumatoid arthritis (RA) and the GI tract

GI manifestations of the disease

Temporomandibular arthritis can impair chewing. Esophageal dysmotility results from low-amplitude peristalsis and reduced lower esophageal sphincter pressure. Vasculitis affects 1% of rheumatoid patients: in 10% of these GI involvement results in cholecystitis, colitis, or ruptured visceral aneurysm. Amyloidosis can result in pseudo-obstruction or malabsorption (see Malabsorption and steatorrhea). See also Felty's syndrome and Still's disease.

GI problems of drug therapy for RA

Endoscopic lesions are seen in 20–40% of rheumatoid patients who take NSAIDs: risk is increased by age over 60, history of peptic ulcer, use of steroids, and extra-articular manifestations. _Helicobacter pylori_ is probably an independent risk factor for peptic ulceration in rheumatoid patients. In the past, use of gold was associated with GI toxicity, especially colitis. METHOTREXATE can cause hepatic fibrosis in cumulative doses over 1.5 g.

Scleroderma and the GI tract

Connective tissue proliferation with fibrosis in the GI tract results in GI manifestations in 80% of scleroderma patients, often with more than 1 site affected. Treatment is symptomatic and supportive only, and often very difficult.

- **Esophagus.** Abnormal peristalsis results in gastro-esophageal reflux (GERD), intermittent dysphagia, and often stricturing. Esophageal manometry shows lack of propagated swallows and low-amplitude contractions. High dose PPIs needed to control reflux: dose–response curve is better for omeprazole than other PPIs in this context. Omeprazole 40 mg bid may be needed. Prokinetics theoretically increase lower esophageal sphincter tone and speed gastric emptying but may not work.
- **Stomach.** Reduced gastric emptying is common and aggravates GERD. Prokinetics should be tried. Erythromycin is a motilin agonist and can speed gastric emptying. If there is intractable early satiety, low volume overnight PEG feeding can be very helpful: one useful maneuver is to place a jejunal extension through the PEG.
- **Small bowel.** Reduced motility, jejunal diverticulae, and consequent bacterial overgrowth may cause bloating, cramps, or signs of malabsorption. Barium studies useful (follow-through shows a classical "stacked coin" appearance). Bacterial overgrowth can be treated with low-dose antibiotics (tetracycline 250 mg bid for 10 days or metronidazole 500 mg bid). Bacterial culture and sensitivities rarely useful. Prokinetics can be tried. Pseudo-obstruction sometimes seen

and in worst cases parenteral nutrition needed. Malabsorption may be aggravated by <u>pancreatic insufficiency</u> (pancreatic exocrine output ↓ in 30%).
- **Large bowel.** Colon may be atonic and severe constipation is common. Thinning and fibrosis of anal sphincters is common and may explain an increased incidence of passive fecal incontinence.

Sickle cell anemia (SCA)

May be linked with a range of GI problems, due to the effects of hemolysis and ischemia, or the consequences of recurrent transfusion.

Clinical features
- Chronic asymptomatic jaundice in SCA may relate to hemolysis and intrahepatic cholestasis.
- <u>Acute abdominal pain</u> due to range of causes (see Box 8.6).
- Sickling or sequestration within liver presents with severe right upper quadrant pain, tender hepatomegaly, jaundice.
- Splenomegaly may occur due to sequestration or <u>portal hypertension</u>, but splenic infarction and hyposplenism usually develop by adulthood.
- <u>Gallstones</u> in > 30% of adults, with increased rates of <u>cholecystitis</u>, <u>choledocholithiasis</u>, and <u>acute pancreatitis</u>.
- <u>Hepatitis B</u> , <u>hepatitis C</u>, and <u>HIV</u> at increased frequency.
- Secondary <u>hemochromatosis</u> may result from recurrent transfusion.

Investigations
Diagnosis of SCA usually established in childhood. Specific investigations depend on clinical presentation. In those with jaundice, general rules apply (see <u>Recent onset jaundice</u>).
- CBC. Typical Hb 6–8 g/dl, reticulocytes 10–20%. Sickling test detects HbS. Marked decrease in Hb with abdominal pain may suggest sequestration crisis.
- LFTs. Bilirubin may be massively ↑ (> 35 mg/dl); AST/ALT usually <1000 U/l unless hepatic ischemia/infarction or acute hepatitis.
- U/S or CT useful to exclude biliary obstruction, hepatic infarction, or vascular occlusion (e.g., <u>Budd–Chiari syndrome</u>, <u>portal vein thrombosis</u>).
- Iron studies (e.g., serum ferritin) may suggest overload (see <u>hemochromatosis</u>).
- <u>Liver biopsy</u> rarely necessary, but may show sinusoidal dilatation and sickling and/or fibrosis with <u>cirrhosis</u>.

Management
- Seek expert hematology input.
- Acute sickling crisis or sequestration treated with exchange transfusion (with aim to reduce HbS to < 30%), IV fluids, and adequate <u>pain control</u> (usually <u>OPIATES</u>). Keep warm, well oxygenated, and treat precipitant to crisis (e.g., infection).
- Specific management depends on diagnosis (e.g., see <u>hepatitis B</u>, <u>hepatitis C</u>, <u>hemochromatosis</u>, <u>gallstones</u>, <u>choledocholithiasis</u>).

Box 8.6 Causes of acute abdominal pain in sickle cell anemia

- Hepatic sickling/sequestration
- Splenic sickling/sequestration
- Cholecystitis
- Acute pancreatitis
- Renal vein thrombosis
- Budd–Chiari syndrome
- Hepatic artery thrombosis/hepatic infarction
- Portal vein thrombosis
- Mesenteric ischemia/infarction

Sjögren's/sicca syndrome

Lymphocytic infiltration of salivary glands causes keratoconjunctivitis and dry mouth. Dysphagia occurs in 75%: mostly due to esophageal dysmotility but there is also an increased incidence of esophageal rings/webs. Chronic atrophic gastritis can occur, as can acute and chronic pancreatitis (perhaps as association with autoimmune pancreatitis); exocrine pancreatic secretion is often impaired. Primary biliary cirrhosis is more common in patients with Sjögren's.

Still's disease

The adult form of rheumatoid arthritis often has GI manifestations such as weight loss (75%), sore throat, hepatomegaly (45%), abnormal liver blood tests (75%), and abdominal pain (50%). Liver failure can be associated with aspirin or NSAID therapy.

Systemic lupus erythematosus (SLE) and the GI tract

Clinical features

- Anorexia, nausea, and vomiting occur in 50% but may be due to disease or treatment. Mouth ulcers are common and usually painless. Sjögren's syndrome and dry mouth occur in 20%.
- Esophageal symptoms are common, but do not correlate well with results of esophageal manometry. In contrast to scleroderma, lower esophageal sphincter is rarely involved.
- Risk of peptic ulceration is increased by combined NSAID and steroid use. PPIs are indicated for gastroprotection.
- Most dangerous manifestation of intestinal involvement is vasculitis (2% prevalence, mortality 50%: commonest in territory of superior mesenteric artery, though classically small vessels are involved), which

can progress to ulceration, hemorrhage, perforation, and infarction. Although rare overall in SLE, an acute abdominal presentation may often reflect vasculitis, especially if there is active disease elsewhere. A smaller proportion of acute abdominal presentations is caused by intra-abdominal thrombosis, either secondary to vasculitis or to antiphospholipid syndrome (see portal vein thrombosis). There is an increased incidence of inflammatory bowel disease in patients with SLE, most often ulcerative colitis. Protein-losing enteropathy and fat malabsorption can also occur.

Investigation. Look for thumbprinting on a plain X-ray which suggests ischemic bowel. Check inflammatory markers. A CT can show abscesses, lymphadenopathy, serositis, bowel-wall thickening, pancreatic pathology, and hepato-splenomegaly. Visceral angiography usually does not help but colonoscopy with biopsy can diagnose vasculitis.

Management. Treatment of vasculitis with IV pulsed steroids can be effective, but vital to exclude infection (e.g., with stool and blood cultures) beforehand.

Systemic mastocytosis

Results from excessive histamine and prostacyclin release from inappropriate mast cell proliferation in skin, bones, lymph nodes. The classic skin sign is multiple red-brown papules or urticaria pigmentosa. 80% have GI symptoms of nausea, vomiting, diarrhea, or abdominal pain. May present with steatorrhea (see Malabsorption and steatorrhea). Symptoms are often brought on by alcohol. There may be hepatomegaly and portal hypertension. Diagnosis is by measuring urinary histamine levels.

Tylosis

- Autosomal dominant disease characterized by hyperkeratosis of palms and the soles of feet.
- Associated high incidence of esophageal, bronchial, and laryngeal cancer, often at a younger age than usual (esophageal cancer in > 90% of cases by 65 years—see esophageal tumors).
- Endoscopic surveillance suggested from age 30\, repeating every three years.

Vasculitis and the GI tract

- Inflammation and necrosis can affect splanchnic blood vessels of all sizes from capillaries to larger arteries. Involvement of medium or large arteries (by e.g., polyarteritis nodosum, rheumatoid arthritis) may be confused with ischemic insults (thrombosis or embolism) but look for systemic features (renal involvement, cutaneous nodules, rheumatoid factor).
- Typically vasculitis is caused by deposition of immune complexes in the walls of vessels, leading to complement activation and an inflammatory reaction that can result in aneurysm formation, vessel rupture, vascular occlusion, and fibrosis.

Box 8.7 Diseases involving GI vasculitis

- Behçet's syndrome
- Polyarteritis nodosa
- Rheumatoid arthritis
- Scleroderma
- Systemic lupus

Visceral arteridides: Churg-Strauss, Henoch–Schönlein Purpura, Wegener's granulomatosis, cryoglobulinemia, familial Mediterranean fever.

Veno-occlusive disease (VOD)

- Hepatic VOD occurs in 10–50% of patients following bone marrow transplantation, usually within first 20 days, and severe cases carry a 90% mortality. Pathogenesis involves fibrosis and obliteration of terminal hepatic venules, due to deposition of coagulation factors, red cells, and hemosiderin-laden macrophages.
- Presentation may be similar to that of acute Budd–Chiari syndrome (BCS), with jaundice, tender hepatomegaly, and ascites. Acute liver failure and multiorgan involvement may occur.
- Liver function tests often show ALT/AST (deranged LFTs >20 days post-BMT also require consideration of graft versus host disease (GVHD)). Doppler U/S may show reversal of portal vein flow, but hepatic venous flow is normal. Transjugular liver biopsy (with portal pressure measurements) may make the diagnosis.
- Treatment has traditionally been supportive, but defibrotide shows considerable promise. This drug binds to vascular endothelial cells, enhancing factors that contribute to fibrinolysis and suppressing those that promote coagulation.

Wernicke's encephalopathy (WE)

- Results from <u>vitamin</u> B1 (thiamine) deficiency. Predominantly found in malnourished patients with <u>alcohol dependency</u> or <u>alcohol-related liver disease</u> (reduced hepatic thiamine storage capacity). May be mistaken for drunkenness.
- Clinical triad (only present in 30%) of ophthalmoplegia (horizontal nystagmus, conjugate gaze palsy, fixed pupils, paralysis of lateral rectus muscles), ataxia (wide based cerebellar gait, with vestibular dysfunction), and cognitive impairment (apathy, spatial disorientation, global confusion).
- Diagnosis is usually clinical, but red-cell transketolase low.
- Potentially fatal if untreated, and 80% subsequently develop Korsakoff psychosis, characterized by retrograde and antegrade amnesia.
- Give parenteral vitamins B and C for rapid correction of severe depletion.
- Acute WE may be precipitated by high carbohydrate load (e.g., IV dextrose in hospital), so vital to administer thiamine if any clinical suspicion of deficiency. Check serum magnesium, and treat if low as thiamine may be ineffective with hypomagnesemia.

Whipple's disease

George Whipple, 1878–1976. Described disease in 1907. Suggested role of bacteria, but this was not proven until 1997. Won Nobel prize for work on <u>pernicious anemia</u>.

- A systemic infection caused by the Gram-positive bacterium *Tropheryma whippelii*. A rare disease (incidence about 0.5 per million per year), it tends to affect middle-aged men: 30% are in farming-related trades. Acquisition is presumed to be oral but this has not been proven.
- The nature of the bacterium was obscure until the 1990s when 16S ribosomal sequencing revealed bacterial DNA related to actinomycetes. The doubling time of the bacterium is very long (18 days).
- Infected people have subtle immune defects in Th1 function, but whether this predisposes them to disease or is a consequence of infection is unclear.

Clinical features

Whipple's disease may affect several organ systems.

- **GI tract.** Malabsorption syndrome with gradual weight loss, diarrhea (steatorrhea or watery stool), and abdominal pain. Occult blood loss is common. Mesenteric and retroperitoneal lymphadenopathy are common.

- **Central nervous system.** Progressive dementia, ophthalmoplegia, and psychiatric symptoms. (Of note, CSF usually normal on examination, although PCR for *T. whippelii* can be positive.)
- **Cardiovascular system.** Endocarditis, myocarditis, or pericarditis.
- **Musculoskeletal system.** Seronegative polyarthralgia is common.

Investigation

Endoscopy. White or yellow patches due to lipid deposits may be seen at upper GI endoscopy. Multiple duodenal biopsy essential, and biopsy shows swollen macrophage cytoplasm, which contains many lysosomes stuffed with *T. whipplei*; these stain positive with PAS. Specific PCR-based assays have been developed. Disorders mimicking the histology of Whipple's are uncommon and include infection with *Mycobacterium avium* and histoplasmosis.

Treatment and prognosis. Initial response to antibiotics is rapid (diarrhea resolving within days, arthralgia within weeks, weight gain within one to two months). Tetracyclines were initially used, but CNS relapses were common and difficult to treat: current recommendations are for benzylpenicillin plus streptomycin or a third-generation cephalosporin to induce remission (success rate over 90%), followed by an antibiotic that crosses the blood–brain barrier for at least one year. Relapse rate approximately 5% in retrospective studies.

Vaccine use in the immunocompromised

- In general, live vaccines should not be given to immunocompromised people or pregnant women.
- Immunocompromised people should probably not receive yellow fever vaccine because of a (theoretical) risk of vaccine-induced encephalomyelitis. This includes patients with HIV (see <u>HIV and the gut</u>).
- Inactivated <u>hepatitis A</u> vaccine is safe and effective and should be given to all travelers to endemic areas, all patients with chronic liver disease, injection drug users, patients requiring clotting factors, and men who have sex with men (MSM).
- If indicated (health care workers, long stay in endemic area, high risk of sexual transmission, high risk of hospitalization in endemic area), <u>hepatitis B</u> vaccine is safe in immunocompromised persons.
- In general cholera vaccination is not recommended for most travelers: exceptions are those with reduced gastric acid or the immunocompromised.

Procedures

Anorectal manometry

An important technique in the evaluation of problems with defecation. Perfused probes or pressure-sensitive transducers are introduced into rectum to record anal sphincter pressures, sensitivity to rectal distension, and the presence of the recto-anal inhibitory reflex.

Clinical assessment of anal sphincter tone by digital examination is very inaccurate, so manometry is indicated in patients complaining of <u>constipation</u> or <u>fecal incontinence</u>, where clinical assessment of sphincter function is important. Resting anal pressures and maximal voluntary squeeze pressures can be measured. If there is a high resting pressure, the normal reflex relaxation response to rectal distension is assessed; this is absent in <u>Hirschsprung's disease</u>. High threshold for initiation of reflex anal relaxation may indicate a problem with rectal compliance (e.g., Hirschsprung's megarectum) or afferent sensory pathways (e.g., spinal cord injuries). Defects in voluntary squeeze suggest abnormal innervation of the external sphincter. A normal voluntary squeeze but low resting pressure suggests a problem in the internal sphincter, which can occur after hemorrhoid surgery or in conditions such as diabetes and systemic sclerosis. In constipated patients with normal resting pressure and normal recto-anal inhibitory reflex, anatomical abnormalities, such as accentuated puborectalis angulation or internal <u>rectal prolapse,</u> should be considered.

Antibiotic prophylaxis in endoscopy

Antibiotic prophylaxis solely to prevent infective endocarditis (IE) is no longer recommended before endoscopic procedures (ASGE 2008, AHA 2007). Only patients with an established source for enterococcus infection, and who have a cardiac condition associated with the highest risk of an adverse outcome from IE (see Box 9.1.1), should be considered for IE prophylaxis.

Indications for antibiotic prophylaxis prior to endoscopy to prevent *other* infectious complications include:
- Biliary obstruction with anticipated incomplete drainage at <u>ERCP</u> (e.g., <u>primary sclerosing cholangitis</u>).
- <u>Sterile pancreatic fluid collection drainage via ERCP or transmural puncture.</u>
- <u>Endoscopic ultrasound</u>-guided aspiration of cystic lesions.
- Percutaneous Endoscopic Gastrostomy placement.

Box 9.1.1 Conditions associated with higher risk of adverse outcomes from endocarditis:

- A prosthetic cardiac valve
- A history of previous IE
- Cardiac transplant recipients who develop cardiac valvulopathy
- Patients with congenital heart disease (CHD), including:
    (a) those with unrepaired cyanotic CHD (including palliative shunts and conduits)
    (b) those with completely repaired CHD with prosthetic material or device, placed surgically or by catheter, for the first six months after the procedure
    (c) those with repaired CHD with residual defects at the site or adjacent to the site of a prosthetic patch or device.

Box 9.1.2 Suggested antibiotic regimens for prevention of infectious complications in GI endoscopy:

IE prophylaxis
Amoxicillin 2 g (or vancomycin 1 g) one hour before procedure

Incomplete biliary drainage
Amoxicillin 2 g and gentamicin 1.5 mg/kg one hour before procedure (or vancomycin 1 g if penicillin-allergic), and repeat amoxicillin 1 g six hours after the procedure

EUS-FNA of cystic lesion
Flouroquinolone e.g., ciprofloxacin 500 mg

PEG
Cefuroxime 750 mg IV 30 minutes before procedure

Antireflux procedures

In those patients with persistent problems related to gastro-esophageal reflux, despite maximal medical therapy (see Dyspepsia and gastro-esophageal reflux), a range of mechanical interventions are available. These aim to reverse mechanical and physiological abnormalities of gastro-esophageal reflux disease (which should be proven by esophageal manometry). Endoscopic and surgical options are available.

Endoscopic approach

Endoscopic gastroplication is currently the only commercially available endoscopic antireflux device (Endocinch, BARD). It involves placing a series of sutures at the gastro-esophageal junction via an endoscopic suturing device. Although modestly effective, long-term efficacy results are limited to two years, and up to half of all patients resume antacid therapy. Other approaches to endoscopic antireflux have been discontinued due to safety concerns or poor uptake.

Surgical approach

Procedure performed laparoscopically or as open operation, and involves mobilization of lower esophagus, reduction of hiatus hernia, and wrapping of gastric fundus around lower esophagus, either totally (e.g., Nissan 360° fundoplication) or partially (e.g., Toupet 270° fundoplication). Re-establishes competence of antireflux barrier and increases resting lower-esophageal sphincter pressure.

Patient selection difficult, because there is no direct comparisons of medical therapy versus antireflux surgery, but indications may include:

- Failed medical therapy, with persistent symptomatic <u>esophagitis</u>.
- Young healthy patient who responds to medical therapy, but unable/ unwilling to take long-term medication.
- Recurrent reflux complications (e.g., laryngitis, asthma, pneumonia).

Complications include dysphagia and air trapping, which may require reoperation, and have been reported in >10% following laparoscopic fundoplication. Mortality rate of 0.2%, is of significance in a condition that runs a benign course in the great majority. No good evidence that surgical fundoplication reduces risk of <u>esophageal tumors</u>.

Argon plasma coagulation (APC)

An approach for the endoscopic treatment of bleeding and superficial mucosal lesions. Allows controlled noncontact electrocoagulation by means of high-frequency energy delivered to tissue through ionized gas. Application and control is easier than for free-beam lasers, but depth of tissue injury is more superficial and not sufficient to effect relief of dysphagia associated with esophageal carcinoma. Particular use for angiodysplasia, gastric antral vascular ectasia, and bleeding related to radiation damage.

Balloon dilatation

See: <u>endoscopic dilatation</u>.

Barium contrast studies

Contrast studies of the GI tract can be performed using single- or double-contrast techniques. Barium is the agent of choice unless there are worries about bowel viability or perforation, in which case barium is avoided because free barium in the peritoneal cavity causes an inflammatory reaction. Single contrast uses low density barium to look for filling defects or contour abnormalities. Double contrast uses smaller amounts of high-contrast barium with gas and gives much better resolution of fine mucosal detail.

Barium swallow and contrast examination of the upper GI tract

Traditionally a barium swallow was the initial investigation of dysphagia but with the use of endoscopic intubation under direct vision most clinicians now use endoscopy as first choice of investigation. However, video fluoroscopy with water-soluble contrast is the preferred method of assessing swallowing dysfunction.

Contrast studies can be useful in demonstrating a sliding hiatus hernia or gastro-esophageal reflux, and in giving information about strictures that may be impassable endoscopically, e.g., in the esophagus or duodenum.

Small-bowel studies

The traditional techniques of small-bowel meal and small-bowel enteroclysis remain very useful in evaluating a variety of small-bowel diseases including tumors; inflammatory pathology, such as Crohn's disease; and Meckel's diverticulum. CT or MRI enterography are supplanting the traditional small-bowel series in many centers. Contrast studies can be useful in diagnosing the level of small-bowel obstruction, although, in this situation, water-soluble contrast should be used. The diagnostic yield of small-bowel contrast studies in obscure GI bleeding is poor and techniques of enteroscopy or capsule endoscopy are preferred.

Barium studies of the colon

This technique is becoming less common because of the availability of colonoscopy and the development of CT colonography, but the barium enema remains a commonly used technique for evaluating the colon. Contraindications include toxic megacolon, ischemic colitis, or other diseases in which the bowel wall is friable and more likely to perforate.

Biofeedback

A process of behavioral retraining (usually applied in gastroenterology to toileting behavior) using sensory training, electromyographic feedback, or manometric feedback. The sensory component teaches the patient to perceive smaller volumes of rectal distension, which are often insensible to constipated patients. The motor component is performed with a pressure probe in the anal canal, to monitor anal sphincter pressure. Patients become accustomed to visual feedback of sphincter activity on voluntary sphincter contraction. This can demonstrate failure of sphincter relaxation or failure of pelvic floor function and many patients can be taught to improve this. About two-thirds of patients with long-term intractable constipation report improvement with the technique. Technique is less successful in patients with psychiatric co-morbidity or poor compliance with home practice.

Bone densitometry

See also <u>osteoporosis</u>. A method of measuring bone mineral density (BMD) to detect osteopenia or <u>osteoporosis</u>, which can be expressed as the number of standard deviations (SD) above or below the mean BMD for young adults (T score) or the mean BMD for age-matched controls (Z score). The risk of fracture increases two to three times for each SD decrease in BMD. WHO criteria for defining osteoporosis includes a T score in the hip and/or spine that is 2.5 or more SD below young adult mean value. Osteopenia is a T score of 1 to 2.5 SD below mean value. The best technique currently involves dual energy X-ray absorptiometry (DEXA). Note that lumbar spine measurements are unreliable in the elderly due to presence of osteophytes, extraskeletal calcification, and vertebral or spinal deformity.

Bougies

General term used for dilators of luminal strictures in the GI tract. Derived from the Algerian town of Bouginhay, medieval capital of the wax candle trade, because wax dilators were used in the middle ages for food impaction. A cork-tipped whalebone was used to dilate an achalasia patient in the sixteenth century. Bougies are widely used in <u>endoscopic dilatation</u>.

Bowel preparation

Bad bowel prep is the bane of colonoscopy. Some sort of bowel preparation is almost always needed. For examination of the left colon a phosphate enema should be given 15–60 minutes pre-procedure but, in patients with diverticular disease or strictures, full bowel prep may be needed. Frail, ill, and elderly may need inpatient preparation.

- **Modification to diet and medication.** Iron should be stopped 1 week prior to colonoscopy. Constipating agents should be avoided for 24 hours preprocedure: some centers suggest stopping antiplatelet agents, including aspirin, for seven days to reduce the risk of immediate or delayed bleeding after polypectomy, but this is not evidence based and not part of current guidelines. Colon cleansing is aided by a liquid diet for 24 hours prior to examination.
- **Purgative regimens** – see Table 9.1.1.

Table 9.1.1 Bowel cleansing regimens for colonoscopy

Preparation	Advantages	Disadvantages	Notes
Nonabsorbable carbohydrate (mannitol, lactulose sorbital) act as osmotic laxatives)	Avoids cramping effects of purgatives	Sweet, unpalatable in large volume needed	Not recommended— hydrogen gas produced by fermentation gives risk of explosion during electrosurgical procedures
Polyethlylene glycol based solutions (e.g., Golytlely)	Safe, effective	Large volume (4 l) often difficult for patients to manage	Widely used
Magnesium salts—have strong purgative and osmotic effects	Magnesium citrate has a milder flavor than magnesium sulphate	Need to drink 2 l of fluid	Should be avoided in patients with renal impairment
Low volume sodium phosphate	Well tolerated—2 x 45 ml aliquots of sodium phosphate taken orally the evening before and 4 hours prior to conlonoscopy produce a vigorous catharsis	Fluid balance shifts or hyper-phosphataemia can be significant, especially in the presence of cardiac or renal disease	Should be avoided in elderly patients, especially those taking ACE inhibitors or with diabetes. Has been reported to cause renal failure in these populations

---

Box 9.1.3 General advice given to patients on preparing for colonoscopy

- Stop Iron tablets seven days before the exam; continue all other medications and laxatives until the procedure.
- Taka a low residue diet for one to two days before the examination (no cereals, nuts, or muesli).
- No solid food after lunch on the day preceding the colonoscopy, but take plenty of clear fluids to avoid dehydration.
- After the exam, it is better not to use public transport, but if essential the patient MUST be accompanied.
- No alcohol or operation of heavy machinery for 24 hours after procedure.
- No driving on day of procedure if sedation has been given or signing of legal documents.

Breath tests

A wide variety of volatile compounds in expired air relate to aspects of digestive function. For urea breath tests, see _Helicobacter_.

Hydrogen breath tests. Sole source of hydrogen in mammals is bacterial fermentation. Increased breath hydrogen can be easily detected using a hand-held meter and does not involve radioactive substrates. A rise of breath hydrogen of > 20 parts per million (ppm) compared with baseline after oral ingestion of 50 g lactose identifies lactose intolerance.

An early rise in breath hydrogen is seen within two hours of glucose or lactulose ingestion in patients with small intestinal bacterial overgrowth (all people show a late rise due to colonic fermentation); conventional testing uses a rise of 20 ppm, which has good specificity but poor sensitivity especially if low doses (< 20 g) of test carbohydrate are used. Sensitivity can be improved by ensuring the dinner preceding the overnight fast contains readily absorbed carbohydrates to avoid a high basal level on the day of the test, measuring the increase at six hours rather than at four and having a cutoff of 10 ppm over baseline for diagnosing malabsorption. Despite these precautions and the attractions of ease of performance and avoidance of a radioactive tracer, many authorities regard hydrogen breath tests as insufficiently sensitive or specific.

Carbon breath tests. The ^{14}C-triolein breath test measures $^{14}CO_2$ in breath after ingestion of labeled trigyceride. The test utility is insufficient to justify the equipment expense and radiation exposure, and the test is not widely used. The sugar xylose is catabolized by aerobic Gram-negative overgrowth flora; following a 1 g oral dose of ^{14}C-D-xylose, elevated $^{14}CO_2$ is found in 85% of people with small-bowel bacterial overgrowth.

Capsule endoscopy

Wireless capsule endoscopy has been a significant advance in recent years, providing the possibility of visualizing areas of the bowel inaccessible to conventional flexible endoscopy (i.e., most of small bowel). The 11 x 26 mm capsule is swallowed and video images are transmitted to a data recorder worn on patient's belt for approximately eight hours. Precise role relative to other diagnostic modalities is being investigated, but diagnostic yield of capsule endoscopy is superior to push enteroscopy for defining obscure small-bowel bleeding in those with negative endoscopy and colonoscopy (68% compared to 32%).

Detailed comparisons of capsule endoscopy with a combined approach of push enteroscopy and radiological examination of the small bowel are ongoing, and further developments in flexible enteroscopy (e.g., double-balloon enteroscopy (DBE)) may also influence relative merits of techniques. Capsule carries disadvantage of not allowing biopsy, and technique is contraindicated in patients with suspected significant intestinal strictures, as capsule may precipitate mechanical obstruction. The International

Consensus on Capsule Endoscopy (Mergener et al. Endoscopy 2007) has published recommendations for the use of this test in different clinical scenarios.

Chromoendoscopy

Endoscopic spraying of the gastrointestinal tract with contrast dyes can highlight subtle irregularities in mucosa, improving sensitivity of endoscopic examination, particularly to identify preneoplastic and neoplastic lesions. Common dyes include indigo carmine as a contrast stain (0.1–0.4%) and methylene blue (0.1%) as an absorptive stain. Narrow Band Imaging (NBI) is emerging as an alternative optical technique to the use of such dyes.

Recent developments in high-resolution and magnifying endoscopy appear to enhance the diagnostic usefulness of chromoendoscopy. Different staining patterns of <u>colon polyps</u> have been categorized (e.g., the five pit patterns described by Kudo), and appear to allow improved endoscopic prediction of histology.

These enhanced imaging methods show promise for detection of esophageal cancers and <u>Barrett's esophagus,</u> gastric neoplasia, and for targeting surveillance biopsies in ulcerative colitis.

Colonic transit studies

See: <u>colonic inertia</u>.

Colonoscopy

First used in the early 1960s, now a standard technique for assessing and treating colonic disease, because most colonic disease starts on the inner mucosal aspect. Cecal intubation is possible in 98% of colonoscopies in expert hands. Current areas of discussion include the following.

Making colonoscopy easier

Because of the tortuosity and lack of landmarks, this remains an issue. Most significant recent developments are the introduction of the variable stiffness colonoscope and magnetic endoscope imaging. The variable stiffness instruments can help negotiate difficult sigmoid loops and splenic flexures, and magnetic endoscope imaging has been shown to facilitate negotiation of loops, improve success rates, and shorten procedure times.

See: <u>bowel preparation.</u>

Sedation

The need for and practice of sedation varies widely and depends on patient expectation as well as local practice. Some countries use general anesthesia. Although some stretching of peritoneal attachments is almost inevitable, with a resulting visceral discomfort, total colonoscopy in unsedated patients is possible with expert endoscopists and motivated patients. In the United States routine practice involves intravenous administration of a benzodiazepine to provide anxiolysis and anterograde amnesia together with an opiate for analgesia. If this combination is used, the opiate should be given first and doses kept to a minimum. A common protocol is to use meperidine hydrochloride 25 mg and midazolam 2.5 mg. Some centers now provide propofol anesthesia with appropriately trained staff.

Monitoring
Current guidelines include routine use of pulse oximetry and supplemental oxygen (2 l/min via nasal cannulae) given to all sedated patients.

Contraindications. See Box 9.1.4.

Risks. See <u>endoscopic complications</u>.

Comparison with barium enema and virtual colonoscopy
Miss rate of colonoscopy for lesions <1 cm can be substantial (up to 25%). Barium imaging using double contrast barium enemas can provide high quality imaging of the colon but operator skill is an important variable and poor prep, air bubbles, muscle spasm, diverticular disease, or convoluted loops may impair the view. Colons difficult to examine by colonoscopy are also those difficult to examine by barium. Colonoscopy is impossible in the presence of barium, so it is logical to attempt colonoscopy first. Barium enema or CT pneumocolon are effective in assessing colon morphology when there are strictures or fistulae that may be impassable to the endoscopist.

Box 9.1.4 Contraindications to colonoscopy

- Avoid if possible for four to six weeks after proven myocardial infarction
- Because of the risk of perforation, colonoscopy is contraindicated in acute or abscess-associated diverticulitis
- Crohn's, ischemic, or ulcerative colitis mandate particular care, but colonoscopy can provide valuable information in these situations, and benefit may outweigh risk.

CT pneumocolon ("virtual colonoscopy")

Technique of imaging the colon using helical CT scanning. Colon is usually cleansed using the same <u>bowel preparation</u> as in conventional colonoscopy, although there is interest in "tagging" intestinal contents with orally ingested contrast agents and then subtracting tagged material at the image-processing stage to enable colonic imaging without bowel prep.

CT images can be reconstructed to give a "virtual colonoscopy" that can include views behind folds that can be difficult with conventional colonoscopy. The role of CT pneumocolon is still being evaluated, but it may have an important role in screening for colorectal disease, particularly in the setting of incomplete colonoscopy; in this area CT pneumocolon is often used as an alternative to barium enema. There is a wide variation in results of clinical trials investigating CT as a screening tool for colon cancer. At least one of these trials reports similar sensitivity of virtual and conventional colonoscopy in detecting colon polyps over 6 mm diameter. CT pneumocolon will have a significant effect on the practice of gastroenterology but the magnitude of this effect is unclear.

CT (computed tomography) scanning

Collimated X-rays through the patient produce a series of attenuation profiles that are computed into cross-sectional images (usually 3–8 mm cuts dependant on machine/clinical indication). More recently continuous motion (helical or spiral CT) has replaced sequential acquisition. Tissue contrast achieved by the fact that tissues attenuate X-ray to differing degrees. Whole abdomen may be scanned within one breath hold. Adiposity improves definition on CT (in contrast to ultrasound). Sequentially timed imaging after injection of iodine-based IV contrast may produce characteristic appearances of lesions/disease in arterial, venous, or portal venous phases. Specific acquisition protocols used dependent on organ/clinical question.

Indications for CT in GI disease wide-ranging, including investigation of acute abdominal pain, cancer diagnosis and staging (e.g., pancreatic and esophageal cancer), assessment of pancreatic, biliary, and liver disease, and investigation of intra-abdominal collections. CT pneumocolon is discussed separately. Targeted biopsy of lesions may be performed by CT or U/S, dependent on anatomical site/local expertise.

Contraindications are few, but include iodine allergy (discuss with radiologists if any useful information to be gained from unenhanced CT).

Radiation dose during abdominal CT is large (equivalent to 500 chest X-rays, or 3.3 years background radiation), so careful consideration of alternatives in young and in those needing repeated imaging. Avoid in pregnancy, especially first trimester.

Defecography studies

A method of evaluating defecation in patients who complain of excessive straining, or who employ digital manipulation to facilitate evacuation. Barium, thickened to a consistency that approximates stool, is introduced into the rectum. Evacuation of the barium is monitored by fluoroscopy. This allows assessment of anorectal anatomy, and measurement of the anorectal angle (the angle made between the axis of the rectum and the axis of the anal canal: usually about 90 degrees) at rest and during defecation. Rectoceles and intussusceptions not seen at rest may be seen during evacuation. The degree of perineal descent can also be assessed, which gives information on the integrity of the puborectalis and other muscles of the pelvic floor. Despite its utility in the assessment of defecation, the interpretation of defacography studies is highly user dependent and may suffer from poor intraobserver reproducibility.

Magnetic resonance imaging (MRI) using an endoanal receiving coil can give good anorectal imaging and also dynamic information about rectal emptying.

Dye spraying

See: chromoendoscopy.

Electrocoagulation

The principle of using electrosurgical or diathermy currents in therapeutic endoscopy is to cause heat with resultant coagulation of blood vessels and to facilitate tissue transaction. There is a difference between cutting and coagulating current, and between monopolar and bipolar electrodes.

- **Cutting current** has an uninterrupted waveform of low voltage. It has relatively high power, but because it is low voltage it is less able to cross dessicated tissue and does not penetrate deeply.
- **Coagulating current** has intermittent high-voltage spikes with intervening off periods lasting 80% of the time. This allows deeper spread of current and less local tissue destruction.
- **Monopolar current** involves current flowing between the wire of a snare loop or the jaws of biopsy forceps and a patient plate.
- **Bipolar current** involves all current flowing from one side of the snare to the other, with the attraction of much more localized effect.
- Local current density is critically important and higher for bipolar electrosurgery, which is why bipolar current is favored for local hemostasis, e.g., from bleeding peptic ulcers, while monopolar current with a "slow cooking" effect (essential on an adequate length of polyp stalk) is favored for polyp surgery.
- The heat produced relates directly to the power settings on the unit dial. Current recommendations are to perform polypectomy at a low power setting (15–25 W) to allow time to react to what is happening and to avoid 'cheese-wiring" the stalk.
- Monopolar electrocoagulation of upper GI bleeding lesions is uncommon, having been replaced by bipolar electrocoagulation or thermal coagulation using a heater probe, often in conjunction with adrenaline injection. See endoscopic hemostasis.

Endoscopic complications

Endoscopy is an invasive procedure, carrying definite risk.

- Cardiorespiratory adverse events (aspiration pneumonia, hypoventilation, vaso-vagal attack, arrhythmias) account for >50% of complications: risk correlates with age and co-morbidity.
- Respiratory depression is a particular risk with the widely used combination of sedative benzodiazepines and opiate analgesics.
- Risk in an individual patient relates to:
  - Patient factors (age, co-morbidity, anesthetic risks).
  - GI disease-related factors (large polyp, malignant stricture).
  - Endoscopic-technique issues (e.g., endoscopist experience, inherent risk of specific intervention).

Upper GI endoscopy

Diagnostic EGD: morbidity 0.1%, mortality of approximately 0.01%. Perforations in 0.01% (usually due to (unsuspected) anatomical abnormality, e.g., pharyngeal pouch, esophageal stricture).

Certain **therapeutic procedures** are associated with specific risks.

- Esophageal dilatation. Overall perforation rate 2.6%, mortality 1%, with increased risk in elderly and malignant strictures (see endoscopic dilatation and esophageal rupture).
- Variceal banding ligation (VBL)/endoscopic sclerotherapy (EST). During acute variceal bleeding, endoscopy-related aspiration of blood/gastric contents is a serious complication (which may be avoided by prior endotracheal intubation—see Acute upper GI bleed). Complications of EST reported in 10–15%: fever, retrosternal discomfort, and dysphagia usually resolve in < 48 hours. EST-induced esophageal ulceration is common, but esophageal perforation, mediastinitis, broncho-esophageal fistula, and stricture formation rarely occur. Bacteremia may lead to endocarditis in patient with prosthetic/diseased heart valves (see antibiotic prophylaxis). VBL appears to carry a significantly lower risk of esophageal ulceration, mediastinitis, and perforation than EST.
- Percutaneous endoscopic gastrostomy (PEG) insertion. 30-day mortality of 20% largely reflects the underlying disease (e.g., advanced dementia, stroke), and immediate PEG-related mortality <1%. Excoriation and infection of the skin around the stoma are common. Peritonitis and gastroenteric fistulae may arise from intra-abdominal migration of the intragastric bumper.

Colonoscopy

Diagnostic colonoscopy has a morbidity of approximately 0.25%, mortality 0.02%. Therapeutic procedures involve a morbidity of 1–7% with a mortality of 0.04%.

Perforation may relate to:

- Direct tip trauma (e.g., into colonic diverticulum) or endoscope looping during scope insertion. The rectosigmoid is the site of >60% of perforations; the splenic flexure is a relatively common site of injury.

Avulsion of the ligaments attaching the colon to the spleen can result in significant hemorrhage.

- Intervention (0.3–1% of polypectomies). A 4–5% perforation rate is associated with balloon dilatation of colonic strictures.
- Free perforation into the peritoneal cavity may occasionally be recognized during the procedure, but usually the diagnosis is suggested by marked persistent abdominal distension or pain after the procedure. Fever, and signs of shock and peritonitis may develop.
- Retroperitoneal perforation may present with subcutaneous emphysema.
- Management. Plain abdominal and erect chest X-rays should be performed, and may show pneumoperitoneum. If they are normal, but clinical suspicion remains, abdominal CT scan may give the diagnosis. Conservative management is sufficient for most small perforations (nil by mouth, IV fluids, IV antibiotics), but close in-patient review necessary, and surgery required in 25% of cases (particularly if perforation large).

Bleeding

- Immediate bleeding is the most common complication of polypectomy. Most cases of immediate bleeding resolve spontaneously. Management includes injecting 5–10 ml of 1:10,000 epinephrine (adrenaline) solution into the stalk/submucosa or hemoclip placement (see also <u>endoscopic hemostasis</u>). Angiography, and even laparotomy are occasionally required.
- Delayed bleeding can occur up to two weeks after colonoscopy.

Postpolypectomy coagulation syndrome presents with pain, peritonitis, and fever, and needs to be differentiated from perforation, as it invariably settles with conservative management.

Splenic rupture is rare, but may present with pain, peritonitis, and hypovolemic shock, with bloods showing acute anemia and raised white cell count. Diagnosis made on CT, and laparotomy often required.

ERCP

Overall complication rate about 5%. For severity grading, see Table 9.1.2.

- <u>**Pancreatitis**</u> is the most common complication of ERCP (3–5% of cases). A severe course is followed in 1%, with mortality rate from sphincterotomy-induced pancreatitis 0.5%. A number of risk factors are associated with post-ERCP pancreatitis (see Box 9.1.5). Careful patient selection for ERCP is vital, because ERCP is most dangerous for people who need it least (20–30% risk of pancreatitis in young woman with abdominal pain, normal bilirubin, and nondilated bile duct).
- **Retroperitoneal perforation** occurs in <1% of sphincterotomies. It may present acutely with surgical emphysema, but pain in the absence of a rise in serum amylase may also provide a diagnostic clue. In those patients in whom the diagnosis cannot be made on a plain abdominal X-ray, CT scanning may be required. Most cases settle with IV antibiotics and a strict nil-by-mouth policy, but close

Table 9.1.2 ERCP complications and severity grading

	Mild	Moderate	Severe
Bleeding	Clinical evidence of bleeding, but Hb fall < 3 g/dl, and no transfusion required	Transfusion required, but < 5 units, and no angiographic or surgical intervention	> 4 units transfused, or angiographic/ surgical intervention
Retroperitoneal perforation	Possible, or only very slight leak, with < 4 days of treatment required	Proven perforation treated medically for 4–10 days	Medical treatment for > 10 days, or intervention (percutaneous or surgical)
Pancreatitis	Amylase > 3 x ULN more than 24 hours after ERCP, with hospital stay extended by 2–3 days	Hospitalization for 4–10 days	Hospitalization for > 10 days, or hemorrhagic pancreatitis, phlegmon, pseudocyst, or intervention (percutaneous or surgical)
Cholangitis	Temp > 38°C for 24–48 hours	Septic illness requiring > 3 days of hospital treatment, or endoscopic/ radiographic intervention	Septic shock or need for surgery

Reproduced from Cotton PB, Lehman G, et al. Endoscopic sphincterotomy complications and their management: an attempt at consensus. Gastrointest Endosc. 1991; 37(3):383-93, with permission from Elsevier.

observation is required in view of the risk of retroperitoneal sepsis and abscess formation, which may require percutaneous or surgical drainage.
• **Bleeding** relating to sphincterotomy usually settles spontaneously, but endoscopic hemostasis techniques may be needed. Angiographic embolization, or surgery are rarely required.
• Cholangitis occurs in approximately 2% of patients following ERCP, usually when the intrahepatic ducts have been filled with contrast, but effective biliary drainage has not been obtained. It is managed with broad spectrum IV antibiotics, and further efforts to establish effective drainage (e.g., percutaneous transhepatic drain (PTD)).

Box 9.1.5 Risk factors for post-ERCP pancreatitis

- Young
- Female
- Suspected <u>sphincter of Oddi dysfunction</u> (SOD)
- Normal serum bilirubin
- Previous ERCP-related pancreatitis
- Difficult common bile duct (CBD) cannulation
- Pancreatic duct filling
- Precut (needle–knife) sphincterotomy
- Pancreatic sphincterotomy
- Balloon sphincter dilatation

Endoscopic dilatation

Mechanical dilatation of GI tract obstruction has been attempted for hundreds of years. The most common site for endoscopic dilatation is the esophagus, with indications including: benign peptic strictures (see <u>Dyspepsia and gastro-esophageal reflux</u> and <u>caustic ingestion</u>); <u>esophageal tumors</u>; <u>Schatzki's rings</u>; <u>achalasia</u>. A course of dilatation provides good relief in > 85% of patients with benign strictures due to reflux, but less effective if stricture due to radiation or corrosives. Most gastric strictures occur at pylorus; causes include peptic ulceration, <u>gastric cancer</u>, and <u>caustic ingestion</u>. Duodenal strictures are usually due to external compression (e.g., <u>pancreatitis</u>, <u>pancreatic cancer</u>) and rarely due to duodenal carcinoma. The most common indication for small-bowel or colonic endoscopic dilatation is <u>Crohn's disease</u>.

Types of dilator

- Fixed diameter dilators ("<u>bougies</u>") have long been used to dilate esophageal strictures. Most dilators (e.g., Savary–Gillard) are inserted over an endoscopically placed wire. May have 20 cm tapered tip, but gradually widen to 5–20 mm fixed diameter. For benign strictures usual dilatation to 16–18 mm, but wider dilatation may be needed for Schatzki's rings.
- Endoscopic dilatation in sites other than esophagus almost exclusively performed using over-the-wire balloons. Balloons are more expensive than push dilators, in part because of their single use. They can be inserted over a wire and positioned either under imaging control or directly at endoscopy through the scope (TTS). Balloon diameters vary from 4 to 40 mm. Larger balloons (30–40 mm) reserved for treatment of <u>achalasia</u>. Balloons exert a direct circumferential pressure rather than the shearing force exerted by bougies. Radial force exerted is less than with bougies and very rigid fibrotic strictures may be difficult to dilate with balloons.

Practice points

- Fluoroscopic screening may be needed with both techniques if the stricture cannot be passed endoscopically. Balloons exert only radial force and probably are less effective than bougies. Both methods safe in hands of experienced endoscopist familiar with their use.

- Anticoagulation should be discontinued prior to endoscopic dilatation, either by discontinuing oral anticoagulants if low risk of thromboembolism, or transferring to intravenous heparin, and discontinuing this four to six hours prior to dilatation, if at high risk of thromboembolism. Aspirin not of significant risk. Antibiotics should be given to patients with higher risk of cardiac lesions (see antibiotic prophylaxis in endoscopy).
- Overall esophageal perforation rate 2.6%, mortality 1%, with increased risk for malignant strictures (6.4% perforation, 2.3% mortality). Other complications include bleeding and pulmonary aspiration.

Endoscopic hemostasis

Endoscopic treatment reduces rebleeding and mortality in patients with significant upper GI bleeding, but must be used in conjunction with effective resuscitation and additional medical therapies (see Emergencies: Acute upper GI bleed). Range of hemostatic modalities used for different clinical indications.

Esophageal varices

See emergencies and portal hypertension.

Variceal band ligation (VBL)

- a varix is sucked into a short plastic sleeve at tip of endoscope, and a tight rubber ring is applied around base (see Color Plate 9).
- Varix thromboses and sloughs off in < seven days. Up to seven bands may be applied.
- Complications include "banding ulcers," but fewer side effects than sclerotherapy, and it is the endoscopic treatment of choice for gastro-esophageal varices.

Injection sclerotherapy

- Longer established than VBL.
- Involves injection of 1–4 ml of sclerosant (e.g., 5% ethanolamine) into or adjacent to varix.
- Like VBL, controls acute bleeding in 85–95% of cases, but risk of sclerotherapy ulcers, esophageal stricture, mediastinitis, and perforation (see endoscopic complications).

Gastric varices

- VBL and standard sclerotherapy not effective.
- Injection of other tissue adhesives (e.g., 2-cyanoacrylate) or thrombin may be effective.
- If bleeding not controlled, Sengstaken–Blakemore tube insertion (see "how to") and TIPSS (transjugular intrahepatic portosystemic shunt) may be necessary, as for esophageal varices.

Bleeding peptic ulcers

Endoscopic therapy is required for patients with: active bleeding, a visible vessel in ulcer base, or adherent clot. Techniques include:

- Injection: approx 4–10 ml adrenaline 1:10,000 injected around and then into bleeding point. Thrombin or fibrin injection also effective, but not widely used. Another modality, in addition to injection, gives best hemostatic results.
- Heat: options include heater probe, multipolar coagulation (BICAP; see electrocoagulation), or argon plasma coagulation (APC). Heater probe includes powerful water jet to clear blood clot, and achieves hemostasis via combination of compression of bleeding point and heat.
- Mechanical clips: range of products available, and may be very effective at clipping clearly visible vessels.

Postpolypectomy bleeds

As with ulcers, injection of adrenaline into the base of polyp stalk, followed by heater probe, may be effective, as may clip placement.

Angiodysplasia/vascular malformation/gastric antral vascular ectasia (GAVE)

Application of heat, with heater probe or argon plasma coagulation (APC), may be effective.

Endoscopic retrograde cholangiopancreatography (ERCP)

Technique

Side-viewing duodenoscope allows selective cannulation of biliary system, and insertion of cannulae into pancreatic/common bile ducts, with pancreatobiliary system delineated with contrast injection and X-ray imaging.

Indications

Smaller role now for ERCP as a primarily diagnostic technique, because of risks of procedure and because of alternative less invasive modalities to investigate pancreaticobiliary system (MRI/MRCP, CT scanning, transabdominal and endoscopic ultrasound). Indications include relief of biliary obstruction with endoscopic stenting (e.g., for pancreatic carcinoma, cholangiocarcinoma), removal of stones from common bile duct, and biopsy or cytological brushing of biliary strictures/lesions. ERCP is required to perform biliary manometry in patients with suspected sphincter of Oddi dysfunction.

Complications

Higher complications in units doing < 200 ERCPs/year, and endoscopists doing < 40/year, but patient-related factors probably even more important. Post-ERCP pancreatitis rate 3–5%, with highest rates (> 20%) in those who need procedure least (e.g., young female patient without jaundice, a nondilated bile duct, and intermittent right upper quadrant pain—also see sphincter of Oddi dysfunction). Post-sphincterotomy bleeding and retroperitoneal perforation less common. Also see endoscopic complications.

Endoscopic ultrasound (EUS)

EUS is becoming more important in diagnosis and management of GI disorders. Echoendoscopes use sound waves for imaging tissue consistency and interfaces between tissue planes, and typically use higher frequencies than those used in transabdominal ultrasound (this results in better definition, but reduced penetration). Three main types of echoendoscope are in use.

* **Radial echoendoscope** has a rotating ultrasound probe integrated into its tip, and 270° or 360° images obtained in a circumference perpendicular to the endoscope tip. Fine needle aspiration (FNA) not currently possible with radial EUS. Main indications include staging of GI tract tumors in terms of local invasion and regional lymphadenopathy (especially <u>esophageal</u>, <u>gastric</u>, and <u>rectal cancer</u>); and diagnosis in pancreaticobiliary disease (exclusion of <u>choledocholithiasis</u>, characterization of pancreatic lesions not seen on CT, and assessment of <u>neuroendocrine tumors</u>). In experienced hands, EUS for detecting mediastinal lymphadenopathy in esophageal cancer has sensitivity 80%, specificity 90%.
* **Linear array echoendoscope** also has an ultrasound probe in tip, but images are obtained along a plane parallel to the endoscope axis. FNA, and even Trucut biopsies, may be obtained using linear EUS, allowing therapeutic functions in addition to the diagnostic uses of radial EUS, including: mediastinal lymph node sampling in lung cancer; FNA of submucosal GI tract lesions, particularly pancreatic masses and <u>pancreatic cystic tumors</u>; endoscopic drainage of <u>pancreatic pseudocysts</u>; EUS-guided celiac plexus nerve block in patients with pain due to <u>chronic pancreatitis</u> or <u>pancreatic cancer</u>. Doppler ultrasound capability allows vascular structures to be missed by the needle, and blood flow to be assessed (e.g., <u>portal vein thrombosis</u>).
* **Ultrasound probes** are thin and need to be advanced through the channel of a regular endoscope. These probes generally provide a high-resolution circumferential view along the same plane as the radial echoendoscope. Miniprobe U/S may be used in the assessment of <u>biliary strictures</u>.

Endoscopy in anticoagulated patients

* The GI tract is the most common site of bleeding in patients on anticoagulants and antiplatelet drugs.
* Previous GI bleeds are a risk factor (30% incidence at three years therapy in those with a history of bleeding compared to 5% in those with no bleeding history).
* The risk of bleeding caused by the endoscopic procedure has to be balanced against the risk of a thrombo-embolic event related to stopping anticoagulation.

Recommendations (see Tables 9.1.3 and 4)

1. Low-risk procedures

No adjustments to anticoagulation needed whatever the underlying condition. Avoid elective procedures when the level of anticoagulation is above the therapeutic range.

2. High-risk procedures in patients with low-risk conditions

Stop warfarin three to five days before the procedure. There may be a need to obtain a preprocedure INR.

3. High-risk procedures in patients with high-risk conditions

Stop warfarin therapy three to five days before procedure. There may be a need for IV heparin once the INR is subtherapeutic. If used, discontinue heparin four to six hours preprocedure and restart two to six hours after procedure. Restart warfarin on the night of the procedure (but note risk of major bleed postbiliary sphincterotomy 10–15% if anticoagulation restarted within three days).

Aspirin and other NSAIDs

Cyclo-oxygenase inhibition by NSAIDs results in suppression of thromboxane A2-dependent platelet aggregation. Limited data suggests aspirin and other NSAIDs do not increase the risk of significant bleeding after endoscopy, polypectomy, or sphincterotomy.

Patients on antiplatelet therapy

Currently antiplatelet therapy includes:

• Antagonists of the adenosine diphosphate receptor (P2T) such as ticlopidine and clopidogrel.
• IIb/IIIa receptor antagonists such as abciximab and tirofiban.

Both classes are associated with increased bleeding risk, particularly in association with aspirin. Recurrent GI bleeding is more common with clopidogrel than aspirin plus a PPI.[17]

Data regarding GI bleeding after endoscopy in these patients are not adequate to make recommendations. For elective high-risk procedures, temporary discontinuation is desirable, especially if the patients is also on aspirin.

Reversing anticoagulation

• The degree of reversal needs to be individualized.
• Supratherapeutic INR may be treated with fresh frozen plasma.
• Correcting the INR to 1.5–2.5 allows successful endoscopic diagnosis and therapy at rates comparable to those in non-anticoagulated patients.
• If vitamin K is used, give small aliquots (0.5–1 mg) intravenously. **Do not give large intramuscular doses of vitamin K** unless permanent reversal of anticoagulation is the goal: the onset of action of vitamin K is delayed and prolongs the time needed to re-establish effective anticoagulation.

It is generally safe to restart warfarin on the evening of the procedure, **but** the benefits of immediate anticoagulation must be balanced against the risks (risk of bleeding is > 10% if anticoagulation restarted within 3 days of sphincterotomy).

Table 9.1.3 Procedure risks

High-risk	Low-risk
Colonoscopic polypectomy (1–2.5%)*	Diagnostic EGD and enteroscopy
Gastric polypectomy (4%)*	Flexible sigmoidoscopy and colonoscopy with or without biopsy
Laser ablation and coagulation (< 6%)*	Diagnostic ERCP
Endoscopic sphincterotomy (2.5–5%)*	Biliary stent without sphincterotomy
Pneumatic dilatation, PEG placement, EUS-guided needle aspiration or biopsy	Endoscopic ultrasound (EUS)

[1]Chan, FKL et al. (2005) N. Engl J. Med. 352: 238
*bleeding risk without anticoagulation

Table 9.1.4 Condition risk

High-risk	Low-risk
AF and valvular heart disease (risk is 5–7% annually, higher in dilated cardiomyopathy or after recent thrombo-embolic events)	DVT
Mechanical valve in the mitral position	Uncomplicated or paroxysmal nonvalvular AF
Mechanical valves of any type in patients with prior thrombo-embolic event	Bioprosthetic valve. Mechanical valve ion the aortic position

Enteroclysis

- A radiological method of examining the small intestine that involves intubation of the duodenum or proximal jejunum, usually combined with metaclopramide to accelerate small bowel transit. 200–250 ml of barium is injected into the small bowel, followed by 1.5–2 l of 0.5% methylcellulose.
- Enteroclysis provides better luminal distension than a small bowel meal and there is less flocculation of barium. However, intubation is not pleasant for the patient, and the technique requires extra time and expertise from the radiologist. Enteroclysis can be helpful in diagnosing small-bowel obstruction (especially intermittent obstruction), mucosal irregularities (e.g., lymphangiectasia or scleroderma), the anatomical extent of small-bowel <u>Crohn's disease</u>, and small-bowel tumors such as <u>carcinoid</u>.
- CT enteroclysis is a similar technique using cross-sectional imaging instead of barium radiology; there is some evidence that this is particularly helpful in diagnosing high-grade intestinal obstruction from abdominal tumor recurrence.
- In general, enteroclysis has poor diagnostic yield in cases of suspected small-intestinal bleeding; current evidence suggests that combination of endoscopic and video capsule enteroscopy is significantly superior.

Enteroscopy

There are three endoscopic methods currently available to image the 5 m of the human small intestine.

- The least used is **sonde enteroscopy**, which uses a 2.75 cm dedicated instrument to examine the whole of the small intestine. The instrument is carried down by peristalsis so that the examination takes several hours to perform. Biopsy and therapy are not possible. Patient discomfort, expense, and time taken have all prevented widespread use of this technique.
- **Push enteroscopy** is a useful method of examining the upper small intestine but its range is limited to the proximal 50–75 cm of jejunum. Biopsy and therapy are possible through a standard-size operating channel, and the technique is carried out using a dedicated 240 cm enteroscope or often a pediatric colonoscope that approximates to the enteroscope in length and handling characteristics.
- **Capsule endoscopy** ("wireless enteroscopy") has been a significant advance in recent years, providing the possibility of visualizing areas of the bowel inaccessible to conventional flexible endoscopy (i.e., most of small bowel). The 11 x 26 mm capsule is swallowed, and video images are transmitted to a data recorder worn on patient's belt for approximately 8 hours. Precise role relative to other diagnostic modalities is being investigated, but diagnostic yield of capsule endoscopy is superior to push enteroscopy for defining obscure small bowel bleeding in those with negative endoscopy and colonoscopy (68% compared to 32%). Detailed comparisons of capsule endoscopy with a combined approach of push enteroscopy and radiological examination of the small bowel are still awaited (see Swain, P and Fritscher-Ravens, A. (2004) Gut 53: 1866), and further developments in flexible enteroscopy (e.g., double-balloon enteroscopy (DBE)) may also influence relative merits of techniques. Capsule carries disadvantage of not allowing biopsy, and technique is contraindicated in patients with suspected significant intestinal strictures, as capsule may precipitate mechanical obstruction.

Extracorporeal shock-wave lithotripsy (ESWL)

ESWL utilizes ultrasound shock waves to fragment stones. In gastroenterology the main (but rare) indications are for gallstones, bile duct stones, or pancreatic duct stones that require dissolution, which cannot be achieved endoscopically and when surgery is not an option.

- Gallstone destruction with ESWL requires a patent cystic duct and single < 2 cm radiolucent stone. URSODEOXYCHOLIC ACID is given after fragmentation to aid dissolution.
- In patients with choledocholithiasis and impacted common bile duct stone, ESWL (and endoscopic laser lithotripsy) may induce sufficient fragmentation to allow endoscopic stone removal. Biliary stent/ nasobiliary drain may improve localization of stone for ESWL.

- Pancreatic duct stones that cannot be removed endoscopically may be treated with ESWL, followed by further attempts at stone fragment clearance.

Complications include biliary colic and <u>acute pancreatitis</u>.

Fecal occult blood tests (FOBT)

- Qualitative tests that rely on oxidation of a colorless compound to a colored one in the presence of pseudoperoxidase activity of hemoglobin and a developer solution of hydrogen peroxidase in alcohol. Cheap, readily available, and convenient, but distasteful for patients to carry out. Relatively high incidence of both false positives and false negatives (see Table 9.1.5). Most tests become positive when about 2 ml blood is lost per day.
- Positive predictive value of FOBT is about 20% for adenomas and 5–10% for cancers. Rehydration of slides with a drop of water before processing results in an increase of positivity and sensitivity but a fall in specificity and positive predictive value.
- New tests that decrease the false positive rates of FOBT while maintaining sensitivity include Hemeselect (an immunochemical test for human hemoglobin), HemoQuant (quantitative assay based of fluorescence of hem-derived porphyrins), and Hemoccult SENSA, a guaiac-based test with greater sensitivity. There is emerging evidence that screening strategies using an immunochemical test rather than a guaiac-based test may be most effective.
- See also <u>colorectal cancer screening and surveillance.</u>

Table 9.1.5 Limitations of fecal occult blood tests and recommendations for correct use

False positive test	False negative tests
Endogenous peroxidase (e.g. vegetable peroxidase in broccoli, turnips, cauliflower, radishes and melon)	Hemoglobin degradation by storage or fecal bacteria
Non human hemoglobin: red meat.	Vitamin C interferes with indicator dye
Any source of GI bleed (epistaxis, gingival bleeding, hemorrhoids)	Lesion not bleeding at the time of sampling
Apirin and NSAIDs, which increase upper GI bleeds.	
Recommendations: Patient should avoid red meat, peroxidase containing vegetables, vitamin C, and NASIDs for 3 days before and during testing. Avoiding iron is recommended but evidence for this is weak.	Recommendations: Develop slides within 4-6 days. Do not rehydrate slides for average risk screening. Two samples of each of three consecutive stools should be tested.

Gastrograffin

A water-soluble contrast medium. Safer than barium in radiological contrast examinations, especially where there is a suspicion of peritonitis if examining the lower bowel or mediastinitis if performing a contrast swallow.

Gastrostomy

The commonest method of nutritional support in patients requiring tube feeding for over two weeks. Can be placed endoscopically (see <u>percutaneous endoscopic gastrostomy (PEG)</u>), radiologically, or (rarely) surgically.

Complications of both percutaneous and radiological endoscopy can be major (leakage with peritonitis, necrotizing fasciitis, and hemorrhage) in about 3% or minor (minor leaks, wound infection, ileus, fever) in about 20%. Peristomal infection is reduced by a single dose of IV <u>CEPHALOSPORIN</u>.

Heater probe

Useful for treating actively bleeding ulcers in the GI tract within reach of an endoscope and also for lowering risk of bleeding of high-risk lesions. Keys to successful use include direct probe pressure to tamponade the vessel, use of 25–30 Joule setting, and repeated applications.

Hepatobiliary scintigraphy (e.g., HIDA scan)

Hepatobiliary iminodiacetic acid (HIDA) scan employs radioactive tracer that is excreted by liver into bile. Sequential scanning over two hours performed. Main uses include the diagnosis of:
- Acute <u>cholecystitis</u> (95% accuracy reported).
- Bile-duct leak post<u>cholecystectomy</u>.
- Cystic duct patency (e.g., blocked due to stone, tumor).
- Hepatic dysfunction (impaired excretion into bile).
- <u>Sphincter of Oddi dysfunction</u>.

In practice, HIDA scanning largely replaced by other imaging modalities.

Hydrogen breath test

See: <u>breath tests</u>.

Ileal pouch–anal anastomosis (IPAA)

The procedure of choice for patients requiring proctocolectomy for ulcerative colitis or familial adenomatous polyposis. Advantages include:

- Removal of nearly all mucosal disease (in contrast to ileorectal anastomosis).
- Preserves normal flow of stool.

A pouch needs to be constructed from ileum because direct anastomosis of ileum to anal verge results in excess stool frequency and anal seepage. There are several forms of pouch (see Figure 9.1.1); the J pouch is the easiest of these to construct and has functional outcomes identical to those of the more complex designs.

Clinical results. Average postpouch stool frequency is six times a day and one to two at night. Incontinence occurs in 10% during the day and 20% at night. Up to 50% need to wear a pad to protect against seepage. 50% require medications to bulk/decrease stools.

Long-term results. Overall morbidity is 25–30%. Failure is rare provided the operation is not done in error in patients with Crohn's disease. The most important factor is probably an experienced surgeon. Complications are shown in Table 9.1.6.

Pouchitis: see separate entry.

Technical issues

Staged procedure. Reported rates of pelvic sepsis vary from 0 to 25% but are higher in patients undergoing a one-stage procedure. Most patients should undergo a 2-stage procedure with diverting ileostomy rather than a 1-stage IPAA. Patients with severe colitis may require a 3-stage procedure: 1. subtotal colectomy and ileostomy; 2. creation of the ileal pouch and diverting ileostomy; 3. Takedown of diverting ileostomy.

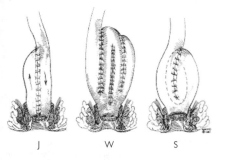

J   W   S

Figure 9.1.1 Three types of ileal pouch. Reproduced from Feldman M, Friedman LS, and Sleisenger MH (2003). *Sleisenger and Fordtran's Gastrointestinal and Liver Disease*, with permission from Elsevier

Table 9.1.6 Complications of ileal pouch–anal anastomosis (IPAA)

Complication	Rate
Pelvic infection	5%
Abdominal sepsis	6%
Small bowel obstruction	17%
Pouchitis	50%
Anastomotic stricture	Very high: usually easy to dilate digitally
Impotence and retrograde ejaculation	1.5% and 4% men
Infertility	3-fold risk
Dyspareunia	7%

Stapled vs hand-sewn anastomosis. A debate arising because of the opposing benefits of removing all colonic mucosa (mucosectomy and technically demanding hand-sewn anastomosis) and preserving a cuff of colonic mucosa to improve functional outcome. A randomized trial at the Mayo clinic found no difference in complication rate, but less night-time incontinence and better anal pressures in the stapled group. Most surgeons use a stapled anastomosis.

Risk of cancer and dysplasia. There is a small risk of cancer in the retained rectal mucosa, estimated at less than 1% at two years post-op. This risk is higher if there was cancer or dysplasia in the original colectomy specimen.

Ileostomy

Operations that expose the ileal serosa to ileal effluent result in serositis. The **Brooke ileostomy** invented in the 1950s involves everting the mucosa and suturing it to the skin. This ileostomy is incontinent: a variation, called a Koch pouch, features an ileal pouch, a nipple valve, and an ileal conduit leading to a cutaneous stoma that can be flush with the skin. Koch pouches are rarely performed due to poor function.

All ileostomies should discharge between 300 and 800 g material per day: 90% of this is water.

Sequelae of ileostomy. Urine is more concentrated. Incidence of urolithiasis is about 5%. Resection of terminal ileum may lead to <u>bile acid malabsorption</u> and <u>vitamin B12</u> deficiency.

Complications of ileostomy. Stomal obstruction, increased ileal discharge, and fluid and electrolyte depletion. Mechanical problems with poorly fitting stomal appliances can cause skin excoriation or even fistula formation.

Liver biopsy (LBx)

No investigation in medicine should be performed unless the result might change management (especially if it carries risk), and LBx demonstrates this point *par excellence*. Studies show that the results of LBx affect subsequent management in only 30% of cases.

Indications

- LBx has a central role in diagnosis of wide range of diffuse parenchymal and focal liver disease.
- Chronic viral <u>hepatitis B and C</u> (histological grade (inflammation) and stage (fibrosis) may determine need/timing of treatment); genetic <u>hemochromatosis</u> (enables cirrhosis to be excluded, but improvements in genetic, biochemical, and imaging assessment are reducing need for LBx); unexplained hepatitis/abnormal liver function tests (where noninvasive tests, such as serology, are nondiagnostic); <u>autoimmune hepatitis</u> (role during initial work-up, and probably in assessing treatment response); <u>nonalcoholic fatty liver disease (NAFLD)</u> (allows identification of steatohepatitis, which may show histological progression); <u>alcoholic liver disease</u> (especially exclusion of <u>alcoholic hepatitis</u>, as clinical diagnosis wrong in >20% of cases); focal liver masses (e.g., liver metastases, <u>focal nodular hyperplasia</u>, <u>hepatocellular carcinoma</u> [but see comments below *re:* seeding]).
- Routine use of LBx, where diagnosis has been established by other modalities, remains unclear for <u>primary biliary cirrhosis</u>, <u>primary sclerosing cholangitis</u>, <u>Wilson's disease</u>.
- Rarely needed in proven acute viral hepatitis.

Contraindications to percutaneous LBx

- Uncooperative patient (sudden movement may lead to liver laceration).
- Biliary obstruction ± <u>cholangitis</u>.
- Deranged clotting. Usual advice is to avoid percutaneous LBx if INR > 1.3, but little clear data, and 90% of biopsy-related bleeds occur in patients with INR < 1.3. If INR 1.4–1.6, may give fresh frozen plasma (FFP), and perform LBx if INR reduces to <1.4. If coagulopathy present, and cannot be corrected sufficient to allow safe percutaneous LBx, consider transjugular LBx.
- Low/dysfunctional platelets. Minimum safe lower limit of platelets 60 × 109/l for percutaneous LBx (but recommendations vary). If platelets 40–60 × 109/l, LBx may be performed immediately after platelet transfusion, if count increased to safe level. Bleeding time should be considered in patients with suspected impaired platelet function (e.g., renal failure, recent antiplatelet drugs), as bleeding time >10 minutes associated with increased risk of bleeding.
- Significant ascites. Drain ascites first (see <u>paracentesis</u>), but transjugular LBx is alternative.
- <u>Amyloidosis</u>. Historical data suggests an increased risk of intraperitoneal bleeding.

- Cystic liver lesions. If communicate with biliary tree biopsy may precipitate biliary leak. Risks of anaphylaxis if inadvertently biopsy hydatid cyst.
- Confirmatory LBx generally avoided in presumed resectable hepatocellular carcinoma, in view of risk of needle track seeding (but reported incidence from diagnostic LBx <2%).

Preprocedure care

- Informed written consent.
- Stop antiplatelet medication at least a week prior to procedure, if clinically possible. Anticoagulation must be stopped prior to percutaneous LBx.
- Preprocedure blood tests, as discussed earlier (within last two weeks if stable chronic disease, more recent if change likely (e.g., recent onset jaundice).
- Imaging. U/S or CT scanning of liver is essential prior to LBx, in part to exclude unexpected pathology that may increase risks (e.g., intrahepatic gall bladder, liver cyst). Debate continues about whether "untargeted" LBx should be performed under U/S guidance in all cases (as argued by most radiologists). Seems reasonable.
- Prophylactic antibiotics should be given for patients at high risk of endocarditis, or if there is a risk of biliary sepsis.

Box 9.1.6 Procedure

- Patient lies supine, with right hand behind head.
- Liver identified by percussion or ideally U/S. Usual approach in midaxillary line, between the lower ribs.
- Aseptic technique, with skin cleaned with iodine-based solution, and skin infiltrated down to the liver capsule using 22G needle and lignocaine 1–2% 4–6 ml. Line of infiltration just above edge of lower rib (to avoid neurovascular bundle running on underside of upper rib). 5 mm scalpel cut into skin to allow advancement of biopsy needle.
- Biopsy performed with patient having been instructed to stop breathing after full expiration (this raises diaphragm, so reducing risk of pneumothorax).
- Two types of biopsy needle used: cutting needle (e.g., Trucut) provides good cores of tissue, but may carry slightly higher complication rate than suction needle (e.g., Menghini). It is important that those undertaking LBx gain confidence and experience using one needle type.
- After biopsy patient lies in right lateral position for 1 hour, then supine for 2 hours, and stays in hospital for 6 hours. Vital signs monitored quarter hourly for 2 hours, then half hourly for 2 hours, then hourly (> 80% of complications occur within first 10 hours, and > 60% within 2 hours).

Complications/risks

Mortality 0.1–0.3%, morbidity 5.9% following liver biopsy. > 80% of complications occur within first 10 hours, and > 60% within two hours. Pain seen in 25%. Complications and death most commonly related to intraperitoneal bleeding or bile peritonitis following gallbladder perforation. Risk factors for bleeding include increasing patient age, intrahepatic malignancy, and > 2 needle passes. Puncture of lung (pneumothorax), colon, and kidney are all recognized. Small subcapsular hematomas are seen on U/S in > 20%, but are rarely symptomatic.

Manometry

- Measuring intraluminal pressure in the gastrointestinal tract is one way of studying motility abnormalities, which cause a number of common clinical problems. See separate entries under esophageal manometry, anorectal manometry, and sphincter of Oddi dysfunction.
- Gastroduodenal manometry is established as a research tool but is not widely used, partly because mild to moderate symptoms correlate poorly with manometric findings and partly because the techniques are somewhat invasive and prolonged.

Esophageal manometry and motility studies

Commonly used techniques to investigate esophageal motility disorders include:

- Intraluminal manometry.
- Radiological studies using barium swallows or video fluoroscopy.

Radionuclide imaging to quantify bolus transit through the esophagus is largely a research tool and will not be further described. Standard endoscopy is a poor method for assessing esophageal function, although there is some interest in using small caliber endoscopes passed transorally or transnasally to diagnose tracheobronchial aspiration and test sensory thresholds.

Radiological assessment (barium swallow with videofluoroscopy) is essential to study the oropharyngeal phase of swallowing and the upper esophageal sphincter and offers a less invasive alternative to manometry in some patients. It can be used by speech therapists working with radiologists to develop compensatory strategies to minimize tracheobronchial aspiration in patients with oropharyngeal swallowing disorders. Limitations of radiological examination of motility include subjective evaluation, study of only a small number of swallows, a lack of standardization of details of swallowing technique such as bolus size, and time delays between swallows.

Manometry is the gold standard for assessing esophageal body motility, because of its quantitative approach. Equipment includes transnasally passed catheters with multiple water-perfused small caliber lumens or more high-tech solid-state devices using pressure transducers embedded into the probe at various levels. Developments in telemetry allow temporary fixation of pressure transducers at the level of the lower esophageal sphincter and recording of data on a belt device. Esophageal manometry is most useful in evaluating patients with dysphagia, noncardiac chest pain, and prior to antireflux surgery.

Reading a manometry report. Four aspects of function need to be characterized to enable most disorders to be diagnosed:
1. Peristaltic performance: percentage of swallows with progressive contraction sequences.
2. Contraction wave configuration (amplitude and duration).
3. Lower esophageal sphincter basal and peak pressures.
4. Lower esophageal sphincter relaxation with swallowing.

Limitations of manometry
- Poor toleration of probe by some patients.
- Longitudinal muscle contraction can result in axial displacement.
- Manometry cannot distinguish muscular from neural problems.

Impedance testing is a newer technique designed to detect intraluminal bolus movement without the use of radiation. It is usually performed with manometry or pH testing. When combined with manometry, it provides information on the functional (i.e., bolus transit) component of manometrically detected contractions. When combined with pH, it allows for detection of gastroesophageal reflux independent of pH (i.e., both acid and nonacid reflux). Indications are similar to those for esophageal manometry.

Esophageal pH monitoring

Ambulatory 24 h pH monitoring is the most widely used test to investigate gastro-esophageal reflux and to correlate symptoms with reflux. The test involves positioning a transnasal pH probe 5 cm above the lower esophageal sphincter (determined manometrically). The patient then conducts life as normally as possible while recording symptoms, meals, and sleep in a diary. The test can also be performed by a wireless capsule-shaped device that is affixed to the distal esophageal mucosa. Esophageal acid exposure is defined as pH less than 4. This should occur for less than 3.5% of total recording time (this is an arbitrary threshold; there is no value that reliably identifies GERD patients).

It is not necessary in most patients with typical reflux symptoms but can be useful in patients with refractory or atypical symptoms not responding to empiric treatment.

Recent technology allows measurement of alkaline reflux from the duodenum into the esophagus, using a different probe positioned in exactly the same way. This can allow rational prescribing with prokinetics such as DOMPERIDONE or mucosal protective agents such as SUCRALFATE in patients with symptomatic reflux not responding to empirical acid suppressant treatment.

Nasogastric tubes

Indications for passing a nasogastric tube include:
- Decompression of the stomach with aspiration of gastric contents in the case of gastric outlet or small-bowel obstruction.
- Reduction of risk of aspiration pneumonia in at-risk patients e.g., prolonged vomiting, reduced conscious level.
- Occasionally in the patient with upper GI bleeding.
- To provide temporary (usually less than two weeks) nutritional support in patients with a functioning GI tract but who cannot or will not eat. Longer periods of enteral nutrition can be provided by percutaneous endoscopic gastrostomy (PEG) tube placement.

Most tubes for feeding are thin (about 5 F) made of silicone or polyurethane and contain weighted tips with a stylet for easy placement. Tubes for gastric decompression or drainage are larger (about 12 F).

Complications of tube placement:
- Intubation of the bronchial tree is not uncommon.
- Intracranial placement is a risk in patients with skull fractures.
- Erosive tissue damage can produce nasopharyngeal trauma, pharyngitis, sinusitis, otitis media, pneumothorax, GI tract perforation, and esophageal ulceration.
- Tube occlusion can occur through inspissated feedings or pulverized medications.

Paracentesis (large volume)

Refers to the drainage of fluid in the peritoneal cavity (i.e., ascites; see Ascites).

Most common indication is for diuretic-resistant ascites related to portal hypertension, but other causes include malignant ascites. TIPSS (transjugular intrahepatic portosystemic shunt) may occasionally be alternative to recurrent paracentesis for diurectic-resistant ascites.

Technique
- As with most procedures in medicine, best way to perform safely and effectively is to watch and learn from experienced colleague.
- Ensure clotting optimized prior to drainage (e.g., INR < 1.4, platelets > 60 × 10^9/l), although normalization of clotting parameters may be impossible to achieve in end-stage liver disease, even with FFP and platelet infusions.

- Patient supine or with head of bed elevated approximately 30° degrees. Examine abdomen, particularly noting lower margin of liver and spleen. Moving laterally from umbilicus, percuss into flanks, until area of stony dullness is reached (usually anterior axillary line). On rolling patient, confirm that area of dullness related to fluid (see GI examination). Use hub end of needle to mark site of planned needle insertion. If in doubt, ask radiologists to perform ultrasound, and mark skin at point of safest and most effective insertion.
- Perform under sterile conditions (i.e., wear sterile gloves + gowns, sterile drapes around "surgical field"). Clean around insertion point with betadine/iodine solution (> 8 cm radius). Using 22G needle and 5 ml syringe, raise a subcutaneous bleb with lidocaine 2%, and then inject further anesthetic through skin, until peritoneal cavity is reached. Using 20 ml syringe, send fluid for analysis (see Ascites and spontaneous bacterial peritonitis). Using pointed-tip scalpel, make 5 mm incision through skin. Drainage catheter inserted over trocar (or use Barcelona needle), at 90° to skin. Depending on patient adiposity, peritoneal cavity entered approximately 4 cm from skin, often indicated by ascitic fluid seeping back along catheter. At this point, advance further 1 cm, then withdraw trocar while advancing catheter (should occur without resistance or discomfort). Tape catheter securely to skin (no need to stitch), and attach bladder drainage bag to catheter (or use vacutaners). Keep bag/container below level of patient, and leave on free drainage.
- Reduced circulating blood volume, with secondary hyperaldosteronism and sympathetic drive may occur 12–24 hours post large volume (e.g., > 4 liter) paracentesis. To prevent this, most hepatologists advise use of albumin as plasma expander. For those patients in whom 5 liters or >5 liters of ascites is removed, 25% human albumin solution (HAS) (8–10 g/l of removed fluid) should be administered. Alternatives to HAS are being sought (see albumin (use in liver disease)), but trials of dextran 70 and hemaccel show that they are less effective in this setting.
- Rare complications include intraperitoneal bleeding, bowel perforation (particularly if history of abdominal surgery i.e., possible adhesions), and infection.

Percutaneous endoscopic gastrostomy (PEG)

- PEG insertion increasingly widely performed when enteral feeding required for > four weeks (10% of nursing home residents in United States have had PEG).
- Main indications include neuromuscular disease (e.g., stroke, motor neuron disease, dementia), and oropharyngeal cancer.
- Ongoing debate surrounds maintenance of enteral feeding in patients with end-stage progressive disease, but PEG tubes are certainly better tolerated than long-term nasogastric feeding.

Technique

"Pull technique" entails:

1. Endoscopy to exclude any lesions within upper GI tract.
2. Endoscopic localization of anterior gastric wall, with corresponding point on anterior abdominal wall identified by transillumination.
3. Sterilization of skin, local anesthetic infiltration, and 5 mm incision into skin at site of planned insertion.
4. Insertion of trocar, followed by looped string, percutaneously into stomach, under endoscopic vision.
5. String grabbed endoscopically with endoscopic snare, and drawn retrogradely out of mouth on removal of endoscope. 9–16F feeding tube attached to string, and drawn into position by traction at skin.
6. Button of PEG tube keeps it lightly impacted against gastric wall.
   - Preprocedure antibiotics (e.g., Cefuroxime 750 mg IV) reduce risk of peristomal infection.
   - PEG can be modified with jejunal feeding tube, which may reduce risk of reflux and gastric aspiration.
   - Alternatives to endoscopic gastrostomy insertion include percutaneous radiological approach or surgical. These may be considered for patients undergoing planned curative surgery for oropharyngeal cancer, as gastric stoma metastases due to endoscopic insertion rarely reported.

Contraindications to PEG Include:

- Inability to bring the anterior gastric wall in apposition to the anterior abdominal wall (e.g., subtotal gastrectomy, ascites, hepatomegaly, severe obesity). Transillumination and finger palpation to choose appropriate PEG site necessary.
- Gastrointestinal-tract obstruction.
- Malignant gastric/peritoneal infiltration.
- Gastric varices.
- Uncorrectable coagulopathy.

Complications

- Major complications in 3%, minor in 20%: infection (wound, peritoneal, abdominal wall abscess, necrotizing fasciitis), local peritonitis, bowel perforation, tube displacement, hemorrhage, "buried bumper," ileus, bleeding, colocutaneous fistula.
- Procedure-related mortality 0.5–2%, overall 30-day mortality 10–15% (largely reflecting underlying disease, but emphasizes need to be sure that patient not put through futile, unnecessary intervention in last few days of life).
- Pneumoperitoneum in 20%, but rarely of significance.

Photodynamic therapy (PDT)

PDT involves the intravenous administration of a photosensitizing drug (e.g., porfimer sodium (Photofrin®), meso-tetrahydroxyphenyl chlorine (Foscan®)), which is taken up by all dividing cells. Drug activated on exposure to low-power red light (630–675 nm) from a laser, leading to nonthermal local tissue destruction (usually to depth of 1–5 mm). Oxygenated tissue particularly affected, and connective tissue largely spared.

- PDT has been used for range of GI diseases, with laser inserted either percutaneously or endoscopically, including:
  - Barrett's esophagus.
  - Esophageal cancer.
  - Palliation of cholangiocarcinoma, and maintenance of biliary patency (with prolonged survival reported in a large single-center study).
  - Palliation of pancreatic cancer reported with PDT.
  - Ablation of endoscopically accessible, small, inoperable tumors.
- Severe cutaneous photosensitivity may occur (patient kept in darkened room for five days after drug given, and direct sunlight avoided for >three weeks, dependent on photosensitizer used). Viscus perforation and hemorrhage are rare.

Positron emission tomography (PET) scanning

Background

- Most tumor imaging relies on demonstrating abnormal anatomy (e.g., a mass). Size is a limiting factor, as is homogeneity with surrounding tissue, and primary or secondary lesions < 1 cm often missed on CT/MRI/transabdominal U/S.
- PET scanning provides information on function, relying on the increased metabolic rate common to most malignancies. Glucose analogue (^{18}F)2-fluoro-2-deoxy-D-glucose (FDG) most commonly used as tracer.
- Combining FDG PET with CT allows functional and anatomical assessment.

Indications

- In GI disease, increasing role for PET CT in primary staging of colon cancer and esophageal cancer, in particular identification of metastases.
- As well as primary staging, PET CT in colon cancer used for:
  - Differentiating local recurrence from posttreatment changes.
  - Excluding extrahepatic metastases in patients with apparently isolated (and, therefore, resectable) liver recurrence post-primary tumor resection.
  - Identifying site of recurrence in patients with rising tumor markers, and no sign of recurrence on anatomical imaging.

- Routine role in staging of <u>pancreatic cancer</u> less well defined. May be of use in characterizing benign versus malignant pancreatic lesions.
- PET using FDG of less use in <u>carcinoid</u> and <u>pancreatic endocrine tumors</u>, probably due to lower metabolic rate, but other tracers (e.g., ^{11}C-L-dopa, ^{11}C-5-HTP) provide better yields.

Limitations

- Differentiation between reactive and malignant lymph nodes difficult.
- False-negatives in tumors with low metabolic rate.
- False-positive uptake in colon (although may sometimes be first indication of undiagnosed colitis or colonic polyps).
- As with other imaging modalities, may fail to characterize lesions <1 cm.

Schilling test

Used in <u>vitamin</u> B12 (<u>cobalamin</u>) deficiency to distinguish between causes due to <u>intrinsic factor</u> (IF) deficiency (i.e., gastric causes—<u>pernicious anemia</u>, post<u>gastrectomy</u>), and those due to impaired uptake of vitamin–IF complex (e.g., ileal <u>Crohn's disease</u>, small-bowel <u>bacterial overgrowth</u>, <u>chronic pancreatitis</u>). Test not affected by vitamin B12 replacement therapy.

Technique

- **Stage I.** Small dose of radiolabeled vitamin B12 (0.5–2.0 mCi) given orally in glass of water, followed one hour later by unlabeled vitamin B12 1 mg IM to saturate vitamin B12 carriers (so that radiolabeled dose is excreted in urine, if absorbed). Vitamin B12 malabsorption diagnosed if < 7% of radiolabeled dose excreted in urine over subsequent 24 hours.
- **Stage II.** Needed to differentiate IF deficiency from other causes. Stage I repeated, but 60 mg of active IF administered orally with the oral test dose. Normalization of vitamin B12 excretion confirms IF deficiency.
- If vitamin B12 excretion low after stage II test, repeating stage I after five day course of antibiotic therapy (normalization suggests <u>bacterial overgrowth</u>), or with <u>pancreatic supplements</u> (normalization suggests <u>pancreatic insufficiency</u>), may help distinguish terminal ileal disease from other causes of malabsorption.
- False positive results due to incomplete urine collection or renal impairment, and interpretation of excretion results may be difficult.

Sedation for endoscopy

- The degrees of sedation used for endoscopy include no sedation, conscious sedation, deep sedation, and general anesthesia.
- Diagnostic upper GI endoscopy may be well tolerated with local anesthetic throat spray only (e.g., lidocaine spray), but conscious sedation (patient able to make purposeful responses to verbal/tactile stimuli, with spontaneous ventilation) is used for most endoscopies.
- The following required in patient undergoing conscious sedation:
  - Supplemental oxygen via nasal cannulae (e.g., 2 l/min).
  - IV access throughout procedure.
  - Pulse oximetry (but demonstrates only hypoxemia, not hypoventilation, so clinical assessment remains vital).
  - Cardiac monitoring.
- Conscious sedation usually involves use of **benzodiazepine** (e.g., IV midazolam 2–10 mg) and **opiate** (e.g., IV meperidine hydrochloride 25–50 mg, fentanyl 50–100 μg), administered by endoscopist. Opiate given first, because of slower rate of action, and careful titration of drug dosages to patient response is essential. In some countries, and for complex procedures (e.g., ERCP), anesthetist-administered deep sedation with propofol (rapid action and recovery, but narrow therapeutic window) increasingly used.
- Sedation implicated in > 50% of <u>endoscopic complications</u>, including aspiration, oversedation, hypoventilation, and airway obstruction. Risks crudely correlate with preprocedural American Society of Anesthesiology (ASA) score (see Table 9.1.7), and involvement of senior endoscopist and anesthetist essential in patients with ASA >3.
- Management of hypoxemia/hypoventilation includes protection of airway (including "jaw thrust"), administration of reversal agent (flumazenil 250–500 μg IV for benzodiazepines, naloxone 400 μg IV/IM for opiates), continued supplemental oxygen (via mask), and emergency mechanical ventilation as necessary. Jaw thrust and flumazenil sufficient in most cases, and addition of naloxone rarely needed, when combination of benzodiazepine and opiate have been used.
- Important that "day case" patient warned before sedation that they must not drive, operate heavy or dangerous machinery, or sign any legally binding documents for rest of the day, and that they will require an escort home.
- General anesthesia for endoscopy generally reserved for situations where cooperation is difficult (e.g., children), or where airway protection with endotracheal tube is important (see comments on variceal bleeding in <u>Acute upper GI bleeding</u>).

Table 9.1.7 American Society of Anesthesiologists (ASA) status

Class 1	Patient has no organic, physiological, biochemical, or psychiatric disturbance. Condition for which procedure is to be performed is localized, with no systemic disturbance.
Class 2	Mild to moderate systemic disturbance caused either by the condition to be treated, or by other pathological processes
Class 3	Severe systemic disturbance or disease from whatever cause, even though it may not be possible to define the degree of disability with finality
Class 4	Severe systemic disorders that are already life-threatening, not always correctable by intervention
Class 5	The moribund patient who has little chance of survival but is submitted to intervention/operation in desperation

Sengstaken–Blakemore tube (SBT)

Background

- Bleeding from gastro-esophageal (GE) varices is primarily controlled by endoscopic and pharmacological therapy (see acute variceal bleeding in emergencies. Acute upper GI bleeding and portal hypertension). If these approaches are ineffective/unavailable, mechanical compression of varices at GE junction should be instituted.
- SBT insertion is one of the most effective emergency interventions in gastroenterology—**done right it saves, done wrong it may hasten the patient's demise.**

Technique

- Essential to be fully prepared before attempting SBT insertion:
  - ICU/HDU setting.
  - Enroll senior nursing/medical staff if available.
  - Anesthetist in attendance, with very low threshold for endotracheal intubation and ventilation prior to insertion (in view of risk of aspiration, difficult insertion, bitten fingers).
- Mouthpiece in, lubricant jelly on SBT. Double glove (especially if any risk of hepatitis C). Left forefinger between mouthpiece and side of mouth, to guide tube. Slow, steady insertion, to limit of tube.
- Inflate gastric balloon to 50 ml with air, using 50 ml bladder syringe and then seal balloon port with two clamps. This should not elicit distress (if it does, this may suggest gastric balloon in esophagus—risk of esophageal rupture). Confirm placement of the gastric balloon in stomach by CXR. Inflate gastric balloon with a further 200 ml of air.

- Slow traction on tube, expecting resistance at about 35 cm from teeth.
- Secure tube under light tension. The correct tension to apply is that exerted by hanging a 500 ml bag of IV fluid to the end of the SBT. The tube can be secured to face guard on a football helmet or baseball catcher mask. The bag of IV fluid can then be removed. This prevents trauma to the lips/mouth. Mark tube to detect slippage.
- Check CXR (see gastric balloon in stomach, with "nipple effect" due to slight traction into distal esophagus).
- Aspirate esophageal port (not balloon) every 15 minutes, gastric port (not balloon) every half hour.
- Aim to deflate and remove SBT < 18 hours and rescope/watch response.

Lack of control of bleeding
- May be due to:
  - Ineffectively deployed SBT + gastric balloon. Check a CXR. Attempt repositioning.
  - Varices feeding into midesophagus (i.e., not controlled by pressure at GE junction). This may be treated by inflating esophageal balloon to a pressure equivalent to 40 mmHg.
  - Gastric or ectopic varices.
- Contact liver center and consider emergency <u>TIPSS</u>.

Seton suture

A seton is a suture, wire, or tubing that is used in the surgical management of anorectal fistulae (e.g., in <u>perianal Crohn's disease</u>). It is threaded through the fistulous tract, and secured outside the anus usually with a knot. It can be left loose to allow for drainage and subsidence of local infection, or tied tightly to slowly cut through the muscle—in theory maintaining muscle fiber alignment, allowing healing, and preventing abscess formation. Treatment with a seton should be reserved for cases refractory to medical therapy.

Stool microscopy

A very useful test to establish an inflammatory cause of diarrhea. Invasive pathogens such as *Shigella* and *Campylobacter* produce many polymorphs and red blood cells. Toxigenic organisms, viruses, and food poisoning bacteria produce a watery stool containing few formed elements. An acute exacerbation of <u>ulcerative colitis</u> can also produce leucocytes and erythrocytes in the stool, giving appearances that resemble bacillary dysentery.

TIPSS (transjugular intrahepatic portosystemic shunt)

Technique

- Involves formation of artificial track between portal vein and hepatic vein, through liver, using radiologically placed mesh metal stent (see Figure 9.1.2).
- Used in treatment of complications of portal hypertension, and aims to reduce hepatic venous pressure gradient (HVPG) to < 12 mmHg.
- Procedure usually performed in specialist liver units. Stent insertion does not preclude liver transplantation, provided not sited too far down portal vein.

Indications

- Uncontrolled acute variceal bleeding (see: Acute upper GI bleeding), where drug/endoscopic therapy has failed, is main indication for TIPSS. Sengstaken–Blakemore tube may be inserted prior to TIPSS. Especially useful for gastric and ectopic (e.g., rectal) varices.
- Secondary prevention of recurrent variceal bleeding (but only where medical/endoscopic prophylaxis has failed).
- Refractory ascites (see Ascites). Reduces need for large volume paracentesis , but no comparative reduction in mortality, and increases risk of hepatic encephalopathy.
- Efficacy of TIPSS reported in Budd–Chiari syndrome, type 2 hepatorenal syndrome, and portal hypertensive gastropathy, but few controlled studies.

Contraindications

- Intrahepatic lesions (e.g., cysts, tumors).
- Vascular obstruction (complete hepatic or portal vein thrombosis).
- Cardiopulmonary disease (severe pulmonary hypertension, congestive cardiac failure).
- Severe bleeding risk (INR > 1.5, platelets < 20 K/µl—but consider in clinical context).
- Biliary obstruction (risk of biliary puncture/fistula).

Complications

- TIPSS blockage. Early thrombosis in 10–15%, but dysfunction in 80% by one year (thrombosis or intimal hyperplasia). Covered stents may reduce TIPSS dysfunction. Blockage clinically suggested by further portal hypertensive complications. Doppler U/S within one week of insertion, and formal venography at one year suggested to exclude occlusion.
- New/worsened hepatic encephalopathy in 10–44% limits use of TIPSS (particularly in Child–Pugh C disease). May necessitate stent occlusion.
- Direct procedure-related complications (e.g., hemobilia, intraperitoneal bleed, hepatic infarction, arteriovenous fistulae, sepsis) in <15%, but major complication in < 3%.
- Hemolysis in 10–15%, due to flow through shunt, but usually resolves in < four weeks.

Ultrasound

- Widely available imaging modality with the great and unique property of enabling imaging of blood flow and soft tissues in real time. It is a complex and challenging technique and results are dependent on user expertise, particularly for specialist work. Extracorporeal (transabdominal) ultrasound is not very useful in imaging the gastrointestinal wall (this is also true of CT) because resolution is insufficient to reveal the cause of wall thickening or the depth of localization of a specific abnormality. This led to the development of combining endoscopy with ultrasound and more recently the capability of EUS-guided tissue sampling to differentiate benign from malignant lesions (see <u>endoscopic ultrasound (EUS)</u>).
- Technique works by sending out high-frequency (1–20 MHz) sound waves from a transducer. These waves reflect back to differing degrees dependent on underlying tissue, are converted into electric pulses, and sent back to analyzer, which provides image of tissues and distance from skin. Higher frequency waves produce more detailed images, but penetrate less deeply into the body (2–5 MHz generally used for abdominal U/S, with 7.5–12 MHz used for EUS). Doppler sonography, integral in modern machines, allows real time information on flow within the morphological image.
- Most useful information provided when a specific question is asked (e.g., "is there biliary dilatation?" rather than "abdo U/S").

Indications
Hepatobiliary
- U/S used as first-line imaging modality for most diffuse and focal hepatobiliary abnormalities. Ideal for studying cystic lesions, and > 90% sensitive and specific in identifying <u>gallstones</u>.
- Many advocate <u>liver biopsy</u> to be done under U/S control, and widely used (alternative is CT) for targeted biopsies in general.
- Doppler facility allows flow in large blood vessels (e.g., see <u>portal vein thrombosis</u>, <u>Budd–Chiari syndrome</u>) and even vascularity of large lesions to be assessed.

Pancreatic
- In <u>acute pancreatitis</u>, U/S can help with detecting gallstones and biliary dilatation, although CT is more sensitive in evaluating pancreatic disease overall.

Luminal GI tract
- Useful for evaluation of the patient with right lower quadrant pain and possible <u>appendicitis</u>. U/S may also help in diagnosis of terminal ileal inflammation or stricturing, diverticulitis, small-bowel obstruction, and bulky mesenteric nodes or GI neoplasms.
- Excellent in diagnosing intraperitoneal fluid collections, such as ascites, abscesses, or hemorrhage, and also in guiding percutaneous needle, aspiration for definitive diagnosis.

Box 9.1.7 **Strengths and weaknesses of ultrasound as an imaging modality**

Strengths
- Unique ability to display flow and soft tissue in real time
- Spatial resolution superior to CT and MRI
- Safe and well tolerated: no ionizing radiation
- Can be performed at the bedside

Weaknesses
- Technically challenging
- Not good in fat or gaseous patients
- Inability to see beyond gas/soft tissue or bone/soft tissue interface
- Relatively poor contrast resolution—this may improve with the development of media for contrast-enhanced ultrasound
- Findings less reliable the farther area of interest is from skin probe (e.g., retroperitoneal structures, pancreas)

Urea breath tests

See: *Helicobacter pylori* (HP).

Whipple's procedure

Allen Oldfather Whipple (1881–1963). American surgeon. Medical historian on Middle East after retirement. Also reported Whipple's triad in insulinoma (see pancreatic endocrine tumors), but did not describe Whipple's disease.
- Procedure (also called pancreatoduodenectomy) involves excision of head of the pancreas, gallbladder, distal common bile duct, duodenum and distal stomach. Anastomoses result in gastrojejunostomy, choledochojejunostomy, and pancreaticojejunostomy (see Figure 9.1.2).
- Indications include ampullary, duodenal, and pancreatic cancer (procedure possible in < 15% of patients with pancreatic cancer, with subsequent approximate 25% five-year survival), cholangiocarcinoma of distal bile duct, duodenal familial adenomatous polyposis, and occasionally chronic pancreatitis.
- Surgical morbidity > 30% (e.g., biliary leak, pancreatic fistula, secondary hemorrhage, postgastrectomy syndrome), surgical mortality 3–5%.
- Pylorus-preserving pancreaticoduodenectomy (PPPD) has been advocated as alternative to Whipple's procedure, as means of reducing early satiety and biliary reflux. Analysis to date suggests no significant differences in surgical morbidity/mortality, or prognosis with pancreatic cancer after PPPD or Standard Whipple's procedure.

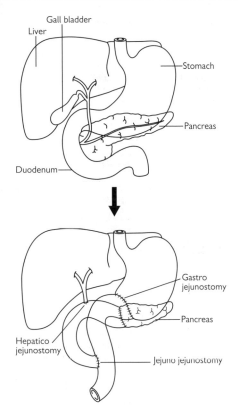

Figure 9.1.2 Whipple's procedure (pancreatico-duodenectomy).

Nutrition

B vitamins

See: vitamins and cobalamin.

Cobalamin (vitamin B12)

Found in animal sources: vegetarians/vegans may have inadequate intake. Deficiency can be caused by disease at a number of sites.

Box 9.2.1 Causes of cobalamin (vitamin B12) deficiency

- Inadequate dietary intake
  - Vegans
  - Alcoholics
- Inadequate release of food bound cobalamin
  - Achlorhydria
  - PROTON PUMP INHIBITORS
- Loss of active intrinsic factor (IF)
  - Pernicious anemia
  - Gastrectomy
  - Congenital lack/abnormality of IF
- Proximal small-bowel disease and pancreatic disease
  - Pancreatic insufficiency
  - Gastrinoma
  - Tropical sprue
  - Small-bowel bacterial overgrowth
  - Fish tapeworm *diphyllobothrium latum* (rare)
- Ileal disorders
  - Mainly loss of absorptive mucosa through surgery or mucosal disease
  - Crohn's disease
  - TB (see TB and the GI tract)
  - Lymphoma
  - Dysfunctional uptake and use of cobalamin by cells: R binder deficiency, transcobalamin II deficiency, some drugs (colchicine)
- Miscellaneous (rarely lead to clinical anemia)
  - Pregnancy
  - Thyrotoxicosis
  - Erythroid hyperplasia
  - Drugs
  - PAS
  - Colchicine
  - Neomycin
  - Metformin

Investigation. If not vegan, do parietal-cell antibodies and intrinsic-factor antibodies to exclude pernicious anemia. Remember that severe vitamin B12 malabsorption can damage mucosa and affect absorptive capacity, so either wait two months before doing Schilling test or repeat after treatment.

Treatment is usually by IM hydroxycobalamin (1 mg 3 ×/week for two weeks, then 1 mg every 3 months), although high dose oral cobalamin (1–2 mg/day) may be effective.

Elemental diets

- Originally designed for the U.S. manned space program, they were used in preparing some patients for surgery and a coincident benefit in <u>Crohn's disease</u> was noted. Possible modes of action include effect on endogenous flora or mucosal permeability. Their use is attractive in children where <u>CORTICOSTEROIDS</u> affect growth, and in pregnancy where drug usage is minimized.
- Several studies have purported to show equivalence between elemental diets and steroids in achieving short-term remission in Crohn's disease. Subsequent meta-analyses tend not to confirm this, but patients with small-bowel disease may benefit. Those with perianal disease or who relapse quickly should avoid it. Efficacy is higher in children than adults.
- Dietary composition varies: elemental diets include polymeric feeds using whole protein and complex carbohydrate, peptide-based diets (containing di- and tripeptides, thought to be better absorbed than amino acids), and true elemental feeds containing amino acids, glucose, and short-chain triglycerides. Available data suggest little difference between elemental and polymeric feeds. There has been concern that the fat content of enteral diets may influence response, but there is little evidence to support this. Compliance is an issue: 85% can manage sip feeding but 15% require a nasogastric tube.

Enteral feeding

In patients who need supplemental feeding, enteral feeding has many advantages over parenteral nutrition—see Box 9.2.2.

Enteral feeding regimens use defined **liquid formula feeds**. Although pure sources of protein, carbohydrate, and lipid are available (so-called feeding modules), these are rarely used in our experience.

Monomeric feeds contain nitrogen as free amino acids, carbohydrates as glucose polymers (providing most of the calories), and minimal amounts of fat as long chain triglycerides (LCT). These feeds are often unpalatable and expensive. There are theoretical disadvantages (dipeptides and tripeptides are absorbed more efficiently than free amino acids) and controlled trial evidence does not show a clear benefit in many situations.

Oligomeric feeds contain hydrolyzed proteins as small peptides together with simple sugars or starch and fat as LCT or a mix of LCT and medium chain triglycerides (MCT). The protein is theoretically better absorbed than free amino acids or whole protein. Although there is some support of this from clinical studies, no clinical benefit has been demonstrated in outcome studies, apart from some reduction of diarrhea and GI side effects in patients receiving cytotoxic chemotherapy.

Polymeric feeds contain nitrogen as whole protein, carbohydrates as glucose polymers, and fat as LCT or a mix of LCT and MCT. They can be made from blenderized food (e.g., beef or milk as protein source; cereal, fruit, and vegetables as CHO source; and corn oil or soy oil as a fat source) or made from milk as a source of protein and fat with addition of corn-oil solids and glucose as a source of carbohydrate. Most polymeric feeds, however, are lactose-free formulas containing casein or soy as a protein source. Fiber is not present in most lactose-free formulas.

> **Box 9.2.2 Why is enteral feeding better than parenteral nutrition?**
> - Fewer complications of line sepsis
> - Enteral feeding can supply gut-preferred fuels such as glutamine and short-chain fatty acids that are often absent from TPN preparations
> - Enteral feeding can prevent mucosal atrophy, preserves mucosal and pancreatic enzyme function, maintains GI IgA secretion
> - Enteral feeding prevents cholelithiasis by stimulating gallbladder motility
> - Less expensive

Exclusion diets

Systematic exclusion of different foods and the use of a food/symptom diary can help identify foods to which a patient may be intolerant or allergic (also see <u>food allergy</u>). A true elimination diet is difficult to pursue and should ideally involve the help of an experienced dietician. It involves a "washout period" of taking bland food such as boiled rice, fish, and chicken followed by the re-introduction of a favorite food every day. About 30% of patients with irritable bowel can identify foods that aggravate symptoms.

Fiber

Refers to residue of food, usually from structural and matrix components of plant cell walls, that is resistant to hydrolysis by human digestive enzymes. Some fibers can bind ions (calcium, iron, magnesium, zinc) and also adsorb bile salts, proteins, and bacterial cells. Fermentation of fiber by bacteria generate short-chain fatty acids, which are a preferred energy source for colonocytes. Although water insoluble fibers have a greater effect on stool mass than water soluble fibers, ingestion of degradable fiber stimulates bacterial growth and generates a fecal mass largely composed of bacteria.

Effects on GI tract

Fiber affects GI motility: gums and pectins slow gastric emptying, while particulate fibers like wheat bran appear to increase it. Effect on intestinal transit time depends on particle size and bulk-forming capacity: large particle size (e.g., coarse bran) is more effective than small particle size in speeding colonic transit. Increased fiber intake has been proposed to reduce the incidence of various diseases including <u>colonic cancer</u>, <u>diverticular disease</u>, <u>appendicitis</u>, <u>cholelithiasis</u>, constipation, hemorrhoids. The bulk of evidence supports a high- fiber diet, but a direct protective effect against colon cancer or in preventing adenoma recurrence has not been proven.

Folic acid (vitamin B9)

- A complex pterin molecule conjugated to glutamic acid. Found in spinach, liver, peanuts, and beans. Destroyed by prolonged cooking.
- Functions as a carrier of one-carbon groups; necessary for synthesis of nucleic acid, proteins, acetylcholine, and methionine.
- Recommended intake is 400 mg/day. Uptake is by a specific carrier-mediated process that involves a hydrolase. This enzyme is inhibited by exposure to alcohol, which may contribute to the folate deficiency seen in chronic alcoholics. Folate deficiency is seen in small-intestine mucosal diseases such as <u>celiac</u> and <u>Whipple's disease</u>.
- Folate metabolism is affected by methotrexate, pyrimethamine, trimethoprim, and triamterene. Salazopyrine inhibits folate transport. Phenytoin and carbamazepine lower folate levels and may produce a megaloblastic anemia.
- The risk of children born with neural tube defects is reduced by pharmacological doses of folate (4 mg/d) given periconceptually.

Food allergy (food intolerance)

- Food allergy implies an immune-mediated reaction to certain foods; food intolerance is a better term for nonimmune reactions. Food intolerance can be enzymatic (e.g., lactose intolerance due to congenital or acquired lactase deficiency), pharmacological (e.g., sensitivity to vasoactive amines such as tyramine in cheeses), or idiopathic.
- The prevalence of true food allergy can be up to 8% in children < three years, with perhaps 2.5% infants < two years having cow's milk allergy. The rate falls to 2.5% of the population after the first decade.
- Risk factors include an immature mucosal immune system, early introduction of solid food, IgA deficiency, and inadequate challenge of the mucosal immune system with commensal flora.

- Pathogenesis of true food allergy in most cases is thought to involve failure of tolerance mediated by gut-associated lymphoid tissue. Both IgE- and cell-mediated process can occur.
- Food allergy is the commonest cause of anaphylactic reactions; peanut allergy has a prevalence of 0.5 to 7% of adults in the United States and UK. Other common causes are cow's milk, eggs, seafood, and fish.
- IgE-mediated hypersensitivity reactions.

Iron

Dietary iron comprises heme (meat, fish, poultry) and nonheme iron (vegetables, grains, and fruits). Poor intake alone rarely causes anemia but may deplete stores and combines with any cause of malabsorption or blood loss to produce anemia. Absorption and losses are about 1 mg/day in adults; menstrual loss in women is 5–50 mg per month.

Absorption takes place in duodenum and upper small bowel. Absorption is increased by vitamin C because it maintains iron in the ferrous state which is more soluble. Absorption is increased in hemochromatosis. It can also increase two- to threefold to compensate for increased loss. Absorption is reduced in cases decreased acid secretion (atrophic gastritris, gastric surgery, prolonged PPI) and small- bowel disease (e.g., celiac disease).

Iron deficiency. Common (5–10% of premenopausal women, 1–5% men). In groups other than premenopausal women, the assumption is usually of occult GI bleeding and this underlies the routine search for GI pathology. 12% premenopausal women with iron deficiency anemia have significant GI abnormalities, so investigation in this group is also important.

Diagnosing iron deficiency is a crucial step. Key routine tests are low serum ferritin and low transferrin saturation as assessed by ratio of serum iron to total iron binding capacity (TIBC). TIBC is usually elevated.

Finding the cause. Overall, upper GI lesions are twice as common as colonic lesions (40% compared with 20% respectively in several large series). Trivial lesions such as mild gastritis and small adenomas do not contribute to iron deficiency: *Helicobacter pylori*-associated gastritis has been implicated in iron deficiency, as have large hiatal hernias and gastric achlorhydria and atrophy. Right-sided colon cancers are the classical occult colonic source of bleeding: angiodysplasia and adenomas are nearly as frequent.

Investigations
Symptoms are not a reliable guide. Investigation should include upper GI endoscopy and low duodenal biopsy (undiagnosed celiac disease is an unusual, but important cause), and colonoscopy. Video capsule endoscopy should be performed if initial endoscopies are negative.

Treatment of iron deficiency
Oral iron. If possible, give oral iron 100–200 mg/day, with vitamin C, which improves absorption. Ferrous sulfate 200 mg tablets contain 65 mg elemental iron. Continue treatment for three months to replenish stores.

In general differences in tolerability are due to differences in concentration of iron. Prophylactic iron may be appropriate in malabsorption, pregnancy, postgastrectomy.

Parenteral iron. Reserved for patients who cannot tolerate oral iron, where there is continued blood loss, or malabsorption. Anaphylactoid reactions can occur.

Oral rehydration solutions (ORS)

- Can be life saving in treating children with diarrheal illnesses; in Western countries it can be helpful in treating patients with high output ostomies, <u>short-bowel syndrome</u>, and <u>HIV</u> infection.
- The principle is to stimulate sodium and water absorption by the sodium glucose co-transporter in the intestinal epithelial brush border. Glucose enhances sodium absorption by an active carrier process: water absorption follows passively. For treating severe diarrhea, rehydration solutions should contain an alkalinizing agent to counter acidosis and be slightly hypo-osmolar (about 250 mM/l) to prevent osmotic diarrhea.
- The precise composition is controversial; there is debate about the type of carbohydrate that should be used and the best concentrations of sodium, potassium, chloride, and base.

Components of feed

- Glucose is the most commonly used substrate and should be provided at 70–150 mM: higher concentrations can cause osmotic diarrhea. Replacing glucose with polymeric carbohydrate such as rice syrup solids provides a hypotonic solution that is better in decreasing stool output.
- In developed countries oral rehydration solutions contain lower concentrations of sodium (Na^+ 50–60 mM) than the WHO formulation (75 mM) since patients tend to suffer less severe sodium loss. Stool sodium concentration in <u>cholera</u> is about 90 mM; maximal absorption of sodium occurs at a concentration of 120 mM and this higher concentration may be optimal in patients with <u>short-bowel syndrome</u> and high stoma output.
- The concentration of potassium in ORS is about 20 mM although stool potassium concentrations are often higher and 30–35 mM may be more appropriate.

Table 9.2.1 Composition of oral rehydration solution

Solution	Na (mM)	K (mM)	Cl (mM)	Citrate (mM)	Glucose (mM)	Osmolarity
WHO	75	20	65	10	75	245 mOsm/l

Parenteral nutrition

Indications

Prevention or correction of specific nutrient deficiencies or to prevent malnutrition when GI tract cannot be used (also see <u>nasogastric tubes</u>). It is usually recommended if enteral intake is inadequate for more than seven days, but this is not evidence based, and the duration of tolerable starvation varies.

Techniques for delivery

Parenteral feeds can be given through peripheral catheters (including standard venous cannulae or midlength fine bore catheters), peripherally inserted central catheters (PICC), or skin-tunneled central venous catheters.

The major limitation to using peripheral catheters is the high incidence of thrombophlebitis. This relates to several factors:
- Osmolality, pH, lipid content of nutrition solution.
- Catheter characteristics (diameter, composition).
- Infusion protocol.
- Diameter and position of vein and insertion technique.

The incidence of thrombophlebitis can be minimized by following the principles outlined in Box 9.2.3.

Peripherally inserted central lines (PICC) can be used for TPN and under optimal circumstances show similar incidences of catheter-related complications to those of subclavian lines. PICC lines should be placed by specialists.

Tunneled central venous catheters use a subcutaneous skin tunnel from a point of the anterior chest wall distant from the point of entry of the catheter into the vein. They are indicated when feeding is likely to be for longer than two weeks, when peripheral access is poor, and when the osmolality is higher than 1,000 mOsm/l. The tip of the catheter needs placing as for a PICC.

Calculating requirements and choosing the feed

In most hospitals this will be done by dieticians or members of the nutrition team. The following principles apply:

1 **Calculate the energy requirements.** This can be done by calculating the basal metabolic rate (available from charts developed by Schofield, WN (1985). Hum. *Nutr. Clin. Nutr.* 39 (suppl. 1): 5).
   - Add 10% for each degree C rise in temperature.
   - Adjust for mobility (add 10% if bed bound: 20% if sitting in chair; 30% if mobile on ward).
   - Add up to 600 kCal if weight gain is required.

2. **Calculate the protein requirements.** Most hospitalized patients need 0.8 to 1.5 g protein/kg/day. Any catabolic illness, protein-losing enteropathy, or nephropathy (or dialysis) increases protein requirements. Protein balance can be checked in most patients if necessary by calculating urinary nitrogen loss from urinary urea excretion and comparing this with content of the prescribed feed.

3. **Consider the amount of fat infused.** The optimal percentage of calories that should be infused as fat is not known, but most

Box 9.2.3 Practical principles in peripheral TPN

- Use as large a vein as possible:, use a fine bore (22 or 23 g) polyurethane catheter
- Put a GTN patch over the infusion site
- Add 500–1,000 IU heparin/l of TPN solution
- Add 5 mg/l of hydrocortisone
- Buffer the solution to pH 7.4
- Keep daily infused volume below 3.5 l; use an infusion pump
- Use an inline 1.2 micron filter
- Provide at least 50% of total energy as lipid: this serves to keep the osmolality low

complications occur at rates over 1 kCal/kg/h, so a max of 0.7 kCal/kg/h is usually observed: this translates to 500–1,500 ml of a 10% lipid solution.

4. **Consider infused carbohydrate.** Intravenous carbohydrate, usually dextrose, is a vital source of calories that stimulates insulin secretion and reduces muscle breakdown (reduces hepatic gluconeogenesis, which needs amino acid precursors from skeletal muscle).
5. **Consider parenteral electrolytes, vitamins, and trace elements.** Sodium. Provide patients weight in kg as baseline, and add calculated losses remembering that bile and small intestinal/ileostomy fluid is near isotonic at 150 mM). Monitor potassium but also calcium (5–10 mM required per day) and phosphate (10–30 mM needed per day).

Clinical management of the patient on TPN

1. Daily weight. This contributes to assessing fluid balance.
2. Blood glucose may be raised if there is insulin resistance.
3. Watch for pyrexia. Any spike may indicate line sepsis: take blood from the feeding catheter and peripheral vein; stop TPN until culture results are known.
4. Beware overenthusiastic feeding of critically malnourished: there is a danger of <u>refeeding syndrome</u>.

Complications of parenteral nutrition

- **Mechanical damage** to veins or local structures (pneumothorax, brachial plexus injury, thoracic duct injury, hemothorax).
- **Vascular complications:** air embolism, catheter thrombosis, embolic complications including pulmonary emboli.
- **Metabolic.** Fluid overload, hyperglycemia, metabolic bone disease, hyperlipidemia.
- **Infectious complications:** line sepsis rates should be below 3–5%.
- **GI complications.** Abnormal liver function is common (most commonly cholestatic pattern, but steatohepatitis is seen on histology. Acalculous <u>cholecystitis</u> (5%), <u>acute pancreatitis</u>, <u>gallstones</u> (30%), and gallbladder sludge (approaching 100%) also occur and presumably relate to bile stasis in the absence of enteral feeding.

See sections on nutrition in entries on <u>Crohn's disease</u>, <u>ulcerative colitis</u>, <u>short-bowel syndrome</u>, and <u>hepatic encephalopathy</u>. Parenteral nutrition also has a role in management of gastrointestinal fistulae, and in <u>acute pancreatitis</u>.

Short-chain fatty acids (SCFA)

Contain one to six carbon atoms (acetate, proprionate, butyrate). Produced in the colon by bacterial fermentation of undigested carbohydrate (about 25 g/day: 90% can be metabolized to SCFA and absorbed). An important source of fuel for colonic mucosa; therefore, reduced fiber intake with enteral feeding or diversion of fecal stream in ileostomy or colostomy can result in mucosal atrophy or <u>diversion colitis</u>.

Vitamins

Defined as organic compounds required in small (<100 mg/day) quantities.

Vitamin A (retinol)
The precursor beta carotene contains two molecules of retinol and is found in green vegetables and carrots. Retinol is found in milk, eggs, and fish oils. Retinoids are stored in hepatocytes and hepatic fat storage cells (Ito cells) and function as regulators of many embryonic and adult genes through binding to the RXR and RAR transcription factors. Deficiency causes night blindness because retinol is a precursor of rhodopsin.

Vitamin B
- **B1** is thiamine: see <u>beriberi</u>.
- **B2** is riboflavin: deficiency causes sore tongue and mouth. Measure by red blood glutathione levels.
- **B3** is niacin: see <u>pellagra</u>.
- **B5** is pantothenic acid.
- **B6** is pyridoxine. Deficiency leads to dermatitis and glossitis.
- **B7** is biotin.
- **B9** is <u>folic acid</u>.
- **B12** See <u>cobalamin</u> (and <u>pernicious anemia</u>).

Vitamin C (ascorbic acid)
Water soluble. Dietary source (fresh fruit, liver) essential. Deficiency causes scurvy: look for bent or coiled body hair, peri-follicular hemorrhage and bruising, and gingivitis. Scurvy is common in alcoholics but can occur in severe Crohn's or other mucosal enteropathies.

Vitamin D

Needs bile acids for solubilization and absorption. Enterocytes package it in chylomicrons. Low levels lead to osteomalacia. Apart from low plasma levels, biochemical evidence for low vitamin D includes 24 chylomicrons urinary calcium of less than 100 mg/day, a high PTH level, and elevated urinary hydroxyprolene.

Vitamin E (tocopherol)

Found in grains, vegetables, meats. Absorption requires intraluminal bile salts and pancreatic esterases. The vitamin is packaged in chylomicrons and stored in liver and fat. The main role is as antioxidant. Chronic cholestasis causes clinical deficiency in children and can lead to retinopathy, cerebellar ataxia, reduced vibration sense, and areflexia (abetalipoproteinaemia causes similar syndrome because of failure to secrete chylomicrons). In adults symptoms take years to develop, but any disease impairing fat absorption can lead to deficiency (ileal disease, impaired bile secretion, intrahepatic disease like PBC).

Vitamin K

Main dietary source is green vegetables. About 50% comes from gut bacterial synthesis. Diets deficient in Vitamin K do not cause deficiency unless gut-sterilizing antibiotics are given. Vitamin K deficiency may arise due to a range of GI diseases, including chronic cholestasis (e.g. primary biliary cirrhosis) and celiac disease. Diagnosis suggested by finding elevated prothrombin time (PT) in right clinical setting. In patient with suspected liver failure, vital to give parenteral vitamin K to exclude deficiency of this as cause of elevated PT.

Appendix

BMI calculator

Height in metres

Weight in kilograms	1.36	1.40	1.44	1.48	1.52	1.56	1.60	1.64	1.68	1.72	1.76	1.80	1.84	1.88	1.92	1.96	2.00
125	68	64	60	57	54	51	49	46	44	42	40	39	37	35	34	33	31
123	67	63	59	56	53	51	48	46	44	42	40	38	36	35	33	32	31
121	65	62	58	55	52	50	47	45	43	41	39	37	36	34	33	31	30
119	64	61	57	54	52	49	46	44	42	40	38	37	35	34	32	31	30
117	63	60	56	53	51	48	46	44	41	40	38	36	35	33	32	30	29
115	62	59	55	53	50	47	45	43	41	40	37	35	34	33	31	30	29
113	61	58	54	52	49	46	44	42	40	38	36	35	33	32	31	29	28
111	60	57	54	51	48	46	43	41	39	38	36	34	33	31	30	29	28
109	59	56	53	50	47	45	43	41	39	37	35	34	32	31	30	28	27
107	58	55	52	49	46	44	42	40	38	36	35	33	32	30	29	28	27
105	57	54	51	48	45	43	41	39	37	35	34	32	31	30	28	27	26
103	56	53	50	47	45	42	40	38	36	35	33	32	30	29	28	27	26
101	55	52	49	46	44	42	39	38	36	34	33	31	30	29	27	26	25
99	54	51	48	45	43	41	39	37	35	33	32	31	29	28	27	26	25
97	52	49	47	44	42	40	38	36	34	33	31	30	28	27	26	25	24
95	51	48	46	43	41	39	37	35	34	32	31	29	28	27	26	25	24
93	50	47	45	42	40	38	36	35	33	31	30	29	27	26	25	24	23
91	49	46	44	42	39	37	36	34	32	31	29	28	27	26	25	24	23
89	48	45	43	41	39	37	35	33	32	30	29	27	26	25	24	23	22
87	47	44	42	40	38	36	34	32	31	29	28	27	26	25	24	23	22
85	46	43	41	39	37	35	33	32	30	29	27	26	25	24	23	22	21
83	45	42	40	38	36	34	32	31	29	28	27	26	25	23	23	22	21
81	44	41	39	37	35	33	32	30	29	27	26	25	24	23	22	21	20
79	43	40	38	36	34	32	31	29	28	27	26	24	23	22	21	21	20
77	42	39	37	35	33	32	30	29	27	26	25	24	23	22	21	20	19
75	41	38	36	34	32	31	29	28	27	25	24	23	22	21	20	20	19
73	39	37	35	33	32	30	29	27	26	25	24	23	22	21	20	19	18
71	38	36	34	32	31	29	28	26	25	24	23	22	21	20	19	18	18
69	37	35	33	32	30	28	27	26	24	23	22	21	20	19	18	17	17
67	36	34	32	31	29	28	26	25	24	23	22	21	20	19	18	17	17
65	35	33	31	30	28	27	25	24	23	22	21	20	19	18	18	17	16
63	34	32	30	29	27	26	25	23	22	21	20	19	19	18	17	16	16
61	33	31	29	28	26	25	24	23	22	21	20	19	18	17	17	16	15
59	32	30	28	27	26	24	23	22	21	20	19	18	17	17	16	15	15
57	31	29	27	26	25	23	22	21	20	19	18	17	16	16	15	15	14
55	30	28	27	25	24	23	21	20	19	19	18	17	16	16	15	14	14
53	29	27	26	24	23	22	21	20	19	18	17	16	16	15	14	14	13
51	28	26	25	23	22	21	20	19	18	17	16	16	15	14	14	13	13
49	26	25	24	22	21	20	19	18	17	17	16	15	14	14	13	13	12
47	25	24	23	21	20	19	18	17	17	16	15	15	14	13	13	12	12
45	24	23	22	21	19	18	18	17	16	15	15	14	13	13	12	12	11
43	23	22	21	20	19	18	17	16	15	15	14	13	13	12	12	11	11

BMI <18.5 – underweight

BMI 18.5–24.9 – acceptable weight

BMI 25–29.9 – overweight

BMI 30–39.9 – obese

BMI >= 40 – morbid obesity

Useful links

GI and hepatology journals

Gastroenterology
www.gastrojournal.org

Clinical Gastroenterology & Hepatology
www.cghjournal.org

American Journal of Gastroenterology
www.nature.com/ajg/index.html

Gut
http://gut.bmjjournals.com

Hepatology
www3.interscience.wiley.com

Inflammatory Bowel Disease
www3.interscience.wiley.com/journal/113307010/home

Alimentary Pharmacology and Therapeutics
www.wiley.com/bw/journal.asp?ref—0269-2813&site—1

GI and hepatology societies

American Gastroenterology Association (AGA)
www.gastro.org

American College of Gastroenterology
www.acg.gi.org

American Association for the Study of Liver Disease (AASLD)
www.aasld.org

Patient support and charitable organizations

American College of Gastroenterology Patient Site
www.acg.gi.org/patients/

American Gastroenterology Association Patient Center
www.gastro.org/wmspage.cfm?parm1—478

American Cancer Society
www.cancer.org

Crohn's & Colitis Foundation of America
www.ccfa.org

Clinical information and teaching

National Digestive Diseases Information Clearinghouse
digestive.niddk.nih.gov

Sites with educational material
http://daveproject.org/index.cfm
www.gastrohep.com

Index